MEDICAL
INTELLIGENCE
UNIT 7

TGFβ and Cancer

John R. Benson, M.A., D.M., F.R.C.S.
The Royal Marsden Hospital and
Institute of Cancer Research
London, England

R.G. LANDES
COMPANY
AUSTIN, TEXAS
U.S.A.

MEDICAL INTELLIGENCE UNIT

TGFβ and Cancer

R.G. LANDES COMPANY
Austin, Texas, U.S.A.

Copyright © 1998 R.G. Landes Company

Please address all inquiries to the Publishers:
R.G. Landes Company, 810 South Church Street, Georgetown, Texas, U.S.A. 78626
Phone: 512/ 863 7762; FAX: 512/ 863 0081

ISBN: 1-57059-539-9

Library of Congress Cataloging-in-Publication Data

Benson, John R., 1959-
    TGF beta and cancer / John R. Benson.
        p.   cm. -- (Medical intellignece unit)
    Includes bibliographical references and index.
    ISBN 1-57059-539-9
    1. Transforming growth factors-beta. 2. Carcinogenesis. I. Title. II. Series.
    [DNLM: 1. Transforming Growth Factor beta--physiology. 2. Neoplasms--physiopathology. 3. Neoplasms--etiology. 4. Cell Transformation, Neoplastic. 5. Cell Communication. QU 107B474t 1998]
RC268.5.B45 1998
616.99'407--dc21
DNLM/DLC   98-42195
for Library of Congress   CIP

Publisher's Note

Landes Bioscience produces books in six Intelligence Unit series: *Medical, Molecular Biology, Neuroscience, Tissue Engineering, Biotechnology* and *Environmental.* The authors of our books are acknowledged leaders in their fields. Topics are unique; almost without exception, no similar books exist on these topics.

Our goal is to publish books in important and rapidly changing areas of bioscience for sophisticated researchers and clinicians. To achieve this goal, we have accelerated our publishing program to conform to the fast pace at which information grows in bioscience. Most of our books are published within 90 to 120 days of receipt of the manuscript. We would like to thank our readers for their continuing interest and welcome any comments or suggestions they may have for future books.

Judith Kemper
Production Manager
R.G. Landes Company

CONTENTS

EDITOR

John R. Benson, M.A., D.M., F.R.C.S.
The Royal Marsden Hospital and
Institute of Cancer Research
London, England
Chapters 1, 2, 4, 7, 8

CONTRIBUTORS

Mitchell S. Anscher, M.D.
Department of Radiation Oncology
Duke University Medical Center
Durham, North Carolina, U.S.A.
Chapter 3

Angela Hague, Ph.D.
CRC Colorectal Tumor
   Biology Research Group
Department of Pathology
   and Microbiology
University of Bristol
School of Medical Sciences
Bristol, U.K.
Chapter 6

Mary Helen Barcellos-Hoff, Ph.D.
Lawrence Berkeley National Laboratory
Berkeley, California, U.S.A.
Chapter 3

Susanne Hougaard, M.D.
The Finsen Center, 5074
Section for Radiation Biology
Copenhagen, Denmark
Chapter 8

R.L. Jirtle, Ph.D.
Department of Radiation Oncology
Duke University Medical Center
Durham, North Carolina, U.S.A.
Chapter 3

Feng-Ming Kong, M.D., Ph.D.
Department of Radiation Oncology
Duke University Medical Center
Durham, North Carolina, U.S.A.
Chapter 3

Janis MacCallum, Ph.D.
ICRF Medical Oncology Unit
Western General Hospital
Edinburgh, U.K.
Chapter 5

Anna M. Manning, Ph.D.
CRC Colorectal Tumor
   Biology Research Group
Department of Pathology
   and Microbiology
University of Bristol
School of Medical Sciences
Bristol, U.K.
Chapter 6

Peter Norgaard, M.D.
The Finsen Center, 5074
Section for Radiation Biology
Copenhagen, Denmark
Chapter 8

Christos Paraskeva, D.Phil.
CRC Colorectal Tumor
   Biology Research Group
Department of Pathology
   and Microbiology
University of Bristol
School of Medical Sciences
Bristol, U.K.
Chapter 6

Hans Skovgaard Poulsen, M.D., Ph.D.,
   DSci.
Section for Radiation
   Biology Rigshospitalet,
Copenhagen, Denmark
The Finsen Center, 5074
Chapter 8

PREFACE

Transforming growth factor β has emerged as a pre-eminent negative growth regulator, with anti-proliferative effects upon of a range of epithelial cell types. Much of the evidence in support of the growth inhibitory properties of TGFβ comes from in vitro studies on established cell lines derived from a variety of normal and neoplastic tissues. However, there is complementary, though circumstantial evidence indicating that epithelial inhibitory effects of TGFβ are operative in vivo. This has evoked much interest in the potential role of this growth factor both in processes of carcinogenesis and in the mediation of response to various pharmacological and ablative hormonal interventions. Nonetheless, elucidating the precise role of TGFβ in malignant progression and its quantitative contribution to any anti-tumor effects has been hampered both by conceptual contradictions and empirical discrepancies. Thus it may be surmised that tumor development and progression of cells along a neoplastic continuum is determined by a combination of 'pro-active' oncogenic events acting in conjunction with loss of responsiveness to negative regulatory influences which serve as a 'brake' on proliferation of cells. In the latter case, enhanced proliferative potential would essentially occur by default. Many transformed cell lines retain responsiveness to TGFβ and receptor expression is often constitutive. However, an inactivating mutation affecting a key component of the TGFβ receptor complex has recently been described in carcinoma cell lines, and provides an important piece of evidence not only accounting for loss of responsiveness to TGFβ, but also linking a defect in a negative regulatory pathway with progression of cells towards malignancy.

Clearly any strategy which attempts to exploit these growth inhibitory properties of TGFβ by stimulating production of TGFβ is dependent upon intact functional receptors. Herein lies one of the conceptual dilemmas; at what stage in tumor development does receptor dysfunction occur, and would a combined approach involving local induction of TGFβ together with restoration of cellular responsiveness be most appropriate? Progress in the field of gene therapy may ultimately permit introduction of functional receptors into cells thereby maximizing innate sensitivity to TGFβ.

A further pertinent aspect of TGFβ function relates to its effects on stromal tissue. Promotion of stromal expansion and angiogenesis would tend to favor tumor development by supporting continued proliferation of malignant epithelium. Therefore augmenting endogenous production of TGFβ within cancerous tissue may be counter-productive. Harnessing of the growth inhibitory effects of TGFβ for therapeutic gain may prove a challenging, though not unconquerable quest which will demand novel approaches. Indeed, anti-TGFβ strategies have been successfully applied clinically in non-cancerous conditions.

This book focuses on the theme that the malignant phenotype is associated with an imbalance of growth factors and disordered inter-cellular communication within the micro-environment of cells. The complex issues of functional pleiotropy and changing roles of TGFβ as a tumor evolves will be discussed. Evidence will be presented suggesting that altered expression of TGFβ and /or its receptors is a primary determinant of neoplastic progression in several common cancers, including not only those of the breast, but also colon, lung, stomach and prostate. The first chapter discusses growth factors as central components in regulation of cellular proliferation and differentiation and briefly outlines the features of the more important positive (stimulatory) growth factors before introducing TGFβ in the context of negative growth factors. Chapter 2 moves on to examine the structural aspects of TGFβ together with its mechanisms of activation. Included within this chapter is an account of TGFβ receptors and discussion of our limited knowledge of intracellular transduction mechanisms and control of TGFβ gene expression. The third chapter provides an account of biological functions of TGFβ, including not only its antiproliferative activity upon a variety of epithelial cell types, but also a spectrum of effects upon cells of mesenchymal origin. Chapters 4 and 5 consider the status of TGFβ in relation to stromal-epithelial interactions within both developing tissues and the adult organism. Developmental studies have yielded invaluable insights into the role of TGFβ in vivo—caution must be exercised when extrapolating from in vitro studies on TGFβ as its function is characteristically context dependent.

The remainder of this book is devoted to assessment of the functional significance of alterations in TGFβ expression within cancers affecting various tissues. Emphasis is placed on the breast cancer paradigm as research in areas of TGFβ pathophysiology and cancer has been most extensive for this hormone-dependent tumor. In particular, the role of TGFβ in carcinogenesis is discussed in detail with reference to breast cancer and mediation of response to therapeutic intervention focuses on anti-estrogen therapy. The clinical potential for strategies aimed at boosting local endogenous levels of TGFβ and enhancing response to this negative growth modulator will be discussed at the laboratory-clinical interface.

This is the first book dedicated to TGFβ and cancer, and provides a comprehensive account of the basic biology of TGFβ together with evidence implicating deranged expression of this growth factor in acquisition of malignancy within specific tissues. It is hoped that this volume will be of interest both to basic scientists working within the field of tumor biology in addition to clinical oncologists and those engaged by the pharmaceutical industry.

FOREWORD

In 1977 the breast cancer trials group that I chair launched the first trial to evaluate the role of adjuvant tamoxifen in early breast cancer (NATO–Nolvadex adjuvant trial organization). This trial recruited both pre- and post-menopausal women with operable breast cancer who were randomized between surgery alone or surgery plus two years of tamoxifen. The first major publication from this trial appeared in *The Lancet* in 1983 and was the first to demonstrate that tamoxifen could significantly improve survival within the first five years of treatment. This observation has now been corroborated by many other studies including the World Overview (Meta analysis). As a second order hypothesis within the trial we addressed the question of the role of the estrogen receptor in selecting those patients most likely to benefit from the adjuvant anti-oestrogen. At the time many critics questioned our sanity and for that matter our ethical integrity because it appeared self-evident that the "anti-estrogen" could only work in patients whose tumors expressed the estrogen receptor. Now there is at least one lesson we can draw from the history of science: nothing should be taken as "self-evident" and if science was the same as common sense then we wouldn't need scientific methodology and we would remain comfortable in the knowledge that the sun circled round the earth! Furthermore any individual who has studied the history of science understands the importance of the unexpected result and should go out of the way to cherish the observations which fail to corroborate that which was "self-evident" in the first place.

It was with some perverse glee therefore that when we came to do the first set of analyses we noted that the estrogen receptor was unable to discriminate between two populations of women with early breast cancer that would or would not benefit from adjuvant tamoxifen. At the time those critics who were unhappy in having their prejudices subverted took comfort by criticizing the techniques used for measuring the estrogen receptor within the tumor samples. In retrospect there was some justification for criticizing the particular method of ligand binding assay that was used, but that aside, in the fullness of time we can now state with some confidence that the estrogen receptor negative patients amongst postmenopausal women with early breast cancer may enjoy a clinically important reduction in the risk of death over a fifteen year period.

When these first counter-intuitive observations came to light I persuaded my group of clinicians and scientists to start thinking hard about alternative mechanisms of action of tamoxifen outside the classical estrogen receptor pathway. At the time these first observations were published Dr. Anthony Colletta, a brilliant you PhD student in my laboratories at King's, came up with the suggestion that the so-called anti-estrogen may work indirectly by the induction of transforming growth factor beta from stromal fibroblast, mediating an indirect effect on the malignant epithelial cells in their proximity. I can remember with great clarity getting an excited phone call from Anthony when I was on holiday in Nantucket Island at a time when he was working in Michael Sporn's department in Bethesda. His experiments using fetal fibroblasts cell culture techniques demonstrated unequivocally the capacity of tamoxifen to induce transforming factor beta from cells clearly defined as lacking an estrogen receptor mechanism.

So far this could have been discounted as mere phenomenology, but a short time thereafter I was able to conduct a clinical experiment which demonstrated in a most spectacular manner that tamoxifen and another triphemylethiline class of compound (toremifene) could indeed have a profound effect on human pathology.

Desmoid tumors are rare neoplasms which are composed entirely of fibroblast. A patient of mine who had originally been treated for a desmoid tumor within the breast appeared as an emergency with her abdomen full of desmoid tumors producing multiple sites of intestinal obstruction, making it surgically inoperable. The patient underwent some simple bypass procedures and was closed up again. Bearing in mind the laboratory experiments just described it was felt that there was nothing to lose in offering the patient high doses of toremifene. A month later the patient was readmitted with a surgical emergency, and on reopening her abdomen I observed that all the tumors had undergone massive necrosis. The dead tumor was scraped out and the holes in the bowel were repaired. The patient made an uneventful recovery and went on to live for a further three years. Following that experience I have treated approximately sixty patients with desmoid tumors using either high doses of tamoxifen or toremifene. About a third of these patients have shown spectacular responses, and some of these responses suggested an infarction rather than the conventional endocrine response of a tumor. There could be little doubt therefore that these groups of drugs, perhaps by inducing transforming growth factor beta and perhaps by implicating stromal epithelial interactions have a real and clinically useful effect on human pathology.

In 1990 I was appointed Professor of Surgery at the Royal Marsden Hospital and the Institute of Cancer Research. I recruited Dr. Anthony Colletta to join me as a team leader in the laboratory and the young Mr. John Benson as a Clinical Research Fellow. John worked like a beaver, taking forward the early clinical and laboratory findings at a rapid pace and effectively making the subject of transforming growth factor beta his own. Furthermore his career at that time and subsequently have demonstrated the value of having a clinician working in the laboratory before developing his surgical career and the value of clinical scientists and laboratory scientists working closely together with a relationship based on mutual respect and trust. This cross talk between the clinic and the laboratory is an exemplar of the future of clinical science which will inevitably lead to a better understanding and more rational therapy for chronic disease like cancer. This book on TGF beta and cancer represents a major achievement for John Benson, pulling together all the fascinating clinical and laboratory knowledge about this centrally important autocrine/paracrine compound.

From my own personal perspective therefore the initial observations from the NATO trial involving 1000 patients producing the first counter-intuitive result concerning the anti-estrogen therapy of breast cancer and the spectacular corroboration of an hypothesis with the experience of a single case of a desmoid tumor has given birth to a field of academic enquiry whose importance is only just beginning to be recognized but is given due prominence with the publication of this book.

Professor Michael Baum
University College London Medical School

ACKNOWLEDGMENTS

The author, J.R. Benson, gratefully acknowledges the Cancer Research Campaign and the Committee for Clinical Research, The Royal Marsden Hospital, for supporting work and results thereof cited in this book. He also offers thanks to Susan Hall and Linda Forman in the Medical Art Departments of the Royal Marsden and Chelsea and Westminster Hospitals respectively for assistance with the illustrations employed throughout this publication, including those originally published elsewhere. Professor Michael Baum and Dr. Anthony Colletta have proved an invaluable and constant source of encouragement, faith and inspiration.

CHAPTER 1

Growth Factors and Carcinogenesis

J.R. Benson

i) Introduction

Many biological processes including wound healing, development and carcinogenesis involve defined patterns of cellular growth and differentiation. Rates of proliferation and pathways of differentiation are stringently regulated and dependent upon precise and coordinated networks of intercellular communication. The latter may involve direct cell-to-cell contact, with junctional elements permitting transfer of signals between cells. This form of communication is restricted to cells in contiguous arrangement. By contrast, indirect modes of communication allow interaction between neighboring groups of cells which are not necessarily in direct contact. Thus cells may interact through the extracellular matrix which surrounds all cells in vivo and whose structure and composition is determined by tissue requirements. Alternatively, cells may also communicate indirectly by means of soluble factors which are secreted by a cellular type and diffuse through the extracellular matrix to reach target cells lying at varying distances from the source. It was first suggested over 20 years ago that density-dependent growth inhibition might be mediated by an increase in cellular requirements for macromolecular growth factors. As confluency was reached, with crowding of cells, their innate growth sensitivity to these macro-molecular factors decreased, possibly as a consequence of a reduction in density of cell surface receptors as confluence was reached.[1] Confrontation experiments in which individual groups of cells are separated by a physical barrier which obviates any direct cell-to-cell interaction have confirmed soluble factors to be a principal form of signaling between cells.

The observation that estrogen could modulate levels of secreted proteins led to the original proposal by Rochefort and colleagues in 1980 that breast cancer might be regulated by "auto-stimulatory" mechanisms.[2] This concept was analogous to the autocrine hypothesis proposed earlier that year by Sporn and Todaro (1980), which was based on the finding that some cancer cells, namely Rous sarcoma virus transformed chick fibroblasts, appeared to have reduced requirements for exogenous sources of certain polypeptide growth factors.[3] These authors suggested that malignant transformation might result in part from excessive production of growth promoting polypeptides by cancer cells themselves, which both secrete and respond to these factors. Such cells would therefore be freed from dependency on exogenous sources and achieve a degree of autonomy. Subsequently, several isolated tumor cell types were shown to release a variety of growth stimulatory polypeptides into their conditioned media, and to possess corresponding receptors for these.[4,5] Furthermore, the demonstration of growth inhibitory substances in addition to stimulatory peptides in conditioned media of cancer cells led to a revised autocrine hypothesis. This embodied the concept that "malignant transformation may be the result not only of excessive production,

---

TGFβ and Cancer, edited by J.R. Benson. ©1998 R.G. Landes Company.

expression and action of positive autocrine growth factors, but also of the failure of cells to synthesis, express or respond to specific negative growth factors they normally release to control their own growth".[6]

Therefore some growth factors are stimulatory, whilst others are inhibitory to epithelial proliferation, and this has lead to a conceptual dichotomy of positive and negative growth factors. Growth factors are produced and secreted locally by many cell types, and target cells possess specific transmembrane receptors to which these growth factors bind and subsequently activate intracellular signal transduction pathways. An extracellular stimulus is thus translated into an intracellular response. Growth factors can function either in an autocrine capacity, whereby they act upon their cell of origin, or can interact with adjacent cells (of a similar or different type) in a paracrine action (Fig. 1.1.). The local micro-environment of a cell contains a pool of positive and negative growth factors, which may be functioning in either an autocrine or paracrine manner. It is the balance of these which determines the polarity and intensity of the effective signal delivered to epithelial cells (Fig. 1.2.).

Excessive proliferation of cells which characterizes both preneoplastic states as well as established tumors, could result from a breakdown of these autocrine and paracrine loops (Fig. 1.3.). There may be an excess of stimulatory growth factors derived either from epithelial cells themselves, or stromal cells. Conversely, the production of negative growth factors which normally serve to keep cell proliferation in check may be deficient. Breakdown of these loops could also result from an abnormal response of target cells to normal levels of growth factors. There may be a failure of response to negative growth factors or enhanced sensitivity to positive ones, for which altered levels of cognate receptors or levels of nuclear oncogenes (e.g., c-*myc*, c-*fos* and c-*jun*) are possible mechanisms.[7-9]

Whatever the mechanistic fault, aberrant function of these growth factor loops will lead to excessive epithelial proliferation and promote immortalization of cells and in turn neoplastic development (Fig. 1.4.).

Much of the experimental work on growth factors and cancer pertains to breast malignancy, with various established breast cancer cell lines having been employed for in vitro investigation of growth factor profiles. The majority of growth factors studied in detail are short polypeptides which have been isolated from the conditioned media of breast cancer and certain other cell lines. These include transforming growth factor alpha (TGF alpha), transforming growth factor β (TGFβ), epidermal growth factor (EGF), platelet derived growth factor (PDGF) and insulin-like growth factors I and II. Much interest has focused on breast cancer cell lines because of the potential role of these growth factors as proximate effectors in hormone dependent growth responses; most of the cited growth factors are stimulatory and have been implicated in mitogenic responses. Thus in estrogen receptor (ER) positive hormone dependent cell lines, the synthesis and secretion of these growth factors is modulated by both estrogens and anti-estrogens. Some ER negative hormone independent cell lines constitutively secrete higher levels of these factors. These observations, together with the basic postulates of the autocrine hypothesis and auto-stimulatory concept of Rochefort were assimilated by Lippman into a collection of fundamental hypotheses relating to mechanisms for mediation of estrogen effects upon breast cancer cells.[10] Firstly, estrogens were considered to directly interact with breast cancer cells and to modify gene expression, leading to altered levels of both cellular and secreted proteins. Secondly, these secreted proteins, or growth factors could act in either an autocrine or paracrine manner to effect estrogen mediated tumor progression. Possible actions include both further stimulation of cycling cells and initiation and recruitment of quiescent cells (from G_0). Finally, it was proposed

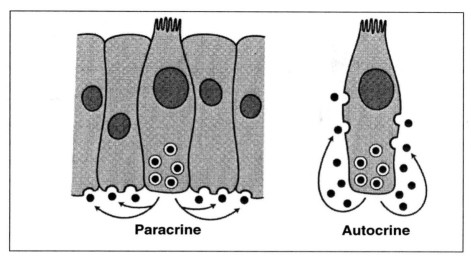

Fig. 1.1. Cells produce and secrete soluble growth factors which enter the extracellular space from where they can act via cognate membrane receptors upon either the same (autocrine) or adjacent cells (paracrine). Reprinted with permission from: Benson JR, Colletta AA. Clinical Immunotherapeutics 1995; 4:249-258. © ADIS International Publications Limited.

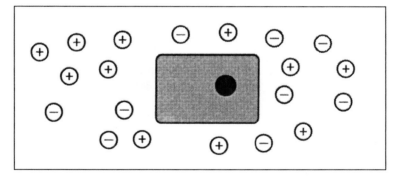

Fig. 1.2. The local micro-environment of a tumor contains a pool of positive and negative growth factors the balance of which determines the polarity and intensity of the effective signal delivered to epithelial cells. Reprinted with permission from: Benson JR, Colletta AA. Clinical Immunotherapeutics 1995; 4:249-258. © ADIS International Publications Limited.

that hormone dependent breast cancer could become hormone independent by the constitutive expression of these same growth factors, thereby acquiring autonomy.

The following section summarizes the evidence for roles of these polypeptide growth factors within this paradigm of hormone dependent breast cancer growth. Though there is much evidence in support of the elegant hypotheses previously set forth, there are some inconsistencies and it is emerging that growth factors may not mediate endocrine effects exclusively via extracellular receptors.

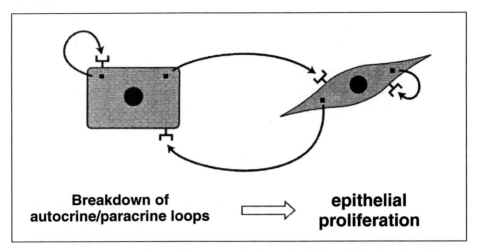

Fig. 1.3. Disordered epithelial proliferation results from a breakdown in the functional interactions between growth factor loops involving both epithelial and stromal cells.

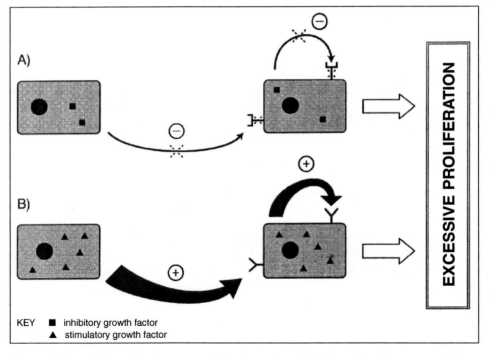

Fig. 1.4. Diagram illustrating the concept of how excessive epithelial proliferation may result from (A) a deficiency in the production/secretion of negative growth factors or cellular response to these or (B) an excess of positive or stimulatory growth factors. In both scenarios, the defect may occur in either the epithelial (autocrine) or stromal (paracrine) cells.

ii) Positive Growth Factors

a) Transforming Growth Factor Alpha

This was one of the factors isolated from fibroblasts transformed with an oncogenic virus.[11] It is a 7 kDal polypeptide with 40% sequence homology to EGF, with which it shares a common receptor. Like many growth factor receptors, the receptor for EGF/TGF alpha possesses an extracellular domain for ligand binding, a short transmembrane segment and an intracellular domain which has intrinsic tyrosine kinase activity and can undergo autophosphorylation (Fig. 1.4). TGF alpha reversibly transforms normal rat kidney fibroblasts and permits anchorage independent growth in soft agar, a feature which forms the basis for assay of both TGF alpha and transforming growth factor β (TGFβ). TGF alpha activity can be found in the conditioned media of several human breast cancer cell lines,[12-14] and cDNA probes have detected corresponding mRNA transcripts in both cell lines and tumor tissue.[15,16] TGF alpha is a potent mitogen for both human epithelial cells (including breast cancer cells) and fibroblasts. When normal cells are transfected with TGF alpha cDNA under the influence of the SV40 promoter, they cause tumor formation when introduced into nude mice.[17,18] This is consistent with an autocrine stimulation of these cells which simultaneously secrete and respond to TGF alpha.

Much interest in TGF alpha has centered on its role as a proximate mitogen in mediation of estrogen stimulation of breast cancer cells. Estradiol has been shown to increase both TGF alpha mRNA levels,[16] and secretion[13,14] of this growth factor from ER positive breast cancer cells, whereas anti-estrogens have the opposite effect. Moreover, the growth inhibitory effects of anti-estrogens could be partially reversed by exogenous TGF alpha.[19] Furthermore, ER negative cells appeared to constitutively express higher levels of TGF alpha.[13] However, it was the experiments from Lippman's laboratory which provided convincing, though not conclusive evidence that TGF alpha might mediate estrogen stimulation of hormone dependent breast cancer cells.[14] These seminal studies demonstrated that conditioned media from estrogen treated MCF-7 cells had elevated levels of TGF alpha and could partially substitute for estrogen in supporting growth of MCF-7 xenograft tumors in mice. Levels of TGF alpha secretion could be augmented between 2 and 14-fold by these ER positive cells.[20] Moreover, v-Ha-*ras* transformed MCF-7 cells, which secreted 3- to 5-fold higher levels of TGF alpha were tumorigenic in more than three-quarters of mice denied estrogen supplementation.[21] These data suggested that TGF alpha might mediate estrogen stimulation of hormone dependent cells, and that high constitutive expression of this growth factor would in turn confer hormonal independence. Tamoxifen, which has estrogen reversible growth inhibitory effects in MCF-7 cells, can antagonize the estrogen induced elevation of the TGF alpha product and its transcript in ER positive breast cancer cell lines.[14] This downregulation of TGF alpha by tamoxifen is consistent with the hypothesis that TGF alpha may participate in a positive autocrine loop mediated via the ER. Limited in vivo data corroborate these in vitro observations and conclusions. Thus a significant reduction in TGF alpha expression has been demonstrated in ER positive breast cancers following tamoxifen treatment for a period of 10 days. Fine-needle aspirates were obtained from 10 patients pre- and post-treatment and TGF alpha levels measured with an enzyme immunoassay.[22] Reduction in TGF alpha expression was associated with reduction in PR which predicts for clinical response.[23] Therefore the growth inhibitory effects of tamoxifen were partly attributable to downregulation of TGF alpha, which was observed in 50% of ER positive tumors. The expression of TGF alpha in ER negative tumors, but its failure to be modulated by tamoxifen suggests that carcinoma cells within these tumors may constitutively produce TGF alpha and escape hormonal regulation. Despite these elegant experiments, evidence has emerged which questions the role of TGF alpha as a proximate mitogen in mediating the effects of both estrogens and anti-estrogens. Several studies have failed to show that blockade of the EGF/TGF alpha receptor abrogates estrogen stimulation. Arteaga and co-workers used both monoclonal and polyclonal antibodies against this receptor, which resulted in both inhibition of EGF binding and elimination of EGF stimulated tyrosine kinase activity. However, though these antibodies could overcome TGF alpha induced growth of MCF-7 cells, they were without effect upon estradiol stimulation of these cells.[24] Similarly, these antibodies had no effect on estradiol induced DNA synthesis in ER positive breast cancer cells.[25] These data imply that other mitogens and growth inhibitory substances are acting upon breast cancer cells in the complex micro-environment of tissues. Functional redundancy may exist, and elimination of one potential growth factor may be insufficient to impact upon estrogen regulated growth. Of interest, provisional data suggests that expression of anti-sense TGF alpha mRNA in MCF-7 cells can completely block estrogen stimulated proliferation.[26] These results could be interpreted as supporting the existence of a possible intracrine pathway which bypasses any extracellular receptors, blockade of which would therefore be inconsequential.

b) Insulin-Like Growth Factors

Other potent mitogens for breast cancer cells exist, amongst which the insulin-like growth factors, IGF-I and IGF-II are prominent.[27-29] Most breast cancer cells, together with breast tumor tissue, possess the type I IGF receptor for which both IGF I and IGF II are functional ligands.[29] Levels of this receptor correlate to some extent with those of ER, but ER negative cells still have significant levels of the IGF receptor. Despite possessing receptors for these growth factors, most breast cancer cell lines do not express the mRNA for either IGF I or II, and probably do not synthesize and secrete these growth factors themselves.[30,31] Therefore though they may respond to IGF's, these cells do not appear to produce them, suggesting that IGF-I and IGF-II may participate in a paracrine rather than an autocrine pathway. This hypothesis is supported by evidence that fibroblasts derived from breast tumor tissue express high levels of IGF-I and II mRNA in vitro. Benign tumor fibroblasts over-express IGF-I, whilst those from malignant tumors over-express IGF-II mRNA. Thus stromal cells are a rich source of IGF's which may act upon neighboring epithelial cells in a positive paracrine manner. Furthermore, not only is there evidence that systemic levels can be modulated by the therapeutic agents such as anti-estrogens, but also for direct modulation of local levels.[32] Tamoxifen treatment of rats leads to reduction of IGF-I expression in tissues which are common sites for breast cancer metastases (liver and lung). Hypophysectomized rats and growth hormone replacement were employed to demonstrate that tamoxifen can mediate these effects in part by a pituitary independent mechanism. Recently, this reduction in IGF-I expression has been shown to occur in the stromal compartment of tissues. An autocrine function for these growth factors however cannot be excluded, and some workers have reported that authentic IGF I[30] and possibly IGF II[33] are expressed by some breast cancer cells. IGF I appears to be increased by estrogen treatment of hormone dependent cells[33] and over-expression of IGF II in MCF-7 cells is associated with phenotypic changes of malignancy and loss of estrogen dependence.[29] An important aspect of regulation by IGF's is the level of their specific binding proteins. Several distinct intracellular and extracellular forms of these exist, and they determine both activity and bioavailability of these growth factors.[34] Furthermore, they are subject to modulation by estrogens[35] and possibly anti-estrogens[36] whose effects may be partly mediated by alteration in levels of these binding proteins.[37] Antibodies directed against the type I receptor should eliminate autocrine and paracrine growth stimulatory effects of IGF I or II upon breast cancer cells. Blockade of this receptor with the monoclonal antibody, alpha IR3 does not inhibit the proliferation of either ER positive or ER negative breast cancer cell lines in a serum-free in vitro system.[38] However, in the presence of serum, this antibody can inhibit growth of most breast cancer cell lines tested, suggesting that the stimulant effect of IGF's upon these cells in vivo is dependent upon the presence of other growth factors.

c) Epidermal Growth Factor

Epidermal growth factor is another mitogenic growth factor which appears to share a common receptor with TGF alpha. The epidermal growth factor receptor (EGFR) is a product of the cerb-B1 oncogene and like many growth factor receptors has an intracellular domain with tyrosine kinase activity. Initial studies on expression of EGF in human breast cancers revealed an apparent dichotomy; a subset of tumors were found to express either ER or EGF. The absence of ER in tumors expressing EGF suggested that this growth factor might be a principle mediator of any mitogenic response.[39] Other studies showed that the EGFR was often coexpressed with ER in breast tumors, but an inverse relationship existed between expression of these two receptors.[16] Human breast tumors generally express high levels of epidermal growth factor receptor (EGFR),[40] and increased EGFR expression is inversely correlated with ER in breast cancer and is a predictor of poor prognosis.[41] In this seminal study of Sainsbury and co-workers involving 135 patients with breast cancer, multivariate analysis revealed EGFR expression to be the most powerful prognostic factor for node negative patients and the second most significant factor for node positive patients.

Similar conclusions have been drawn from in vitro studies using breast cancer cell lines; both ER positive (e.g., MCF-7) and ER negative (e.g., MDA-MB-231) cell lines generally express EGFR with an inverse correlation between levels of these two receptors.[42,43] The density of EGFR on the cell surface does not appear related to response to EGF in a predictable manner. Though cells expressing high levels of EGFR appear to be less responsive to exogenous EGF, tumorogenicity does appear to correlate with levels of EGFR expression.[42] This is consistent with in vivo studies cited above indicating a poorer prognosis in EGFR rich tumors.

iii) Negative Growth Factors

In accordance with the extended autocrine hypothesis,[6] regulation of tumor growth involves not only modulation of stimulatory growth factors, but also of inhibitory ones. Cells which have lost an inhibitory response would have a selective growth advantage, and estrogen stimulation could result from a simultaneous increase in levels of growth stimulators and decrease of growth inhibitors. The principle negative growth regulator characterized hitherto is transforming growth factor β (TGFβ), which represents a family of multifunctional regulatory polypeptides. These will be considered in detail in the next chapter. In brief, these polypeptides are inhibitory to many epithelial cell lines, including breast cancer cells in vitro. Conversely, TGFβ is generally stimulatory to cells of mesenchymal origin, such as fibroblasts. It is the former property which has attracted interest in these factors as important negative regulators of epithelial proliferation both in normal and malignant tissue. Many breast cancer cells both secrete and respond to TGFβ, for which they possess cognate receptors, thus implying the operation of a potential autocrine inhibitory mechanism. Once again in the context of breast cancer, modulation of TGFβ secretion in vitro by estrogens and anti-estrogens has been found to mirror that of positive growth factors such as TGF alpha. However, as will be discussed in chapter 7, some contradictory observations have become apparent, and these may reflect the complexity of TGFβ function which is highly context dependent and may change as a tumor evolves.

iv) Growth Factor Receptors

Endocrine control of tumor growth may be accomplished not only by modulation of growth factor levels, but of their receptors. The EGF receptor for example is regulated by both estrogen and anti-estrogen in MCF-7 cells.[44] Transfection of the EGF receptor into ER positive (ZR-75) cells can lead to hormone independent growth,[45] though this is not a consistent phenotypic change.[46] Estrogen has also been reported to increase phosphorylation of the EGF receptor and thus could 'prime' it for propagation of intracellular signals once activated properly by its own ligand.[47] Levels of type I IGF receptor are increased 7-fold by estrogen treatment, suggesting that receptor upregulation and enhanced sensitization to IGF could be a mechanism for mediation of estrogen stimulated growth.[48]

Control of the cell cycle and hence rate of growth of a tumor is determined by the balance of growth factors acting upon a cell. These growth factors may be either stimulatory or inhibitory, and act in either an autocrine or paracrine manner. Although cells have an inherent program which partly determines rates of proliferation and differentiation, this 'sea' of soluble growth factors represents a principle mechanism for modulation and regulation of cellular activity by exogenous stimuli. The exact function of any individual growth factor depends upon both cellular source and target, together with other coexisting growth factors. The concept that endocrine stimulated growth may be mediated by modulation of these growth factors is both simple and attractive. However, such a sequential or "in series" mechanism is probably over-simplistic.[49] Growth factor pathways exist not just to mediate estrogen regulated growth. Clearly hormone independent ER negative cells can proliferate without prior interaction of ER with its ligand.

The rate of progression of cells through the cell cycle is ultimately dependent upon the expression profile of activator oncogenes and tumor suppressor genes. As a cell evolves from an immortalized to a fully transformed state, a series of events occur at the genetic level which lead to activation of oncogenes or loss of suppressor gene function through point mutations or deletions, gene amplification and translocation. Some of these events may lead to a change in sensitivity to growth factors, with for example an augmented response to EGF and IGF I. Furthermore, some oncogenes code for growth factors or their receptors such as the c-*sis* oncogene which codes for a protein with close homology to PDGF, and the c-erbB2 oncogene which codes for a transmembrane receptor-like protein very similar to the cytoplasmic domain of EGF. Therefore escape from hormone dependence may occur not only from altered levels of and sensitivity to growth factors, but also from constitutive activation of their receptors which can propagate intracellular signals in the absence of bound ligand. Oncogenes coding for aberrant expression of receptors such as c-erbB2 may permit the bypassing of conventional growth factor pathways. About 30% of breast carcinomas over-express this c-erbB2 oncogene which correlates with a poor prognosis.[50]

v) Growth Factors and Regulation of Tumor Growth

Transforming growth factor β is the only negative polypeptide growth factor which has been thoroughly investigated and documented. Others may exist, but TGFβ appears to be functionally pre-eminent with the protein product and its receptor being expressed in a wide range of both normal and malignant tissues. From a teleological perspective, the existence of multiple mitogenic growth factors may guarantee a rapid growth phase during the early stages of embryogenesis thereby maximizing the chances of survival. A degree of functional redundancy may be an evolutionary safeguard to ensure an organisms survival in adverse circumstances where certain specific growth factor pathways may be compromised and would otherwise result in an attenuated mitogenic response and threaten survival.

The price to pay for collective and potent mitogenic capacity of cells may be a lower threshold for development of malignancy. During the 1980s, concepts of carcinogenesis were dominated by the paradigm of the oncogene. The malignant phenotype was considered to arise as a consequence of the accumulation either randomly or serially of alterations in genes derived from activation of normal cellular counterparts termed proto-oncogenes. The latter code for a variety of proteins including growth factors and their receptors together with several nuclear proteins which have a central role in growth regulatory mechanisms. Activated oncogenes represent a positive and dominant change which confers upon cancer cells a selective growth advantage over normal cells in possession of the corresponding inactivated proto-oncogene.

According to the above paradigm, *"evil overrides good"*[51] with oncogenic events within a cell tending to be dominant. Tumor suppressor genes are integral components of a cell's genetic code and serve to regulate cellular proliferation by exerting a negative influence and acting as a brake. Defects in these genes may involve either a deficiency of a negative (inhibitory) growth factor or it's receptor, or a protein which regulates cell division, and thus leads to excessive proliferation and neoplastic progression by default.

Random mutations within the genome are more likely to activate a proto-oncogene and lead to increased rates of proliferation through enhanced expression of mitogenic growth factor pathways, than to influence any negative regulatory pathway. Certainly the chances of any restraint upon cell proliferation through augmentation of a limited spectrum of inhibitory pathways would seem remote. Inhibitory growth factors such as TGFβ are a central component of these negative regulatory pathways. The manipulation of growth factor loops represents a potentially important therapeutic strategy. The malignant phenotype may be associated with an imbalance of growth factors within the micro-environment of cells. Oncogenic sequelae might involve either an excess of positive mitogenic growth factors such as transforming growth factor alpha and insulin-like growth factors, or a deficiency of negative ones such as TGFβ.

Pharmacological intervention, possibly in conjunction with gene therapy, could be employed to augment local endogenous levels of negative (inhibitory) growth factors or suppress levels of positive (stimulatory) ones. Boosting of endogenous TGFβ levels could correct any preexisting or acquired deficiency, or compensate for activation of cellular proto-oncogenes resulting in over production of stimulatory growth factors or other oncogenic activities such as constitutive activation of their cognate receptors. Locally induced TGFβ could derive either from stromal or epithelial sources, with epithelium responding to TGFβ acting in paracrine or autocrine capacity respectively. As discussed in chapter 7, there are innate advantages of strategies aimed at local induction of TGFβ rather than enhancement of systemic levels of TGFβ. However, similar considerations may not pertain to mitogenic growth factors, for which reduction in systemic levels may translate into therapeutic gain. Pollak and co-workers have demonstrated that tamoxifen treatment in vivo is associated with a reduction in serum IGF-I levels and proposed that as IGF-I is not only a mitogen for breast cancer cells, but also stimulates the motility and metastatic potential of malignant cells. This reduction in circulating IGF-I might be an important component of tamoxifen's anti-neoplastic action in vivo.[152] Curiously, Sherwin and co-workers found TGF alpha activity in the urine of more than three-quarters of patients with disseminated malignancy. This contrasted with failure to detect this growth factor in urine of normal controls.[53] Receptor targeting may also be a more realistic strategy for oncogenically activated pathways, rather than those involving defective negative regulatory systems; receptors for TGFβ are ubiquitous and their loss/dysfunction does not appear to be a general mechanism whereby cells escape from restraints on proliferation.[7,54] However, as alluded to earlier, functional redundancy amongst growth factor pathways may limit the efficacy of ablative therapies based on a single receptor type.

Other approaches aimed at maximal exploitation of the growth inhibitory effects of TGFβ include enhancing the sensitivity of target cells. This could increase therapeutic ratios by minimizing the degree of local TGFβ induction compatible with clinical efficacy. As will be discussed in the following chapter, TGFβ is bound to specific components of the extracellular matrix which restrict its bioavailability. If levels of binding proteins can be modulated pharmacologically, then this could provide an indirect means for boosting local levels of functionally active forms of TGFβ. There is provisional evidence that levels of IGF binding proteins can be modified by anti-estrogens.[36]

Recent advancements in understanding of regulatory mechanisms in cell growth and differentiation have contributed greatly to our understanding of neoplastic states. Valuable insights into disordered growth have come from studying developmental processes, and it is becoming apparent that cancerous tissues are a kind of caricature of normal tissues.[55] Many tumors are grossly similar to their tissue of origin, this being most evident in well differentiated lesions. Indeed, less well differentiated tumors may not represent a degree of de-differentiation per se; tumors may arise from malignant stem cells which undergo differentiation like normal stem cells. The proportion of these which have undergone differentiation (and apoptosis) relative to those which continue to proliferate and remain undifferentiated determines the histological grade. Thus a cell may possess the typical features of a malignant phenotype, yet still have gone through a sequential process of differentiation not dissimilar to its nonmalignant counterpart.[55] Furthermore, cancer cells display a finite number of aberrant pathways leading to disordered growth patterns, and alterations in nucleotide sequence and composition which characterize a cancer cell represent only a small fraction of a cell's complete DNA content.

This apparent similarity between normal and malignant cells has been expounded by Schipper[56,57] who has emphasized that cancer cells are not 'alien' and genetically disparate like exogenous pathogens, but rather are rogue internal elements which have achieved some degree of autonomy by dislocation of normal pathways of intercellular communication. However, a cancer cell is not completely autonomous and some channels of communication persist. In effect, a malignant tumor represents a state of regulatory imbalance in which cancer cells have achieved various degrees of escape from mechanisms controlling normal rates of proliferation and differentiation. A central theme of this proposal is that cancer is a potentially reversible process, and that by correcting abnormal cellular expression and transcriptional patterns, aberrant pathways of communication might be restored and in turn 'rogue' cancer cells re-regulated and effectively "tamed". Malignant cells would be controlled rather than killed and survival increased by effectively rendering tumor behavior more benign.

This philosophy of "cell control" as opposed to "cell kill" exploits similarities between cancer and normal cells, in contrast to cytotoxic strategies which rely on presumed qualitative differences between these two cell populations. According to this concept the therapeutic goal shifts from one of cell kill to re-regulation. As this method exploits similarities between cancerous and normal tissues, there may be a fundamental advantage over cytotoxic approaches.

It is now recognized that individual tumors are composed of a heterogeneous population of cells with degrees of phenotypic variability based on subtle differences in patterns of gene expression. These result in different rates of proliferation, invasive potential and response to therapeutic agents. Though a particular tumor may be designated as of a certain histological type and grade, these labels are surrogate classifications, and represent only the dominant morphological type.

It is this biological heterogeneity which underlies the variable natural history of breast cancer, and has hitherto restricted the efficacy of therapies. The potential extent of this cellular heterogeneity within a tumor and its micro-metastases has important therapeutic consequences. It is unlikely that even a combination of chemotherapeutic agents will successfully target the majority of cells. Rather, these agents will serve as a therapeutic probe to select sub-populations or clones of cells which have a similar phenotype and response. Depending on the degree of heterogeneity, a particular combination chemotherapy schedule will target a variable proportion of the total cell population leaving a fraction of cells which are unresponsive to any of the agents employed.

It may be more sensible and rational to use therapeutic agents which can exploit the similarities between these differing clones of cells and hence have a wider 'cellular appeal'. These could include hormonal and other agents which can accomplish re-regulation through modulation of biological response modifiers and natural cytokines to which most cancer cells can still potentially respond. Such a response will depend upon innate similarities which persist between cancer cells and is likely to be witnessed in the majority of malignant cells. By contrast, cytotoxic regimens based on a finite number of drugs with specific actions have more limited scope and are likely to influence a smaller proportion of cancer cells. However, as these regulatory strategies largely rely on normal pathways of cellular communication, therapeutic indices may be small. Nonetheless, control of rogue cancer cells by such methods may not be associated with specific deleterious effects upon nonneoplastic cells.

Neoplastic progression may result in part from loss of negative growth control through autocrine/paracrine interactions, and agents which can restore inhibitory responses would facilitate re-regulation and 'taming' of rogue cancer cells. This is the fundamental rationale for therapies based on local induction of the negative growth modulator TGFβ within tissues. There is now evidence for the pharmacological manipulation of local endogenous levels of TGFβ which may be of relevance to the mode of action of several important agents with proven therapeutic efficacy. This strategy of modulating local endogenous TGFβ production has potential clinical importance both for treatment of established tumors and prevention of malignancy (see chapter 7).

Therefore elucidation of growth factor pathways allows us to decipher the language of intercellular communication, but on the other hand presents a potentially valuable strategy whereby manipulation of growth factor loops can be exploited for maximal therapeutic gain. The role of TGFβ in this scenario is pivotal and local induction of this inhibitory growth factor within tissues by pharmacological intervention possibly in conjunction with gene therapy presents a potentially useful therapeutic approach to 're-regulation' of disordered growth associated with neoplastic states.

References

1. Holley RW. Control of growth of mammalian cells in culture. Nature 1975; 258:487-490.
2. Rochefort H, Coezy E, Joly E et al. Hormonal control of breast cancer in cell culture. In: Iacobelli S, King RJB, Lindren HR, Lippman ME, eds. Hormones and Cancer-Progress in Cancer Research and Therapy. New York: Raven Press. 1980; 14:21-29.
3. Sporn MB, Todaro GJ. Autocrine secretion and malignant transformation of cells. NEJM 1980; 303:878-880.
4. Lippman ME, Dickson RB, Gelmann EP et al. Growth regulation of human breast carcinoma occurs through regulated growth factor secretion. J Cell Biochem 1987; 35:1-16.
5. Lippman ME, Dickson RB, Gelmann EP et al. Growth regulatory peptide production by human breast carcinoma cells. J Cell Biochem 1988; 30:52-61.
6. Sporn MB, Roberts AB. Autocrine growth factors and cancer. Nature 1985; 313:745-747.
7. Kimchi A, Wang X-F, Weinberg RA et al. Absence of TGFβ receptors and growth inhibitory responses in retinoblastoma cells. Science 1988; 240:196-199.
8. Roberts AB, Anzano MA, Wakefield LM et al. Type β-transforming growth factor: A bifunctional regulator of cellular growth. Proc Natl Acad Sci (USA) 1985; 82:119-123.

9. Curran T, Bravo R, Muller R. Transient induction of c-fos and c-myc is an immediate cosequence of growth factor stimulation. Cancer Surv 1985; 4:655-681.

10. Lippman ME, Dickson RB, Knabbe C et al. Autocrine and paracrine regulation of human breast cancer. Breast Cancer Res Treat 1986; 7:59-70.

11. DeLarco EJ, Todaro GJ. Growth factors from murine sarcoma virus transformed cells. Proc Natl Aca Sci (USA) 1978; 75:4001-4005.

12. Salomon DS, Zwiebel JA, Band M et al. Presence of transforming growth factors in human breast cancer cells. Cancer Res 1984; 44:4069-4077.

13. Perroteau I, Salomon D, DeBortoli M et al. Immunological detection and quantitation of alpha transforming activity in human breast carcinoma cells. Breast Cancer Res Treat 1986; 7:201-210.

14. Dickson RB, Bates S, McManaway M, Lippman ME. Characterisation of estrogen responsive transforming activity in human breast cancer cell lines. Cancer Res 1986 (a); 46:1707-1713.

15. Bates SE, Davidson NE, Valverius EM et al. Expression of transforming growth factor alpha and its messenger ribonucleic in human breast cancer: Its regulation by oestrogen and and its possible functional significance. Mol Endocrinol 1988; 2:543-555.

16. Perez R, Betsholtz C, Westermark B, Heldin C-H. Frequent expression of growth factors for mesenchymal cells in human mammary carcinoma cell lines. Cancer Res 1987; 47:3425-3427.

17. Rosenthal A, Lindquist PB, Bringham TS et al. Expression in rat fibroblasts of a human transforming growth factor alpha cDNA results in transformation. Cell 1986; 46:301-309.

18. Watanabe S, Lazar E, Sporn M. Transformation of normal rat kidney cells by an infectious retrovirus carrying a synthetic rat type alpha TGF gene. Proc Natl Aca Sci (USA) 1987; 84:1258-1262.

19. Koga M, Sutherland RL. Epidermal growth factor partially reverses inhibitory effects of anti-oestrogens on T47-D human breast cancer cell growth. Biochem Biophysic Res Comm 1987; 146:739-745.

20. Dickson RB, McManaway ME, Lippman M.E. Estrogen-induced factors of breast cancer cells partially replace oestrogen to promote tumour growth. Science 1986 (b); 232:1540-1543.

21. Kasid A, Lippman ME, Papageorge AG et al. Transfection of v-ras DNA into MCF-7 cells bipasses their dependence on oestrogen for tumourogenicity. Science 1985; 228:725-728.

22. Noguchi S, Motomura K, Inaji H et al. Down-regulation of Transforming growth factor alpha by tamoxifen in human breast cancer. Cancer 1993; 72:131-136.

23. Howell A, Harland RNL, Barnes DM et al. Endocrine therapy for advanced carcinoma of the breast. Relationship between the effect of tamoxifen upon concentration of progesterone receptor and subsequent response to treatment. Cancer Res 1987; 47:300-304.

24. Arteaga CL, Tandon AK, von Hoff DD, Osborne CK. Transforming growth factor β: potential autocrine growth inhibition of estrogen receptor negative human breast cancer cells. Cancer Res 1988 (b); 48:3898-3904.

25. Arteaga CL, Osborne CK. Growth factors as mediators of estrogen/anti-estrogen action in human breast cancer cells. In: Lippman ME, Dickson RB, eds. Regulatory Mechanisms in Breast Cancer. Boston: Kluwer Academic Publishers, 1991:289-304.

26. Reddy KB, Yee D, Coffey RJ, Osborne CK. Inhibition of estrogen-induced breast cancer in autocrine TGF alpha expression. Proc Am Ass Canc Res 1993; 34:1406.

27. Myall Y, Shiu RPC, Bhaumick B. Receptor binding and growth promoting activity of insulin-like growth factors in human breast cancer cells (T47D) in culture. Cancer Res 1984; 44:5486-5490.

28. Karey KP, Sirbasku DA. Differential responsiveness of human breast cancer cell lines MCF-7 and T47D to growth factors and 17β-oestradiol. Cancer Res 1988; 48:4083-4092.

29. Cullen KJ, Lippman ME, Chow D et al. Insulin-like growth factor II over-expression in MCF-7 cells induces phenotypic changes associated with malignant progression. Mol Endocrinol 1992; 6:91-100.

30. Yee D, Cullen KJ, Paik S et al. Insulin-like growth factor II mRNA expression in human breast cancer. Cancer Res 1988; 48:6691-6697.

31. Yee D, Paik S, Lebovic GS et al. Analysis of insulin-like growth factor I gene expression in malignancy: Evidence for a paracrine role in human breast cancer. Mol Endocrinol 1989; 3:509-517.
32. Huynh HT, Tetenes E, Wallace L, Pollak M. In vivo inhibition of Insulin-like growth factor I gene expression by tamoxifen. Cancer Res 1993; 53:1727-1730.
33. Huff KK, Knabbe C, Lindsay R et al. Multi-hormonal regulation of insulin-like growth factor-I related protein in MCF-7 cells. Mol Endocrinol 1988; 2:200-208.
34. Yee D, Rosen N, Favoni RE et al. The insulin-like growth factors, their receptors and their binding proteins in human breast cancer. Cancer Treat Res 1991; 53:93-104.
35. Clemmons DR, Camacho-Hubner C, Coronado EB et al. IGF binding protein secretion by breast carcinoma cell lines: correlation with ER status Endocrinol 1990; 127:2697-2686.
36. Lonning PE, Hall K, Aalvaag A, Lien EA. Influence of tamoxifen on plasma levels of IGF I and IGF BP 1 in breast cancer patients. Cancer Res 1992; 52:4719-4723.
37. Murphy LC. Anti-estrogen action and growth factor regulation. Breast Cancer Res Treat 1994; 31:61-71.
38. Arteaga CL, Osborne CK. Growth inhibition of human breast cancer cells in vitro with an antibody against the Type I somatostatin receptor. Cancer Res 1989; 49:6237 -6242.
39. Fitzpatrick SL, Brightwell J, Wittliff JL. Epidermal growth factor binding by breast tumor biopsies and relationship to estrogen and progesterone receptor levels. Cancer Res 1984; 44:3448-3453.
40. Harris AL, Nicholson S. EGF receptors in human breast cancer. In: Lippman ME, Dickson RB, eds. Breast Cancer-Cellular and Molecular Biology. Boston: Kluwer Academic Publishers. 1988:343-362.
41. Sainsbury JRC, Farndon JR, Sherbet GV, Harris AL. EGF receptors and estrogen receptors in human breast cancer. Lancet 1985; (i) 364 -366.
42. Davidson NE, Gelmann EP, Lippman ME, Dickson RB. Epidermal growth factor receptor gene expression in estrogen receptor positive and negative human breast cancer cell lines. Mol Endocrinol 1987; 1:216-223.
43. Imai Y, Leung CKH, Friesen HG, Shiu RPC. Epidermal growth factor receptors and effect of epidermal growth factor on the growth of human breast cancer cells in long-term tissue culture. Cancer Res 1982; 42:4394-4398.
44. Berthois Y, Dong XF, Martin PM. Regulation of EGF receptor by estrogen and anti-estrogen in the human breast cancer cell line MCF-7. Biochem Biophysic Res Comm 1989; 159:126-131.
45. Van Agthoven T, Van Agthoven TL, Portengen H et al. Ectopic expression of EGF receptors induces hormone independence in ZR-75-1 human breast cancer cells. Cancer Res 1992; 52:5082-5088.
46. Valverius EM, Velu T, Shanker V et al. Over-expression of the EGF receptor in human breast cancer cells fails to induce an estrogen-dependent phenotype. Int J Cancer 1990; 46:712-718.
47. Reddy KB, Mangold GL, Tandon AK et al. Inhibition of breast cancer cell growth in vitro by a tyrosine kinase inhibitor. Cancer Res 1992; 52:3636-3641.
48. Stewart AJ, Johnson MD, May FEB, Westley B. Role of insulin-like growth factors and Type I IGF receptor in estrogen stimulated proliferation of human breast cancer cells J Biol Chem 1990; 265, No. 34:21172-21178.
49. Freiss G, Prebois C, Vignon F. Control of breast cancer cell growth by steroids and growth factors: Interactions and mechanisms. Breast Cancer Res Treat 1993; 27:57-68.
50. Slamon DJ, Clark GM, Wong SG et al. Human breast cancer: Correlation of relapse and survival with amplification of the HER-2/neu oncogene. Science 1987; 235:177-182.
51. Pollak M, Huynh HT, Pratt Lefebre S. Tamoxifen reduces serum Insulin-like growth factor I (IGF I). Breast Cancer Res Treat 1992 (a); 22:91-100.
52. Bishop JM. Molecular themes in oncogenesis. Cell 1991; 64:235-248.
53. Sherwin SA, Twardzik DR, Bohn WH et al. High molecular weight transforming growth factor activity in the urine of patients with disseminated cancer. Cancer Res 1983; 43:403-407.

54. Wakefield LM, Colletta AA, McCune BK, Sporn MB. Roles for transforming growth factors β in the genesis, prevention and treatment of breast cancer. In: Dickson RB and Lippman ME, eds. Genes, Oncogenes and Hormones: Advances in Cellular and Molecular Biology Breast Cancer. Boston: Kluwer Academic Publishers, 1991:97-136.
55. Pierce GB, Spiers WC. Tumours are charicatures of the process of tissue renewal: prospects for therapy by directing differentiation. Cancer Res 1988; 48:1996-2004.
56. Schipper H, Goh CR, Wang TL. Rethinking cancer: Should we control rather than kill? Canadian J Oncol 1991; 3:207-216, 220-224.
57. Schipper H. Shifting the Cancer Paradigm: Must we Kill to Cure? (Editorial) J Clin Oncol 1995; 13, No.4:801-807.

CHAPTER 2

The TGFβ Family

J.R. Benson

i) Introduction

TGFβ is the prototype of a superfamily of homologous regulatory peptides which also include inhibins, activins[1] and Mullerian Inhibitory Substance.[2] Inhibins and activins modulate secretion of the gonadotrophic hormone, follicle stimulating hormone (FSH) from the anterior pituitary gland by either suppressing or stimulating levels of FSH transcript respectively.[3,4] TGFβ can partially mimic the repressive activities of inhibins, but cannot substitute for activins. Conversely, inhibins and activins have some morphogenic properties and can direct patterns of differentiation in human leukemia cell lines.[5] The decapentaplegic (DPP) product of Drosophila[6] which has 25-30% sequence homology to TGFβ, is part of this superfamily, testifying to a high degree of evolutionary conservation and possible origin from a common ancestral gene. The DPP gene product is a key endogenous morphogen in embryonic development, and is related structurally and functionally to the Vgl product of *Xenopus Laevis* with which it shares at least 50% sequence homology. Both DPP and Vgl gene products have strong homology with another group of morphogens termed bone morphogenetic protein (BMP) which orchestrates new bone formation in mammals.[7,8] Indeed, certain human and bovine BMP's exhibit up to 75% sequence homology with DPP. TGFβ exists as 3 mammalian isoforms, TGFβ1,[9] TGFβ2[10] and TGFβ3.[11] A β4 isoform has been isolated from a cDNA library of chick embryo chondrocytes[12] whilst a fifth isoform (TGFβ5) is expressed in *Xenopus Laevis*.[13] No isoforms corresponding to TGFβ4 nor TGFβ5 have yet been identified in mammalian tissues.

TGFβ1 was the first isoform to be isolated and characterized, being initially extracted from human and bovine platelets in which it is contained in abundance in alpha granules.[9] Subsequently it was also found in high concentration in placental tissue (Frolik et al 1983) and finally cloned in 1985.[15] TGFβ2 was also isolated form porcine platelets[10] and has since been identified in several mammalian species including humans, monkeys and rodents. The β3 isoform was initially identified in cDNA libraries derived from cells of porcine (ovarian) and human (ovarian, placenta, brain) origin.[11]

ii) Structure of the TGFβ Molecule

Each isoform is a 25 kDal homodimeric peptide composed of 2 peptide chains, of 112 amino-acids in length and containing a conserved motif of 9 cysteine residues. Of these 9 cysteines, 6 participate in formation of 3 interlocking intramonomeric disulphide bonds which are buried within, and stabilize each monomer. Crystallographic analysis of the β2 isoform reveals that when these peptide monomers are linked together by formation of disulphide bridges, an eight-membered ring structure or "cysteine knot" configuration is formed from these intra- and interchain sulphide bonds, which complement hydrophobic interactions and stabilize the whole molecule at the secondary and tertiary levels.[16] The surface residues involved in direct receptor binding have yet to be determined, but the evolution of a dimeric structure may permit some regulation of ligand activity through complex allosteric interactions.

The TGFβ molecule is synthesized as part of a larger precursor molecule of which the mature moiety constitutes the C-terminal fragment. This is initially covalently linked to a precursor pro-region, consisting of 2 peptide chains of variable length ranging from 249 to 310 amino-acids. During synthesis, the mature molecule is cleaved proteolytically from the pro-region, but remains noncovalently attached. In this loosely bound state, the pro-region is able to fold itself around the mature TGFβ component and render it functionally latent, being thus otherwise known as latency associated peptide (LAP).[17] TGFβ is usually synthesized in a homodimeric form with two identical chains, but heterodimers composed of different monomers have been documented.[10,18] Most cells secrete TGFβ in a latent form[19,20] with the mature TGFβ molecule linked to the pro-region. In turn, this is attached to a latent TGFβ binding protein (LTBP) to form the large latent complex.[21] The mature TGFβ molecule linked to the pro-region in the absence of LTBP is termed the small latent complex. LTBP is a high molecular weight protein which is bound to LAP by disulphide bonding.[22] It contains multiple repeat sequences which are characteristic of extracellular matrix proteins such as fibrillin and basement membrane proteins.[22,23] These typically involve EGF repeat sequences, but LTBP also possesses repeats containing eight cysteine residues.[21] LTBP may therefore represent a component of the extracellular matrix and effectively chaperones the TGFβ molecule as it passes from cell interior to exterior during the process of secretion. LTBP also appears to bind the large latent complex to components of the extracellular matrix, and may therefore be important in both sequestration of TGFβ and determination of its local bio-availability.[24] Pulse-chase studies using the fibrosarcoma cell line HT-1080 have confirmed that both free and TGFβ1 bound forms of LTBP are associated with the extracellular matrix and can only be released proteolytically with plasmin, thus implying a covalent linkage. By contrast, the mature TGFβ moiety is released from the large latent complex by sodium dodecylsulphate (SDS) treatment, consistent with a noncovalent interaction.[17] LTBP rapidly associates with the extracellular matrix following secretion, with low levels being detected in conditioned media. Moreover, this interaction between the LTBP component of the large latent complex is independent of other components (LAP and TGFβ1). Several different immunological types of LTBP have been identified which have different binding affinities for the extracellular matrix.[25] This may permit targeting of TGFβ1 extracellularly and account for observed patterns of immunohistochemical localization.[26,27] In particular, the distribution of TGFβ in immunohistochemical sections may be more a reflection of the pattern of expression of LTBP isoforms rather than cellular origin. This could partly account for some discrepancies and controversy over interpretation of immunohistochemical studies which examine levels of protein product only. Current in situ hybridization techniques may help resolve some of these issues.

Figure 2.1 is a schematic representation of the structure of the large latent TGFβ1 complex. Crystallographic analysis indicates that in the β2 isoform the disulphide bridges within the pro-region are formed between cysteine residues 223 and 225 whilst that within the mature region involves cysteine residue 77.[28,29] As LTBP is strongly bound to the extracellular matrix by covalent interactions, it has been proposed that the latent TGFβ1 complex is released from the ECM by enzymatic cleavage at a hinge region located between the ECM and LAP binding sites of LTBP. Therefore a small fragment of LTBP (approximately 50Kd) remains attached to the ECM following release of the complex.[24]

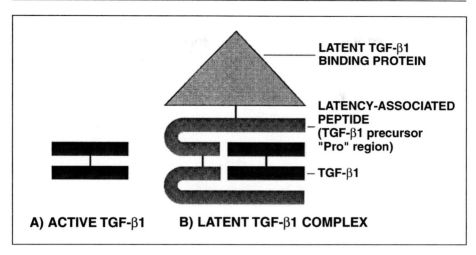

A) ACTIVE TGF-β1   B) LATENT TGF-β1 COMPLEX

Fig. 2.1. Structure of the latent TGFβ complex—see text for explanation. Reprinted with permission from: Wakefield LM et al. In: Dickson RB and Lippman ME, eds. Genes, Oncogenes and Hormones: Advances in Cellular and Molecular Biology. © Kluwer Academic Publishers.

Binding of the large latent complex to the ECM constitutes an important function of LTBP, which indirectly determines local levels of biologically active forms of TGFβ by controlling not only bioavailability but also activation of TGFβ. Though details of activation remain elusive, the dual association of LTBP with LAP and ECM via separate discrete binding sites is no doubt crucial to maintaining TGFβ in a latent form and preventing functional 'ectopism' once the large latent complex has been secreted into the extracellular space. Studies with cocultures of endothelial and smooth muscle cells have provided evidence that the enzyme transglutaminase is required for activation of latent TGFβ. This enzyme facilitates formation of cross-links between ECM proteins and LTBP.[30] Inhibitors of transglutaminase prevent activation of TGFβ1 in endothelial cells treated with retinoids.[31] It is the combined function of LTBP together with its associated proteinases which thus regulate binding to and release from components of the ECM.

A further central role for LTBP involves active participation in pathways of TGFβ secretion. Though evidence has emerged for possible intracrine pathways, most signaling pathways for TGFβ involve interaction with surface membrane receptors for which prior secretion of the peptide is a prerequisite for initiation of any cellular signal. TGFβ1 and LTBP exhibit coordinated induction suggesting that LTBP is vital for the ultimate functional expression of TGFβ. Experiments using the human erythroleukemia cell line, HEL have shown that the magnitude of TGFβ1 induction by the phorbol ester 12-myristate 13-acetate (PMA) correlates with that of LTBP. Increases in levels of both TGFβ1 and LTBP transcripts followed a similar time course and pulse-chase analysis showed that TGFβ1 became associated with LTBP within a short time period after synthesis. This large latent complex is rapidly processed and secreted from producer cells, whereas solitary precursor forms of TGFβ1 (small latent complexes) are retained within cells for a longer time period and secreted very slowly.[32] Other experiments with recombinant TGFβ1 precursor have shown that an anomalous small latent complex is formed in the absence of LTBP which contains abnormal disulphide bridges.[33] The latter prevent release of mature TGFβ1 and therefore LTBP may be essential for the correct assembly, secretion, and ultimately release of functionally active forms of TGFβ1 from cells. Mature TGFβ1 released from intracellular precursor forms by proteolytic cleavage with trypsin have reduced biological activity (growth inhibitory effects) compared with mature TGFβ1 derived from normal extracellular complexes. Therefore the secretion process *per se* may evoke changes in the tertiary structure of TGFβ1 which enhance activity of the mature product.[32] Both TGFβ1 precursor peptide and LTBP contain signal sequences which may interact synergistically to promote optimal channeling of newly secreted TGFβ1 into secretory pathways. Unprocessed TGFβ1 precursor is localized predominantly to the Golgi complex suggesting that absence of LTBP interferes with secretion at the stage of transfer from this cytoplasmic structure.[32]

iii) Mechanisms of Activation of TGFβ

"Activation" is a collective term describing a sequence of events leading to the release of active TGFβ which can interact with receptors to generate an intracellular signal. The mature moeity must be dissociated from both the latency associated peptide (LAP) and LTBP. Though precise details of activation in vivo remain elusive, there is circumstantial evidence that this represents an important step in the regulation of TGFβ action. Thus receptors for TGFβ are widespread and present on most cell types. The interaction of ligand with these receptors is therefore likely to be determined by specific temporal and spatial patterns of activation. Furthermore, levels of the latent form of TGFβ within both tissues and plasma exceed those required for evoking a maximal response from corresponding levels of the active product.[34] An important corollary of this postulate that activation is a major determinant of TGFβ bioactivity is that changes in levels of TGFβ synthesis may not be accompanied by proportional changes in the functional profile of TGFβ. This is further confounded by posttranscriptional control mechanisms which may prevent concordance between measured changes in TGFβ gene expression and levels of protein product.[35] It follows that elevated levels of TGFβ synthesis may not necessarily be accompanied by increased biological activity if the activation process per se is a rate-limiting step.

Most cells in tissue culture secrete TGFβ into their conditioned medium in a biologically inactive form.[36-39] This has permitted investigation of potential mechanisms of activation, but the physiological relevance of such in vitro studies to in vivo processes is uncertain. Changes in the proportion of TGFβ in the biologically active form following exposure to a variety of activating conditions can be assessed using quantitative bioassays which rely on highly sensitive cells lines as response indicators (e.g., mink lung epithelial cells). Notwithstanding certain technical limitations, four principle activating factors have emerged:

   i) Heat
  ii) acidification/alkalinization
 iii) chaotropic agents
  iv) enzymes (proteases)

Thermal activation is not an option in vivo; Lyons and co-workers showed that either mild or extreme changes in pH could activate latent TGFβ from conditioned media of fibroblast cell lines (AKR-MCA and NRK-49F). Exposure of conditioned media to either strongly acidic (pH 1.2) or alkaline (pH 12) conditions produced significant amounts of active TGFβ with almost complete inhibition of ^{125}I-TGFβ binding (indicating a high proportion of TGFβ in the active form). By contrast, mild acidification (pH 4.5-5.5) yields only 20-30% activation, and time course studies suggest that 2 discrete forms of latent TGFβ may exist—one of these is sensitive to mildly acidic conditions and the other to a much lower pH (1.5). It is questionable whether acid activation of TGFβ is physiologically relevant, though mildly acidic conditions (4.5-5.5) may pertain in the micro-environment of cells or within certain protected locations within the extracellular matrix.

Plasmin is a widely distributed cell-associated serine protease. In selected cell lines, this enzyme can produce a comparable degree of activation to mild acidification.[40] Plasmin could have a genuine role in mechanisms of activation in vivo. A more physiological model has been employed involving coculture of endothelial cells and smooth muscle cells to demonstrate that activation in vivo may be dependent upon interactions involving more than a single cell type.[41,42] Though each of these cell types secrete only latent TGFβ in mono-culture, conditioned medium from cocultures contains large amounts of active TGFβ, indicating functional cooperation between endothelial cells and smooth muscle cells. Further investigation of this coculture system has revealed that active TGFβ is released from the latent complex by enzymatic cleavage of LAP by plasmin. Smooth muscle cells are indirectly responsible for production of plasmin by endothelial cells via fibroblast growth factor (FGF) which induces plasminogen activator (PA-1). This cooperative model for TGFβ activation is consistent with an earlier one proposed by Lyons et al.[40] According to this simpler, unicellular model, binding of ligand to cellular receptors results in production of PA-1 which limits activation of plasminogen. This could serve as a negative feedback system to control plasmin-mediated activation of latent TGFβ.

Other candidates for enzymatic activation of TGFβ have been investigated including glycosidases[43] and thrombospondin.[44] Activation by proteases located at the cell surface or in the extracellular matrix at the cell periphery is a feasible mechanism for release of active TGFβ in vivo. Plasmin is associated with activation in several in vitro cell models[45] and the conserved cysteine residues in LAP represent likely substrates for these enzymes. The resultant disruption of disulphide bonds promotes dissociation of mature TGFβ from its precursor peptide (LAP). As discussed above, the enzyme transglutaminase may indirectly be implicated in activation of TGFβ by controlling interaction between LTBP and the extracellular matrix.

Barcellos-Hoff and co-workers have recently used an irradiated murine mammary gland model to study possible mechanisms of activation in vivo.[46] Levels of TGFβ immunoreactivity were measured in tissue extracts following whole body irradiation with ^{60}Co-l (0.5-5 Gy). Despite no changes in *total* levels of TGFβ protein or mRNA, irradiation of tissues resulted in increased expression of collagen type III which is a known target for TGFβ action. Therefore apparent increases in TGFβ bioactivity occurred in the absence of increases in TGFβ synthesis. These authors employed an anti-TGFβ antibody which selectively recognizes activated forms of TGFβ, together with an antibody which specifically recognizes LAP. Exposure of tissues to ionizing radiation led to increased immunoreactivity for active TGFβ, but falls in expression of LAP. This differential immunoreactivity between active and latent forms of TGFβ presumably resulted from enhanced epitope exposure secondary to release of TGFβ from the small latent complex and provided important direct evidence for activation in vivo within intact tissues. The time course of this radiation-induced TGFβ activation in vivo was relatively rapid (within 1 hour), implying that mediation by proteases is unlikely to be involved. Instead, it was suggested that latent TGFβ may be directly subject to redox effects, with activation resulting from the action of reactive oxygen species (ROS).[47] Incubation of latent TGFβ in a cell culture medium containing ascorbate and trace metals, thereby generating oxygen-free radicals, resulted in activation of a significant proportion of latent TGFβ. By contrast, there were no effects on the measured bioactivity of active TGFβ when incubated under similar conditions. Changes in levels of tissue oxygenation accompanying various pathological states, including malignancy, may provide a mechanism for activating latent TGFβ whose redox sensitivity is probably located within the precursor peptide (LAP). The distribution of redox potentials within tissues may partially determine spatial and temporal patterns of TGFβ activation. Other mechanisms of activation such as proteolytic cleavage provide further opportunity for regulation and in particular permit feedback control of TGFβ activation via plasminogen activator inhibitors. Furthermore, though pharmacologically induced TGFβ is secreted in the biologically active form in vitro, this may not pertain in vivo, where pathways of activation may be rate-limiting and thus represent a potential therapeutic target. For example, binding of the latent TGFβ molecule to the mannose 6-phosphate/insulin-like growth factor receptor II is a prerequisite for activation of TGFβ in a coculture system of endothelial and smooth muscle cells.[48] It is unclear whether TGFβ secreted in response to pharmacological intervention can bypass conventional mechanisms of activation, or whether the intrinsic capacity of activation processes can be modulated concurrently with TGFβ synthesis.

iv) TGFβ Receptors

Receptors for TGFβ are ubiquitous, having been detected on most cell types.[49] Two principle forms of TGFβ receptor are recognized (type I and type II), and their mechanism of action has recently been elucidated.[50] These two receptor types appear to functionally cooperate and receptor II is required for binding of TGFβ to receptor I, and both receptors jointly coordinate a cellular response. Unlike most transmembrane receptors for growth factors, these TGFβ receptors do not possess intrinsic tyrosine kinase activity, but instead have a cytoplasmic component consisting of a serine/threonine kinase (Fig. 2.2.). The TGFβ molecule binds to the type II receptor which has a constitutively active kinase domain, whose phosphorylating activity is minimally increased following binding of ligand, but which evokes a conformational change in the receptor leading to the recruitment of the type I receptor into a ternary complex. This results in phosphorylation of the type I receptor by the kinase domain of the type II receptor, which may also be dependent on some interaction between the TGFβ molecule bound by the type II receptor and the type I receptor. Receptor I can be labeled through cross-linking using a bi-functional reagent, implying some physical contact between this receptor and ligand.[50] Proteolytic mapping of receptor I suggests that phosphorylation by receptor II occurs upon serine and threonine residues within the highly conserved GS domain, and mutations within this region preclude generation of intracellular signals. Therefore according to this model, receptor II serves to bind TGFβ and recruit type I receptor into a tertiary complex before directly phosphorylating this receptor. It is the kinase activity of receptor I which propagates the intracellular signal emanating from the complex (Fig. 2.3.). The mechanism by which this signal is generated is unknown. As the GS domain is highly conserved, it seems unlikely that diverse biological responses would result from motifs within this domain orchestrating the association of various substrate molecules with this receptor. The type I receptor has recently been found to interact with the immunophilin designated FKBP-12.[51] This is a cytoplasmic receptor which binds the macrolides (immunosuppressants) FK506 and rapamycin. Mutant FKBP-12 with impaired binding to these immunosuppressants, fail to associate with type I receptor. Receptor I appears to share or overlap this macrolide binding site on FKBP-12, which may thus represent its natural ligand, and constitute a proximal step in the intracellular signaling pathway. Several type I receptor isoforms have been documented, and the pleiotypic effects of TGFβ may partly be due to the particular receptor isoform which is recruited into the complex prior to generation of the intracellular signal by the kinase activity of the type I receptor.

Though receptors I and II are the two principle TGFβ signaling receptors, their exists another membrane glycoprotein termed betaglycan, or type III receptor. This has widespread distribution, often coexisting with type I and II receptors, and which similarly binds all 3 isoforms with relatively high affinities. Transient transfection experiments involving individual receptors have shown that in the presence of labeled TGFβ, betaglycan forms immune precipitate with type II receptors.[52] These observations suggest that betaglycan may form a ligand transfer complex in which it presents ligand to receptor II, thereby

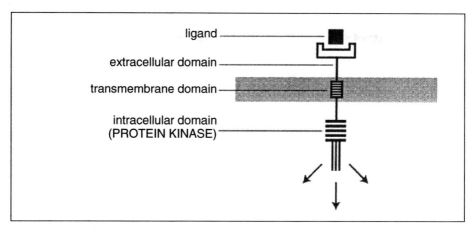

Fig. 2.2. Growth factors generally mediate a response via surface membrane receptors which possess a tripartite structure; an extracellular domain binds ligand whilst the intracellular component is involved in generation of the intracellular signal and usually possess a tyrosine or serine/threonine kinase domain. The two elements are linked by a trans-membrane component which also serves to anchor the entire structure and ensures appropriate functional orientation of the extracellular and intracellular components.

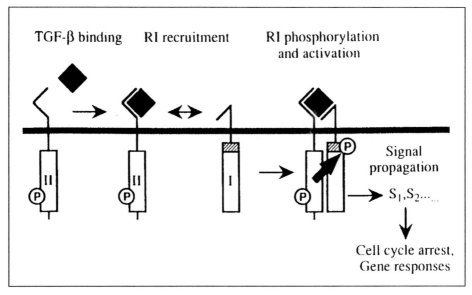

Fig. 2.3. Schematic representation for the generation of an intracellular signal by the coordinated action of types I and II TGFβ receptors. The type II receptor recruits receptor I subsequent to binding of ligand leading to activation of the kinase domain of the type I receptor with propagation of signaling to downstream elements. Reprinted with permission from: Wrana JL et al. Nature 1994; 370:341-346. © Macmillan Magazines Limited.

increasing receptor binding affinity and enhancing cell responsiveness. The rodent mesenchymal cell line L_6E_9 expresses receptors I and II but no betaglycan. Following transfection
of the latter into these cells, the binding affinity of receptor II for TGFβ is increased 50-fold,
this correlating with coprecipitation of betaglycan with receptor II and hence ternary complex formation. In contrast to betaglycan, receptors I and II have relatively low intrinsic
affinities for TGFβ, implying that this presentation of ligand by betaglycan has an important physiological role. Moreover, betaglycan permits receptors to overcome an innate re-
fractoriness to the β2 isoform, and may serve to compensate for the relatively lower intrinsic
binding affinities of the β2 and β3 isoforms to RII.[52] There is some evidence that betaglycan
can function as a dual modulator of TGFβ accessibility which is consistent with the multifunctional character of TGFβ. Membrane bound betaglycan serves to bind TGFβ and present
it to receptor II, but the large extracellular domain of betaglycan may be shed to yield soluble
forms which sequester TGFβ within the ECM and restrict its access to the TGFβ signaling
receptor.[53]

Though loss of TGFβ receptors has been reported in retinoblastomas,[54] this does not
appear to be a general phenomenon in evolution of tumors, and many human tumor cell
lines do respond to TGFβ (Table 2.1).[55] Maintenance of response to TGFβ by tumor cells is
crucial to strategies aimed at augmenting local endogenous levels of negative growth factors. This response is dependent upon both intact receptors and intracellular transduction
pathways. Thus transformed human mammary epithelial cells which have become resistant
to the growth inhibitory effects of TGFβ maintain TGFβ1 production and their receptor
profile remains unaltered.[56] Similarly, when human colonic adenoma cell lines undergo
conversion to a malignant phenotype, their response to the growth inhibitory effects of
TGFβ1 are reduced despite no change in receptor density.[57] Therefore such strategies are
doomed when intact surface receptors can bind ligand, but have become dislocated from
intracellular transduction pathways. The retention of a growth inhibitory response to TGFβ
by neoplastic cells, at least in the early stages of carcinogenesis, has two important implications. Firstly, it suggests that excessive epithelial proliferation may result from a defect in the
functional expression of negative growth factors such as TGFβ, and secondly that effective
therapeutic strategies aimed at boosting local levels of endogenous growth inhibitors might
prove feasible.

v) Intracellular Transduction Mechanisms

Until very recently, there was no evidence that receptor binding of the TGFβ ligand led
to either activation of protein kinases or changes in cyclic nucleotide metabolism, events
which are involved in transduction of many growth stimulatory peptides such as EGF and
TGF alpha. Activation of these tyrosine kinase receptors by mitogenic stimuli leads to initiation of poorly defined intracellular signal transduction pathways culminating in altered
expression of proto-oncogenes such as c-*myc*, c-*fos* and c-*jun*. Massague and co-workers
have confirmed that a primary initial step in propagation of an intracellular signal following binding of the TGFβ receptor to its ligand is the activation of a protein kinase. However,
more distal events involved in generation of a growth inhibitory signal remain to be elucidated, but there is evidence for interaction of TGFβ with cell cycle regulatory systems whereby
TGFβ prolongs the G1 phase or induces cell cycle arrest. Attention has focused on the possible 'mechanistic interfaces' between inhibitory growth factors and the products of tumor
suppressor genes, such as the retinoblastoma susceptibility gene (RB). The product of this
gene (pRB) is a 105 kDal protein which controls progression through the cell cycle and
whose function is determined by it's state of phosporylation (Fig. 2.4.). The unphosphorylated
(active) form occurs in G_1 (and G_0) whilst phosphorylated (inactive) forms dominate S-phase
and G_2M.[58] TGFβ can interact with this system by maintaining pRB in an unphosphorylated

Table 2.1. Effects of TGFβ on growth of cell lines

Cell Line	ER status	(no. of reports documenting effect)		
		None	Inhibition	Stimulation
MCF-7	+ve	4	5	-
T47-D	+ve	3	1	1
ZR75-1	+ve	1	2	-
BT-20	-ve	-	2	1
MCF-7	+ve	4	5	-
MDA-MB-231	-ve	-	1	-
HBL-100	-ve	1	2	-
Hs578T	-ve	-	4	-
MDA-MB-435	-ve	-	1	-
MDA-MB-468	-ve	-	1	-
SK-BR-3	-ve	1	2	-

Table 2.1 Effect of TGfβ on the growth of a selection of human breast cancer cell lines. The figures in the table refer to the number of reports documenting inhibition, stimulation or no effect upon cell lines. Culture conditions were not uniform, involving experiments with anchorage dependent and independent growth. Most experiments were carried out in medium containing serum, but some cells were cultured in serum-free medium.

form which facilitates arrest of cell growth.[59] Thus addition of exogenous TGFβ to mink lung epithelial cells in mid- to late G_1 blocks exit from G_1 and inhibits RB phosphorylation, the extent of which correlates with overall growth inhibitory effects of TGFβ. Furthermore, cells transformed with the SV40 large T antigen, which binds the unphosphorylated (active) forms of pRB are no longer growth inhibited by TGFβ.[60] Phosphorylation of pRB is partly effected by the cyclin-D associated protein kinases, CDK 4 and CDK 6, which oppose the growth inhibitory effects of pRB.[61] TGFβ might therefore reduce levels of pRB phosphorylation by inhibiting activity of CDK 4 and CDK 6. These protein kinases are normally inhibited by a group of proteins collectively termed p16[INK4B]. Recently, Hannon and Beach have found that TGFβ treatment of keratinocytes is associated with a 30-fold induction of a member of this group, protein p15. This inhibits CDK4 and CDK 6 and thus indirectly would favor accumulation of the unphosphorylated form of pRB, and hence cell cycle arrest.[62] It is unlikely that this is an exclusive mechanism for reducing levels of the phosphorylated RB product. Another important cyclin-dependent kinase is E-cyclin/CDK2 which mediates TGFβ arrest of mink lung epithelial cells.[63] This CDK has its own specific inhibitor, p27, but expression of this is unaffected by TGFβ. Though this protein kinase inhibitor could be controlled at a posttranscriptional level, Peters has proposed an elegant model in which the protein kinases CDK4 and CDK6 are considered to bind and sequester p27. TGFβ would induce p15, decrease levels of CDK4 and CDK6 and thus release any bound p27. This in turn would have a growth suppressive effect via inhibition of E-cyclin/CDK2. Thus p27 would operate through a threshold mechanism dictated by levels of p15 (Fig. 2.5.).[64] The active form of pRB may control progression through the G1 phase of the cell cycle by down-regulation of the c-*myc* gene. Growth inhibition by TGFβ in rodent keratinocytes is associated with reduced expression of this gene,[65] and transformation with SV40 renders these cells resistant to growth inhibition by TGFβ with no change in c-*myc* expression.[66] However, modulation of Rb activity may not be a direct, serial and obligatory step in mediation of TGFβ inhibition. Ong and co-workers have shown that breast cancer cell lines lacking a functional RB gene, but which still possess TGFβ receptors, are inhibited to the same degree as RB positive cells.[67] Moreover, though downregulation of c-*myc* expression is associated with growth inhibitory effects of TGFβ in keratinocytes, this is not observed in other cell types such as fibroblasts,[68] and keratinocytes which constitutively express high levels of c-*myc*, are still growth inhibited by TGFβ.[69] Thus neither RB nor c-*myc* have been shown conclusively to be essential elements in some linear sequence of events mediating growth factor inhibition by TGFβ. This conclusion is further supported by experiments demonstrating that exogenous TGFβ1 can induce growth arrest in retinoblastoma gene negative osteosarcoma cells (SA052) which have been pretreated with the cytotoxic agent N-phosphoacetyl-1-aspartate (PALA). This cell line is normally insensitive to growth inhibition by TGFβ1, but in the presence of PALA TGFβ1 appears to exert influence on cell cycle events independently of RB protein.[70] TGFβ1 has recently been found to downregulate another proto-oncogene, c-*myb*, whose product like c-*myc* normally stimulates cell proliferation.[71] In addition to regulation of pRB by TGFβ, reciprocal interactions may occur, whereby the TGFβ gene itself becomes a target for control by pRB. A retinoblastoma control element (RCE) which mediates suppression of c-*fos* expression by RB has also been identified in the promoter regions of all TGFβ genes. This suggests that pRB may directly modulate transcription of these genes via this RCE, though other sequences may also be involved.[72] RB appears able to regulate TGFβ1 transcription in either a positive or negative manner, depending upon cell type; it upregulates TGFβ1 transcription in CCL-64 and A549 cells,[73] both of which are strongly inhibited by TGFβ1. Conversely it downregulates transcription in NIH3T3 and AKR-2B cells in which TGFβ has a weakly growth stimulatory effect.[74] It unknown whether these downstream events are linked to initial activation of receptor kinase domains via cytosolic kinase cascades, but undoubtedly complex interactions between formal transduction pathways occur. Both parallel and sequential interactions will create some degree of functional 'cross-talk', which may ultimately restrict the efficacy of some of the newer therapeutic strategies which target aberrant expression of elements in these intracellular pathways.

The genes coding for TGFβ1, TGFβ2 and TGFβ3 are located on chromosomes 19q, 1q and 14q respectively.[49] The location of genes coding for the 3 mammalian isoforms of TGFβ on multiple chromosomes may be advantageous from an evolutionary viewpoint; thus any chromosomal insult which abrogates expression of one isoform is less likely to affect expression of the other two. A degree of functional redundancy amongst these isoforms may therefore minimize the consequences of potential oncogenic events which disrupt negative signaling pathways.

vi) Control of TGFβ Gene Expression

In vitro studies have confirmed that a wide variety of cell types produce TGFβ and can respond to this growth factor. Furthermore, in vivo work has shown that isoforms of TGFβ have well-defined and predictable patterns of expression during both development as well as pathological states resulting from tissue insult. It is likely that specific changes in the spatial and temporal expression of TGFβ accompany carcinogenesis, though the nature and significance of these have yet to be elucidated.

The activation of TGFβ, with release of the mature, active form which can bind to receptors, represents one modality for controlling expression of TGFβ (section iii). Similarly, preferential sequestration of latent TGFβ within the extracellular matrix serves to restrict its bioavailability and control rates of presentation of active ligand to receptors. Though these are probably important methods of controlling bioactivity of TGFβ, they are likely to

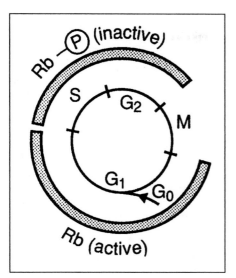

Fig. 2.4. Progression through the cell cycle is accompanied by changes in the state of phosphorylation of the retinoblastoma protein (pRB). TGFβ promotes accumulation of the unphosphorylated, or active form of pRB which acts as a brake to suppress cell proliferation.

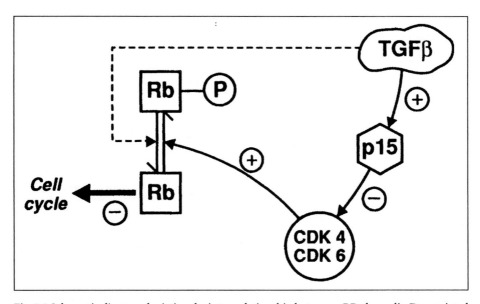

Fig. 2.5 Schematic diagram depicting the inter-relationship between pRB, the cyclin D associated protein kinases (CDK 4 and CDK 6) and TGFβ. The latter mediates effects upon the phosphorylation of pRB indirectly by determining the level of activity of these protein kinases which are critical regulatory elements in cell cycle control.

constitute a fine-tuning mechanism with high sensitivity which can respond rapidly to local tissue demands. More profound changes in expression of TGFβ are likely to involve alteration in the rate of synthesis of both TGFβ and its cognate receptor.

There is evidence from in vitro and in vivo studies for the control of TGFβ expression at both transcriptional and posttranscriptional levels. The latter appear particularly relevant to induction of TGFβ in response to pharmacological intervention, though both mechanisms may be operative under physiological conditions (chapter 7). Moreover, different mechanisms of control may occur in systems of repair and inflammation compared to those involving neoplastic processes. Studies examining changes in TGFβ1 mRNA levels in various in vivo model systems have confirmed increased rates of transcription, though the time course of induction is variable.[75] Thus phorbol ester (TPA) treatment of mouse epidermis results in a rapid increase in TGFβ1 transcript within 2-3 hours following exposure to TPA.[76] By contrast, in other model systems representing a range of pathological processes including myocardial infarction and osteogenesis, induction of TGFβ1 mRNA typically occurs after a minimum period of 24 hours.[77,78] Though precise mechanisms remain unclear, activation of TGFβ1 transcription occurs in response to diverse stimuli and pathological processes. Amongst exogenous factors, TGFβ isoforms are themselves potent inducers of TGFβ transcription. This auto-induction may serve to promote rapid expansion of the extracellular matrix in vivo, and accelerate wound repair and new bone formation. Auto-induction effectively amplifies the response to growth factors which may be particularly pertinent to developmental and neoplastic processes.[79] TGFβ1 induces increased expression of TGFβ1 mRNA in AKR-2B fibroblasts which is maximal at 6-12 hours. Increased levels of transcript (25-fold) were associated with increased levels of TGFβ1 protein in conditioned media. Curiously, there was delayed suppression of TGFβ2 and TGFβ3 expression by TGFβ1. By contrast, treatment of the same cells with exogenous TGFβ2 resulted in induction of all isoforms, albeit not simultaneously. This autoregulation of TGFβ gene expression involves a combination of both transcriptional and posttranscriptional mechanisms, in which the TGFβ mRNA molecule undergoes posttranscriptional stabilization, thereby enhancing rates of translation.

Embryological studies indicate that all 5 isoforms of TGFβ are differentially regulated with defined patterns of expression at particular stages of development. Though these are consistent within taxonomical groups, there is variation between species thereof. Thus expression of TGFβ1 is absent from chick embryos, but present throughout development of mammalian forms.[27] Furthermore, individual cells in vitro can exhibit differential responses to external stimuli with increases in expression of one isoform and decreased expression of others. When keratinocytes are exposed to changes in Ca^{2+} concentration in their surrounding media, there is a 10-fold increase in TGFβ2 mRNA levels, but a concomitant decrease in TGFβ1 expression of 3- to 5-fold. Increased levels of TGFβ2 transcript are associated with corresponding increases in levels of TGFβ2 product secreted into the conditioned medium. Of interest, the magnitude of this increase was approximately 5-fold that of transcript induction, suggesting additional control at a posttranscriptional level. Indeed, studies with v-H-*ras* transformed cells confirm that translational control can occur independently of transcriptional control. These cells exhibit similar changes in levels of transcript as normal keratinocytes in response to changes in Ca^{2+} concentration, but do not secrete TGFβ2 into their conditioned media.[80]

The differential control of individual isoform expression is likely to be mediated via promoter sequences within the respective genes. Transcriptional activity is regulated by binding of regulatory proteins to specific nucleotide sequences within these promoter regions. The TGFβ1 mRNA molecule has a particularly long 5′ untranslated region (UTR) which corresponds to a large 5′ flanking sequence in the cognate gene. Studies with 5′ deletion mutants have revealed the presence of both promotory and inhibitory sequences within this region. Two distinct promoters have been identified within the TGFβ1 gene.[81,82] These contain GC rich sequences including 11 CCGCCC repeats. Three inhibitory regions exist within the 5′ component of the TGFβ1 gene. As with the promoter sequences[81,83] these are located both upstream of the first transcriptional start site and between the first and second start sites (see chapter 7, section ii (c)).[76]

These negative regulatory regions contain sequences which are known to be inhibitory for other genes.[84] Precise details of how these regions mediate promotion and inhibition of transcription remain to be elucidated. However, both TGFβ1 auto-induction and induction by phorbol esters involve binding of the AP-1 complex to specific sequences of the TGFβ1 gene.[85] The AP-1 complex incorporates products of the nuclear oncogenes *jun* and *fos* which have been implicated in control of cell growth and differentiation.[86] The activity of these nuclear oncogenes is in turn regulated by both their corresponding gene products[86] as well as TGFβ1.[88]

At least 3 sequences exist within the promoter regions of TGFβ1 which bind the AP-1 complex. Implication of these sequences in control of TGFβ1 expression is supported by experiments involving mutant constructs in which AP-1 binding sites have been deleted. Cells containing these constructs are unresponsive to inductive effects of TPA and TGFβ1.

Similarly, coexpression of TGFβ1 constructs in A549 cells with anti-sense c-*jun* or anti-sense c-*fos* completely abrogates TGFβ1 induction, indicating that both elements of the AP-1 complex are essential for TGFβ1 auto-induction.[89,90] There appears to be a complex interplay between growth factors and nuclear proto-oncogenes and their products. The interdependence of their expression may render cells vulnerable to oncogenic change as aberrant expression of one factor could reverberate with indirect effects upon expression of other factors, thus providing maximal disruptive influence upon normal regulatory processes.

Transcriptional factors other than AP-1 complex are involved in control of TGFβ gene expression. Studies with a *Drosophila Melanogaster* cell culture system in which expression of TGFβ promotor (*p*TGFβ:CAT) constructs were examined in vivo have shown that the transcription factor Sp-1 strongly mediated induction of the β1 and β3 isoforms, though not TGFβ2.[91] Moreover, specific binding of *p*TGFβ1 and *p*TGFβ3 to pure Sp-1 or nuclear extracts occurred, and subsequently Sp-1 has been shown to bind to the G-C rich promoter sequences of the TGFβ1 gene.[82,85] Activation of the TGFβ2 gene can occur via the transcription factor ATF-2. This provides a mechanism for control of the TGFβ2 gene by the Rb protein.[92] As previously discussed, a retinoblastoma control element (RCE) has been located within the promoter region of all TGFβ genes. This region may interact with other control elements to regulate expression of TGFβ in either a positive or negative manner depending on cell type.[73,74] There is evidence for involvement of AP-1 in mediation of Rb effects upon TGFβ1 gene expression.[85] Moreover, Rb protein can downregulate *fos* expression via the RCE, thus providing opportunity for feedback regulation of the AP-1 complex.[72]

There are complex interrelationships between the promoter regions of TGFβ and various sets of transcription factors and other nuclear proteins involved in cell-cycle control, and ultimately cell growth and differentiation. Caution must be exercised in extrapolating from in vitro studies on gene regulation. Elegant experiments employing growth of mammary epithelial cells on different substrates reveal that the extracellular matrix can regulate expression of the TGFβ1 gene. Streuli and co-workers stably transfected the mammary epithelial cell line CID-9 with a construct containing the TGFβ1 promoter linked to a CAT reporter gene.[93] Cells were subsequently cultured on either plastic or basement membrane rich matrix derived from EHS tumors.[94] Levels of CAT activity were 10- to 13-fold greater in cells cultured on plastic, suggesting that the ECM negatively regulates TGFβ1 expression at the transcriptional level and this is upregulated in isolated cells grown on plastic in vitro. However, when cells were cultured in conditions permitting formation of an endogenous basement membrane, transcriptional activity of the TGFβ1 gene was suppressed. These findings are consistent with the observations that the function and expression of TGFβ is highly context dependent, both in terms of the cellular and matrical environment of an individual cell. (See chapter 7, section ii (c).)

References

1. Mason AJ, Hayflick JS, Ling N, et al. Complementary DNA sequences of ovarian follicular fluid inhibin show precursor structure and homology with transforming growth factor β. Nature 1985; 318:659-663.
2. Cate RL, Mattalanio RJ, Hession C, et al. Isolation of the bovine and human genes for Mullerian inhibiting substance and expression of the human gene in animal cells. Cell 1986; 45:685-698.
3. Attardi B, Keeping HS, Winters SJ et al. Rapid and profound suppression of messenger ribonucleic acid encoding follicle-stimulating hormone β by inhibin from primate Sertoli cells. Mol Endocrinol 1989; 3:280-287.
4. Ling N, Ying SY, Ueno N et al. Isolation and partial characterisation of a Mr 32000 protein with inhibin activity from porcine follicular fluid. Proc Natl Aca Sci (USA) 1985; 82:7217-7221.
5. Eto Y, Tsuji T, Takezawa M et al. Purification and characterisation of erythroid differentiation factor (EGF) isolated from human leukaemia cell line THP-1. BBRC 1987; 142:1095-1103.
6. Padgett RW, St. Johnston RD, Gelhart WM. A transcript from a Drosophila pattern gene predicts a protein homologous to the transforming growth factor-β-family. Nature 1987; 325:81 -84.
7. Wozney JM. Bone morphogenetic proteins. Prog Growth Factor Res 1989; 1:267-280.
8. Kingsley DM. The TGFβ superfamily:New members, new receptors and new genetic tests of function in different organisms. Genes Development 1994; 8:133-146.
9. Assoian RK, Komoriya A, Meyers CA et al. Transforming growth factor beta in human platelets. J Biol Chem 1983; 258:7155-7160.
10. Cheifetz S, Weatherbee JA, Tsang MLS, et al. The transforming growth factor-β system, a complex pattern of cross-reactive ligands and receptors. Cell 1987; 48:409-415.
11. Derynck R, Lindquist PB, Lee A, et al. A new type of transforming growth factor-β, TGFβ3. EMBO J 1988; 7:3737-3743.
12. Jakowlew SB, Dillard PJ, Kondaiah P et al. Complementary deoxyribonucleic acid cloning of a novel transforming growth factor-β messenger ribonucleic acid from chick embryo chondrocytes. Mol Endocrinol 1988; 2:747-755.
13. Kondaiah P, van Obberghen-Schilling, Ludwig RL et al. cDNA cloning of porcine transforming growth factor-β1 mRNA's. J Biol Chem 1988; 263:18313-18317.
14. Frolik C.A., Dart L.L., Meyers C.A. et al. Purification and initial characterisation of a type β transforming growth factor from human placenta. Proc Natl Aca Sci (USA) 1983; 80:3676-3680.
15. Derynck R, Jarrett JA, Ellson YC et al. Human transforming growth factor beta complementary DNA sequence and expression in normal and transformed cells. Nature 1985; 316:701-705.
16. Doapin S, Li M, Davies R. Crystal structure of transforming growth factor β2 refined at 1.8A resolution. Proteins 1993; 17:176-192.
17. Wakefield LM, Smith DM, Flanders KC, Sporn MB. Latent transforming growth factor β from human platelets. J Biol Chem 1988; 263:7646-7634.
18. Ogawa Y, Schmidt DK, Dasch JR et al. Purification and characterisation of transforming growth factor type β2.3 and β1.2 heterodimers from bovine bone. J Biol Chem 1992; 267:2325-2328.
19. Wakefield LM, Smith DM, Tohru Masui et al. Distribution and modulation of cellular receptors for transforming growth factor β. J Cell Biol 1987; 105:965-975.
20. Miyazano K, Hellman U, Wernstedt C and Heldin C-H. Latent high molecular weight complex of transforming growth factor β1. J Biol Chem 1988; 263:6407-6415.

21. Kanzaki T, Olofsson A, Moren A et al. TGFβ1 binding protein:A component of the large latent complex of TGFβ1 with multiple repeat sequences. Cell 1990; 61:1051-1061.
22. Maslen CL, Corson GM, Maddox BK et al. Partial sequence of a candidate gene for the Marfan Syndrome. Nature 1991; 352:334-337.
23. Sasaki M, Yamada Y. The laminin B2 chain has a multidomain structure homologous to the B1 chain. J Biol Chem 1987; 262:17.111-17.117.
24. Taipale J, Miyazono K, Heldin C-H, Keski-Oja J. Latent transforming growth factor β1 associates to fibroblast extracellular matrix via latent TGFβ binding protein. J Cell Biol 1994; 124:171-181.
25. Olofsson A, Miyazano K, Kanzaki T et al. Transforming growth factor-β1, β2 and β3 secreted by a human glioblastoma line. J Biol Chem 1992; 267:19482-19488.
26. Butta A, Maclennan K, Flanders KC et al. Induction of transforming growth factor beta 1 in human breast cancer in vivo following tamoxifen treatment. Cancer Res 1992; 52:4261-4264.
27. Heine UI, Munoz EF, Flanders KC, Ellingworth LR, et al. Role of transforming growth factor β in the development of the mouse embryo. J Cell Biol 1987; 105:2861-2876.
28. Daopin S, Piez KA, Ogawa Y, Davies DR. Crystal structure of TGFβ2:an unusual fold for the superfamily. Science 1992; 257:369-373.
29. Schlunegger MP, Grutter MG. An unusual feature revealed by the crystal structure at 2.2A resolution of human transforming growth factor β2 Nature 1992; 358:430-434.
30. Flaumenhaft R, Abe M, Sato Y et al. Role of latent TGFβ binding protein in the activation of latent TGFβ by cocultures of endothelial and smooth muscle cells. J Cell Biol 1993; 120:995-1002.
31. Kojima S, Nara K, Rifkin DB. Requirement for transglutaminase in the activation of latent transforming growth factor β in bovine endothelial cells. J Cell Biol 1993; 121:439-448.
32. Miyazano K, Olofsson A, Colosetti P, Heldin C-H. A role of the latent TGFβ1 binding protein in the assembly and secretion of TGFβ1. EMBO J 1991; 10:1091-1101.
33. Sha X, Brunner AM, Purchio AF, Gentry LE. Transforming growth factor β1:importance of glycosylation and acidic proteases for processing and secretion. Mol Endocrinol 1989; 3:1090-1098.
34. Miyazono K, Heldin C-H. Latent forms of TGFβ: Molecular structure and mechanisms of activation. In: Clinical Applications of TGFβ. Chichester: Wiley (John) and Sons Ltd., 1991:81-92.
35. Benson JR, Baum M. Transforming growth factor beta isoforms in breast cancer. Br J Cancer 1994; 70:1278-1278.
36. Lawrence DA, Pircher R, Kryceve-Martinerie C, Julien P. Normal embryo fibroblasts release transforming growth factors in a latent form. J Cell Physiol 1984; 121:184-188.
37. Moses HL, Tucker RF, Leof EB et al. Type β transforming growth factor is a growth stimulator and a growth inhibitor. Cancer Cells 1985; 3:65-71.
38. Keski-Oja J, Leof EB, Lyons RM et al. Transforming growth factors and control of neoplastic cell growth. J Cell Biochem 1987; 33:95-107.
39. Wakefield LM, Colletta AA, McCune BK, Sporn MB. Roles for transforming growth factors β in the genesis, prevention and treatment of breast cancer. In: Dickson RB and Lippman ME, eds. Genes, Oncogenes and Hormones: Advances in Cellular and Molecular Biology Breast Cancer. Boston: Kluwer Academic Publishers, 1991:97-136.
40. Lyons RM, Keski-Oja J, Moses HL. Proteolytic activation of latent transforming growth factor β from fibroblast conditioned medium. J Cell Biol 1988; 106:1659-1665.
41. Sato Y, Tsuboi R, Lyons R et al. Characterisation of the activation of latent TGFβ by cocultures of endothelial cells and pericytes or smooth muscle cells:A self-regulating system. J Cell Biol 1990; 111:757-763.
42. Antonelli-Orlidge A, Saunders KB, Smith SR, D'Amore PA. An activated form of transforming growth factor β is produced by cocultures of endothelial cells and pericytes. PNAS (USA) 1989; 86:4544-4548.
43. Miyazono K, Heldin C-H. Role for carbohydrate structures in TGFβ1 latency. Nature 1989; 338:158-160.

44. Schultz-Cherry S, Murphy-Ullrich JE. Thrombospondin causes activation of latent transforming growth factor-β secretedby endothelial cells by a novel mechanism. J Cell Biol 1993; 122:923-932.

45. Flaumenhaft R, Abe M, Mignatti P, Rifkin DB. Basic fibroblast growth factor-induced activation of latent transforming growth factor-β in endothelial cells:Regulation of plasminogen activator activity. J Cell Biol 1992; 118:901-909.

46. Barcellos-Hoff MH, Derynck R, Tsang ML-S, Weatherbee JA. Transforming growth factor-β activation in irradiated murine mammary gland. J Clin Invest 1994; 93:892-899.

47. Barcellos-Hoff MH, Dix TA. Redox-mediated activation of latent transforming growth factor-β1. Mol Endocrinol In press.

48. Dennis A, Rifkin DB. Cellular activation of latent transforming growth factor β requires binding to the cation-dependent mannose-6-phosphate/insulin-like growth factor receptor. PNAS (USA) 1991; 88:580-584.

49. Massague J. The transforming Growth Factor-β Family Ann Rev Cell Biol 1990; 6:597-641.

50. Wrana JL, Attisano L, Rotraud W et al. Mechanism of activation of transforming growth factor β receptor. Nature 1994; 370:341-346.

51. Wang T, Donahoe P.K., Zervos A.S. Specific interaction of type I receptor of the TGFβ family with the immunophilin FKBP-12. Science 1994; 253:674-676.

52. Lopez-Casillas F, Wrana JL, Massague J. Betaglycan presents ligand to the TGFβ signalling receptor. Cell 1993; 73:1435-1444.

53. Lopez-Casillas F, Payne H, Andres JL et al. Betaglycan can act as a dual modulator of TGFβ access to signalling receptors:mapping of ligand binding and GAG attachment sites. J Cell Biol 1994; 124:557-568.

54. Wakefield LM, Sporn MB. Suppression of carcinogenesis:A role for TGFβ and related molecules in prevention of cancer. In: Klein G, ed. Tumour Suppressor Genes. New York: Marcel Dekker, 1990:217-243.

54. Kimchi A, Wang X-F, Weinberg RA et al. Absence of TGFβ receptors and growth inhibitory responses in retinoblastoma cells. Science 1988; 240:196-199.

56. Valverius EM, Walker-Jones D, Bates SE et al. Production of and responsiveness to transforming growth factor β in normal and oncogene transformed human mammary epithelial cells. Cancer Res 1989; 49:6269-6274.

57. Manning AM, Williams AC, Game SM, Paraskeva C. Differential sensitivity of human colonic adenoma and carcinoma cells to transforming growth factor beta:conversion of an adenoma cell line to a tumorigenic phenotype is accompanied by a reduced response to the inhibitory effects of TGFβ. Oncogene 1993:6:1471-1477.

58. DeCaprio JA, Ludlow JW, Lynch D et al. The product of the retinoblastoma susceptibility gene has properties of a cell cycle regulatory element. Cell 1989; 58:1085-1095.

59. Laiho M, De Caprio JA, Ludlow JW et al. Growth inhibition by TGFβ linked to suppression of retinoblastoma protein phosphorylation. Cell 1990; 62:175-185.

60. DeCaprio JA, Ludlow JW, Figge J et al. SV40 large tumour antigen forms a specific complex with the product of the retinoblastoma susceptibility gene. Cell 1988; 54:275-283.

61. Sherr CJ Mammalian G1 Cyclins. Cell 1993; 73:1059-1065.

62. Hannon GJ, Beach D. p15 INK4B is a potent effector of transforming growth factor β induced cell cycle arrest. Nature 1994; 371:257-261.

63. Koff A, Ohtsuki M, Polyak K et al. Negative regulation of G1 in mammalian cell:inhibition of cyclin E-dependent kinase by TGFβ. Science 1993; 260:536-539.

64. Peters G. Stifled by inhibitions. Nature 1994; 371:204-205.

65. Pientenpol JA, Holt JT, Stein RW, Moses HL. Transforming growth factor β1 suppression of c-myc gene transcription:role in inhibition of keratinocyte proliferation. Proc Natl Aca Sci (USA) 1990 (a); 87:3758-3762.

66. Pientenpol JA, Stein RW, Moran E et al. TGFβ1 inhibition of c-myc transcription and growth in keratinocytes is abrogated by viral transforming proteins with pRB binding proteins Cell 1990 (b); 61:777-785.

67. Ong G, Sikora K, Gullick W. Inactivation of the retinoblastoma gene does not lead to loss of TGFβ receptors or response to TGFβ in human breast cancer cell lines. Oncogene 1991; 6:761-763.

68. Chambard J-C, Pouyssegur J. TGFβ inhibits growth factor-induced DNA synthesis in hamster fibroblasts without affecting the early mitogenic events. J Cell Physiol 1988; 135:101-107.

69. Reiss M, Dibble CL, Narayanan R. Transcription activation of the c-myc proto-oncogene in murine keratinocytes enhances the response to epidermal growth factor. J Invest Dermatology 1989; 93:136-141.

70. Smith GH. Transforming growth factor β and functional differentiation. J Mamm Gland Biol Neoplasia 1996; 1 (4):343-352.

71. Satterwhite DJ, Aakre ME, Gorska AE et al. Inhibition of cell growth by TGFβ1 is associated with inhibition of B-myb and cyclin A in both BALB/MK and Mv1Lu cells. Cell Growth Diff 1994; 5:789-799.

72. Robbins PD, Horowitz JM, Mulligan RC. Negative regulation of human c-fos expression by the retinoblastoma gene product. Nature 1990; 346:668-671.

73. Danielpour D, Dart L, Flanders KC et al. Immunodetection and quantitation of the two forms of TGFβ (TGFβ1 and TGFβ2) secreted by cells in culture. J Cell Physiol 1990; 138:79-86.

74. Shipley GD, Childs CB, Volkenant ME, Moses HL. Differential effects of epidermal growth factor, transforming growth factor and insulin on DNA and protein synthesis and morphology in serum-free cultures of AKR-2B cells. Cancer Res 1984; 44:710-716.

75. Roberts AB, Kim S-J, Kondaiah P et al. Transcriptional control of expression of the TGFβ's. Ann NY Aca Sci 1990; 593:43-56.

76. Akhurst RJ, Fee F, Balmain A. Localised production of TGFβ mRNA in tumour promoter-stimulated mouse epidermis. Nature 1988; 331:363-365.

77. Thompson NL, Bazoberry F, Speir EH et al. TGFβ1 in acute myocardial infarction in rats. Growth Factors 1988; 1:91-99.

78. Joyce ME, Jingushi S, Soltero RG et al. Role of TGFβ in fracture healing. Walter Reed Bone Symposium, 1988.

79. Jakobovits A. The expression of growth factors and growth factor receptors during mouse embryogenesis. In: Kahn P and Graf T, eds. Oncogenes and Growth Control. Berlin-Heidelberg: Springer-Verlag, 1986.

80. Glick AB, Danielpour D, Dart LL et al. Induction and autocrine receptor binding of TGFβ2 during terminal differentiation in primary mouse keratinocytes. Mol Endocrinol In press.

81. Kim S-J, Glick AB, Sporn MB, Roberts AB. Characterisation of the promoter region of the human transforming growth factor -β1 gene. J Biol Chem 1989 (a); 264:402-408.

82. Kim S-J, Denhez F, Kim K-Y et al. Activation of the second promoter of the TGFβ1 gene by TGFβ1 and phorbol ester occurs through the same target sequences. J Biol Chem 1989 (b); 264:19373-19378.

83. Kim S-J, Jeang KT, Glick A et al. Promoter sequences of the human transforming growth factor-β1 gene responsive to TGFβ1 autoinduction. J Biol Chem 1989 (c); 264:7041-7045.

84. Distel RJ, Ro SJ, Rosen BS, Groves DL, Spiegelman BM. Nucleoprotein complexes that regulate gene expression in adipocyte differentiation:direct participation of c-fos. Cell 1987; 49:835-844.

85. Kim SJ, Angel P, Lafyatis R et al. Auto-induction of transforming growth factor β1 ids mediated by the AP-1 complex. Mol Cell Biol 1990; 10:1492-1497.

86. Rauscher FJ, Cohen DR, Curran T et al. Fos-associated protein (p39) is the product of the jun proto-oncogene. Science 1988; 240:1010-1016.

87. Schutte J, Viallet J, Nau M et al. Jun-B inhibits and c-fos stimulates the transforming and transactivating activities of c-jun. Cell 1989; 59:987-997.

88. Pertovaara L, Sistonen L, Bos TJ et al. Enhanced jun gene expression is an early genomic response to transforming growth factor type β stimulation. Mol Cell Biol 1989; 9:1255-1262.

89. Angel P, Hattori K, Smeal T et al. The jun proto-oncogene is positively autoregulated by its products, Jun/AP-1. Cell 1988; 55:875-885.

90. Van Obberghen-Schilling E, Roche NS, Flanders KC et al. Transforming growth factor β1 positively regulates its own expression in normal and transformed cells. J Biol Chem 1988; 263:7741-7746.
91. Geiser AG, Busam KJ, Kim S-J et al. Regulation of the transforming growth factor-β1 and β3 promoters by transcription factor Sp1. Gene 1993; 129:223-228.
92. Kim S-J, Wagner S, Liu F, et al. Retinoblastoma gene product activates expression of the human TGFβ2 gene through transcriptional factor ATF-2. Nature 1992; 358:331-334.
93. Streuli CH, Schmidhauser C, Kobrin M et al. Extracellular matrix regulates expression of the TGFβ1 gene. J Cell Biol 1993; 120:253-259.
94. Kleinman HK, McGarvey ML, Hassell JR et al. Basement membrane complexes with biological activity. Biochemistry 1986; 25:312-318.

CHAPTER 3

Biological Functions of TGFβ

Mitchell S. Anscher, Mary Helen Barcellos-Hoff,
Feng-Ming Kong, Randy L. Jirtle

i) Introduction

Transforming growth factor β (TGFβ) is a molecule with varied, and seemingly paradoxical, functions in normal and malignant tissue. It plays an important role in regulating extracellular matrix production and accumulation, cell growth and differentiation, and immunomodulation. Many of these effects are interrelated, and disruption of this intricate web may contribute to the development of malignancy.

In this chapter, five areas of TGFβ function which are important in the carcinogenesis pathway will be reviewed: extracellular matrix effects; cell proliferation; angiogenesis; immunomodulation; and tumor promotion, progression, and metastasis. Mechanisms through which TGFβ affects these processes will be identified and potential strategies for antineoplastic therapies will be discussed.

ii) Extracellular Matrix Effects

a) Interactions Between TGFβ and the Extracellular Matrix

Although it has long been recognized that extracellular matrix (ECM) is necessary for cell adhesion and migration, in recent years other aspects of its biology have been identified and appreciated. In addition to providing the scaffolding on which cells move or are embedded, current concepts of ECM function reflect its integration into models of cell regulation. ECM receptors are now featured as a critical interface by which second messenger pathways are activated. The information conveyed by engaging particular ECM components via specific integrins and adhesion receptors affect growth, differentiation, homing, hormone and growth factor responses and cell death. Thus ECM can transduce information to cells regarding time (while undergoing development), place (during morphogenesis) and function (following differentiation). Another important aspect of ECM is that it mediates the action of soluble proteins like growth factors and cytokines by controlling access, stability, storage and function. Together, insoluble ECM molecules and soluble cytokines are a resilient web that act locally to maintain the differentiated cellular phenotype. Conversely, disruption of this web may promote disregulation and contribute to carcinogenesis.

Thus, the effect of TGFβ on ECM production and accumulation is an important component of its biological effects. This action was documented in one of the first demonstrations of TGFβ activity, when fibrosis was shown to develop at the sites of its local injection.[1] Experimental studies on the regulation of ECM by TGFβ are many and varied, but are in general agreement in supporting a wide role leading to ECM accumulation by stimulating protein production and inhibiting proteases that promote degradation. This general phenomenon is regulated at sundry levels. Fibronectin and collagen type I are ECM proteins that have been particularly associated with the action of TGFβ. Ten- to 20-fold increases in expression of mRNA for these proteins in fibroblasts following exposure to TGFβ are the result of both transcriptional regulation and effects on stability, which result in protein that is subsequently efficiently incorporated into the ECM.[2,3]

Some ECM regulation, however, may be indirect in light of TGFβ's effects on a variety of other growth factors. TGFβ inhibits metalloproteinases and induces proteases inhibitors selectively in the presence of growth factors that would otherwise have the opposite effect.[4] The action of platelet derived growth factor (PDGF), which is also associated with matrix formation, may be augmented by TGFβ induction of its receptor.[5-7] The recently identified connective tissue growth factor (CTGF), which is rapidly induced by TGFβ treatment of a variety of cell types, appears to elicit changes in extracellular matrix generally attributed to TGFβ.[8] TGFβ treated fibroblasts and endothelial cells, in culture and in wounds, produce CTGF, which in turn is mitogenic.[9] Furthermore, CTGF induces fibroblasts to produce collagen, fibronectin and integrins while injection of CTGF alone generates granulation tissue in vivo.[8] CTGF mRNA is associated with the desmoplastic response of breast tumors and is found in the stroma, in contrast to TGFβ mRNA which was localized to tumor cells. Thus, CTGF may be a downstream mediator of TGFβ's effects on matrix deposition and proliferation in connective tissue. Another particularly interesting aspect of TGFβ biology is the demonstration that induction of anchorage independent growth by TGFβ, a signature effect that is the basis for its misleading 'nome de plume', may be an indirect response via CTGF.[10]

Unfortunately, the complex biology of TGFβ is further complicated by the variety of cell culture models in use and the differences between normal and transformed cells. Thus, in a number of transformed cell lines, TGFβ stimulates protease production, thereby potentially contributing to their invasive phenotype. Furthermore, since protease mediated activation of the latent TGFβ complex may be necessary for its biological activity, there is the potential for an autoregulatory loop in which TGFβ stimulates certain proteases like plasmin.[11]

b) Reciprocal Regulation of TGFβ Action and ECM Composition

One of the most basic functions of the ECM is its ability to serve as a reservoir of growth factors, and concomitantly, modify their action. Silberstein and Daniel[12] have suggested that TGFβ contributes to tissue morphogenesis via its effects on stromal ECM deposition. ECM may in turn modulate the production of growth factors.[13,14] Conversely, studies in cultured cells indicate that the association of cells with an ECM alters their response to growth factors[15-17] and hormones.[18] Thus perturbations in the interaction between the ECM and epithelium could also alter the production, concentration, and/or response to growth factors.

This is particularly true for TGFβ, which is secreted as a latent complex. Its storage in the ECM is an important mechanism for bioavailability that is insured by a covalent bond to an extracellular matrix protein prior to secretion in many cell types. The resulting so-called large latent complex is composed of TGFβ noncovalently bound by a dimer of its amino terminus propeptide, which is called latency associated protein (LAP), that is in turn disulfide linked to latent TGFβ binding protein (LTBP).[19] LTBP belongs to a family of large extracellular glycoproteins, structurally similar to fibrillins, that contain epidermal growth factor (EGF)-like repeats and multiple cysteine-containing repeats. LTBPs ensure that the latent TGFβ complex is efficiently bound to the ECM[20,21] by serving as a substrate for transglutaminase mediated cross-linking to other ECM proteins.[22] In the plasmin model of activation, the resulting protein complex must be proteolytically processed before LTBP is released from the matrix, which is a prerequisite for latent TGFβ complex to be activated by plasmin resulting in the release of biologically active TGFβ.[22] Autoregulation of the large latent complex by TGFβ induced LTBP has been observed in osteoblastic cells.[20]

Additionally, the small latent complex, consisting of LAP and TGFβ, may be bound by other extracellular matrix proteins, including collagen type IV, thrombospondin, and fibronectin. Thrombospondin, a multifunctional extracellular glycoprotein induced by TGFβ,[3] is another example of a protein that has complex interactions with TGFβ. It is a heparin sulfate binding protein implicated in cell adhesion, tumor growth and metastasis, angiogenesis and chemotaxis.[23] It is a coresident with latent TGFβ of the alpha-granules of platelets and can bind to active TGFβ.[24] An interesting function of thrombospondin is the ability of a region of the peptide to nonenzymatically activate latent TGFβ.[24,25] This action can be antagonized by the binding peptide, suggesting that finely tuned regulation of activation may occur if this mechanism occurs in vivo.

iii) Cell Proliferation Effects

It was recognized early that the effects of TGFβ are strongly influenced by the context in which it acts. Thus it stimulates mesenchymal cell proliferation but is a profound inhibitor of epithelial cell growth.[26,27] The complex interplay between TGFβ and ECM proteins probably contributes to the context-specific action of TGFβ on cell growth in many cell culture systems,[28,29] and possibly to some of the conflicting data in some cell types. ECM substrata modulates TGFβ effects on differentiation but not on proliferation.[28] Furthermore, cells that no longer respond to growth inhibitory signals may still respond with altered ECM production.[30] ECM modulation has also been attributed a role in the TGFβ effects on angiogenesis.[31]

TGFβ is the most potent known inhibitor of cell cycle progression of normal mammary epithelial cells.[32] Transgenic animal models have demonstrated that TGFβ can specifically inhibit mammary alveolar development.[33,34] It also causes human mammary cells to produce a particular ECM that affects cell-cell and cell-substrate interactions.[30] Nonneoplastic human mammary epithelial cells (HMEC) and breast cancer cells in vitro as well as in vivo exhibit differential sensitivity to the anti-proliferative effect of TGFβ. Immortalization of primary HMEC is not associated with the acquisition of TGFβ resistance.[32] Rather, TGFβ resistance appears concomitant with the development of tumorigenic (i.e., invasive) properties and hormone-independence,[35-37] suggesting that there is a link between resistance and progression. Furthermore, the malignant progression appears to be associated with the increased autocrine production and secretion of TGFβ by breast cancer cells.[38-40]

The simplest way to reconcile these seemingly contradictory experimental results is to postulate that in the early stages of breast cancer development, mammary epithelial cells are sensitive to growth inhibition by TGFβ. However, if acquisition of TGFβ resistance and the associated higher levels of TGFβ production by the tumor cells are late events in breast cancer progression then agents that induce TGFβ activity may be stage specific in eliciting therapeutic effects.[41] Thus, malignant progression that is associated with increased autocrine production and secretion of TGFβ by breast cancer cells,[38-40] may offer a growth advantage in vivo.[41] This may be mediated by TGFβ action on the tumor microenvironment that provides a net positive gain by suppressing immune surveillance, stimulating angiogenesis and disrupting normal stromal function (see below).

a) Growth Regulation by Induction of Apoptosis

TGFβ induces apoptosis in a number of both normal and neoplastic tissues and cell models.[42-46] Thus as a negative regulator of growth, inhibition of the cell cycle is augmented by the elimination of cells from a population. A fascinating example identified by Bauer and colleagues is the potentially crucial process of apoptosis induced in transformed cells by TGFβ treated normal cells.[47] In this cell culture model, as in a number of others, the frequency of transformed foci decrease as the number of cells increases. This effect has been attributed to the large numbers of normal cells, which influence transformed cells by producing inhibitory growth factors or inducing differentiation. However, it has been demonstrated by Langer et al[47] that cells transformed chemically, virally or physically can be preferentially eliminated from a population via TGFβ induced soluble signals that elicit apoptosis. The specific signals are not known in detail but involve reactive oxygen species (ROS) generation.[47]

1) Reactive Oxygen Species in TGFβ Biology

Interestingly, there is mounting evidence that TGFβ may signal certain events through the generation of ROS.[47-51] TGFβ induces the production of hydrogen peroxide in bovine endothelial cells,[52] mouse osteoblastic cells, where it has been shown to be necessary for the transcriptional activation of the EGR-1 gene,[48] and human lung fibroblasts, where it is generated by the activation of NADH oxidase.[51] Recent studies have also implicated ROS as an important signal for TGFβ induced apoptosis.[47,53]

The potential for an autocrine loop has been realized by the recent demonstration that latent TGFβ can be oxidatively activated.[54] ROS-mediated activation would endow latent TGFβ with the ability to act as a sensor of oxidative stress and, in releasing active TGFβ, to signal multiple cell types to change their phenotype, presumably directed towards recovery of homeostasis. The response of mammary gland to ionizing radiation is mediated by the rapid and persistent conversion of latent TGFβ to its active form.[55,56] The exquisite sensitivity of latent TGFβ to in vivo activation following small doses (0.1 to 5 Gy) of ionizing radiation supports the hypothesis that the redox sensitivity of latent TGFβ is a global tissue damage response mechanism that modifies microenvironment composition and cell phenotype.[57] Since TGFβ is implicated in a variety of ROS-mediated tissue pathologies that include acute respiratory distress syndrome,[58] atherosclerosis[59] and radiogenic fibrosis,[60,61] oxidative activation of latent TGFβ may be deleterious to tissue in certain disease states leading to chronic production of ROS. A variety of tumor cells also generate ROS.[62] Thus, in some situations, a self-amplifying cascade could be envisioned in which TGFβ is activated by ROS and then stimulates nonphagocytic cells to produce more ROS, which contribute further to activation via the redox sensitivity of latent TGFβ.[54]

iv) Angiogenesis

Angiogenesis is a vital component of embryogenesis, wound healing and the growth of malignant tumors. It is the process through which new blood vessels are formed in both tumor and nonmalignant tissue. These new vessels originate as sprouts from small venules. The process begins with localized breakdown of the basement membrane of the venule by proteases, followed by migration of endothelial cells. These migrating endothelial cells elongate and align to form a sprout. Subsequently, the endothelial cells begin to proliferate in order to further lengthen the developing vessel. Maturation of the sprout occurs with the formation of a lumen and a basement membrane. Eventually, two hollow sprouts meet and fuse, forming a capillary loop which enables blood to flow. Thus, the major processes involved in new vessel formation are enzymatic breakdown of the basement membrane, endothelial cell migration, proliferation and differentiation.[63,64] In addition to proteases, extracellular matrix and more than a dozen cytokines, including TGFβ, play important roles in this process at the molecular level.[63,65]

The role of TGFβ in angiogenesis is complex and incompletely understood. Paradoxical roles for TGFβ can be demonstrated, depending upon whether one is studying early or late angiogenic events, or using in vivo or in vitro conditions. In vitro models of early angiogenesis (i.e., proteolysis, invasion, migration and proliferation) have shown that TGFβ inhibits these processes. For example, TGFβ inhibits production of plasminogen activator[66] thereby decreasing conversion of plasminogen to the protease, plasmin. TGFβ has been demonstrated to inhibit endothelial cell invasion into both human amniotic membranes[67] and collagen gels.[68] This cytokine also inhibits endothelial cell migration and proliferation in vitro.[68-70] RayChaudhury et al[71] have shown that thrombospondin expression, an extracellular matrix protein which inhibits endothelial cell proliferation, is increased by TGFβ.

In the later stages of angiogenesis, endothelial cells differentiate from a proliferative migratory state into a quiescent phenotype. In vitro models suggest that TGFβ promotes this process. Madri,[29] and later Merwin,[72] showed that endothelial cells grown in collagen gels organize into tube-like structures under the influence of TGFβ, suggesting that TGFβ promotes termination of angiogenesis and maintains the differentiated endothelial cell phenotype.

The effect of TGFβ in vivo, however, is to promote angiogenesis.[1,73,74] To address the seemingly paradoxical effects of TGFβ, Yang and Moses[75] studied the effects of TGFβ in vivo using the chicken chorioallantoic membrane model of angiogenesis. These authors found that TGFβ initially induced a rapid pleiotropic cellular response characterized by an increase in fibroblast and epithelial cell density. This effect, however, appeared to be due to cell migration, rather than an increase in proliferation. Later, capillary cords appeared and grew toward the point of TGFβ delivery. As the cords approached the site of TGFβ delivery, proliferation of endothelial cells within these vessels was inhibited. Finally, a perivascular mononuclear cell infiltrate appeared which correlated with the remodeling of the newly formed cords into larger blood vessels. These findings suggested that the in vivo and in vitro effects of TGFβ were similar, but that in vivo TGFβ could act via paracrine mechanisms to coordinate a program of cellular responses.

Brogi et al[76] demonstrated the importance of the paracrine effects of TGFβ on angiogenesis in vitro. These investigators demonstrated that the addition of TGFβ to cultured human vascular smooth muscle cells resulted in increased expression of mRNA for the angiogenesis promoting cytokines vascular endothelial growth factor (VEGF) and basic fibroblast growth factor (bFGF). Similarly, Petrovaara et al[77] found that the treatment of AKR-2B fibroblasts and A549 lung adenocarcinoma cells with TGFβ resulted in increased expression of VEGF mRNA and protein. In contrast, treatment of endothelial cells with TGFβ had no effect on VEGF expression. Mandriota et al[78] demonstrated an inhibitory effect of TGFβ on VEGF induced angiogenesis in vitro which was due to the downregulation of flk-1, the major endothelial cell signal transducing tyrosine kinase receptor for VEGF. Also, TGFβ is chemotactic for monocytes, which locally release angiogenic factors, such as tumor necrosis factor alpha.[79-82] Thus, there is a growing body of evidence to support the indirect nature of the angiogenic effects of TGFβ.[83] These findings, in part, help to explain why TGFβ had not been thought to be angiogenic in vitro.

Furthermore, the angiogenic effects of TGFβ in vitro depends on its concentration in the microenvironment.[29,63,76,81,84,85] For example, Pepper et al[81] demonstrated that VEGF and bFGF-induced endothelial cell invasion and capillary lumen formation was inhibited by high concentrations of TGFβ (5-10 ng/ml), whereas endothelial cell invasion induced by vascular endothelial growth factor (VEGF) and basic fibroblast growth factor (bFGF) was potentiated by low concentrations ($\leq$ 1 ng/ml).

The regulatory influence of the extracellular matrix on the contribution of TGFβ to angiogenesis is also important.[29,86,87] The extracellular matrix influences the concentration and activity of various growth factors, including TGFβ.[88-93] Conversely, cytokines, in particular TGFβ, can also influence the composition of the extracellular matrix.[94,95]

Iruela-Arispe et al[86] developed a model of in vitro angiogenesis that recapitulates many of the cellular functions involved in capillary formation in vivo. These investigators found that their angiogenic cultures contained high levels of active TGFβ, and that TGFβ stimulated the proliferation of endothelial cells that had adopted an angiogenic phenotype. In contrast, TGFβ was inhibitory for the same endothelial cells at subconfluent densities. Their results suggested that the response of endothelial cells to TGFβ was contingent upon the composition and organization of the extracellular matrix. Sankar et al[93] have shown that changes in the extracellular matrix environment can alter the expression of the type I and type II TGFβ receptors on endothelial cells, altering their responsiveness to TGFβ. Thus, the extracellular matrix appears to impact significantly upon the role of TGFβ in angiogenesis.

v) Immunological Effects

Many cancer patients have an impaired ability to mount an immune response against tumor cells.[96-98] Tumors often produce soluble growth factors with immunosuppressive properties, such as TGFβ.[96,99] Among the important mechanisms through which TGFβ stimulates tumor promotion and progression are impairment of immune surveillance.[100] The effects of TGFβ on the immune system are complex and diverse.[97,100-104] Factors which determine the biological effects of TGFβ on the immune system include whether TGFβ is latent or active, the target cell type, the state of differentiation of the target cell, the activation state of the cell, the number of TGFβ receptors, the influence of other growth factors in the milieu, and the extracellular matrix.[101] In general, however, resting immature cells are stimulated by TGFβ, whereas mature activated cells are inhibited.[105] In this section, the influence that TGFβ exerts on the various components of the immune system will be reviewed, with an emphasis on the impact that this cytokine has on the host's defenses against malignancy.

a) Lymphoid and Myeloid Precursors

TGFβ has bidirectional effects on hematopoietic cell proliferation. This cytokine tends to inhibit early stem cell proliferation while promoting maturation of late stage progenitor cells.[101] For example, TGFβ inhibits the development of early stem cells into lymphoid and myeloid cells under the influence of stem cell factor and/or IL-6, IL-11 and Granulocyte Colony Stimulating Factor (GCSF).[106-109] TGFβ also blocks the proliferation of pre-B cells induced by IL-7,[110] and regulates the clonal expansion of B cells.[110,111] The differentiation of CD3-, CD4-, CD8- (early immature) thymocytes into CD3+ cells is inhibited by TGFβ, but this cytokine will stimulate differentiation into CD8+ (suppressor) cells.[110,111] Mature T lymphocytes themselves also produce TGFβ. The diminished anti-tumor T-cell response in gut associated lymphoid tissue (GALT) may be due to the suppressive effect of TGFβ produced by CD8+ T cells in this tissue, which results in inhibition of stimulation of CD4+ T helper cells.[112]

TGFβ inhibits early myelopoiesis,[113-116] but promotes later granulopoiesis via an enhanced response to Granulocyte-Macrophage Colony Stimulating Factor (GMCSF) or GMCSF plus GCSF.[117-119] Similarly, TGFβ inhibits Macrophage Colony Stimulating Factor (MCSF) induced growth of early macrophage progenitor cells, whereas the growth of more mature cells in the macrophage lineage is stimulated.[116,120]

b) T Cells

TGFβ inhibits the proliferation of T cells. T cells normally proliferate and activate in response to stimulation with cytokines such as IL-2, IL-4, and IL-12.[121,122] TGFβ inhibits the proliferation of T cells activated by these mitogens.[97,101,111,121,123-125] It also suppresses the growth and activation of cytotoxic T cells, Natural Killer (NK) cells, and lymphokine activated killer (LAK) cells.[101,120] As in the case of activated T cells, the inhibitory effects of TGFβ on the proliferation of NK cells, LAK cells and cytotoxic T cells can be overcome by IL-2.[124,126-128] Thus, the growth of lymphoid cells depends upon a balance of positive and negative factors. TGFβ also stimulates the differentiation of immature cells into mature activated T cells, which are growth inhibited by TGFβ.[111,129-131] The ability of T cells (and polymorphonuclear cells) to migrate from the circulation is inhibited by TGFβ.[132,133] This effect is due, in part, to a decrease in E-selectin expression, an endothelial cell specific adhesion molecule, by TGFβ.[105,134]

c) B Cells

As with T cells, TGFβ stimulates immature B cells to mature into specialized B cells, but inhibits the function of these differentiated cells.[135-137] TGFβ inhibits proliferation of B cells in response to mitogens such as IL-7, IL-2, and B cell growth factor (BCGF-12kDa).[107,131,136-140] It inhibits production of IgG and IgM class antibodies, but stimulates the production of IgA by B lymphocytes.[136,141] Peripheral blood B cells stimulated with the Epstein-Barr virus (EBV) results in increased production of IgM, IgG, IgA, and IgE. TGFβ does not block the constitutive expression of these immunoglobulins in EBV transformed cells; B cells not transformed with EBV retain the ability to respond to TGFβ.[142]

d) Macrophages

The effects of TGFβ on macrophage function can be divided into 2 types: indirect and direct.[143] TGFβ indirectly effects macrophage function by suppressing T cell proliferation and/or decreasing production of the macrophage activating cytokine, interferon gamma (IFNγ).[144-147] In addition, TGFβ can stimulate the production of antagonists to cytokines released by macrophages.[147,148]

As is the case with T and B cells, the effect of TGFβ on monocytes is bidirectional.[101] TGFβ directly inhibits proliferation of immature granulocyte-macrophage progenitor cells,[114,140,149] whereas it enhances growth of mature progenitor cells after stimulation with GMCSF.[109,114,119,140] Thus, TGFβ promotes maturation of macrophages, an immunostimulatory effect. In addition, TGFβ exerts positive influences on the immune system in that it promotes chemotaxis for macrophages (and neutrophils) in vitro and in vivo,[150-153] it stimulates macrophages to produce IL-1 (a macrophage and neutrophil chemotactic cytokine)[150,151,153] and increases the expression of adhesion receptors on macrophages;[95,154,155] it has the opposite effect on adhesion of peripheral blood leukocytes, T cells, and PMN's.[132,133,156]

The effects of TGFβ on phagocytosis depend on the system under study. For example, mouse peritoneal macrophages deactivated by TGFβ retained phagocytic function.[157,158] In other systems, TGFβ has been shown to either increase or decrease macrophage surface receptors involved in the process of phagocytosis.[154,159-162]

TGFβ also effects macrophage function through the downregulation of expression of major histocompatibility complex (MHC) antigens and antigen presentation, a system through which macrophages can activate T cell function.[130,163-165] The cell surface expression of MHC antigens is essential for target cell recognition by T cells.[166] In addition, TGFβ has a bifunctional influence on cytokine production by macrophages, which may be crucial in tumor cell killing.[167,168] It stimulates mRNA expression for several cytokines (IL-1α, IL-1β, IL-6, TNFα, PDGF, and bFGF) via increased gene transcription in resting macrophages,[150,151,153,169,170] whereas it has the opposite effect in activated macrophages on the release of IL-1, TNFα and IL-6.[169,171] Furthermore, TGFβ is constitutively expressed by resting macrophages and treatment of human macrophages with TGFβ leads to increased expression of TGFβ mRNA by these cells, suggesting that TGFβ autoregulates its production by macrophages.[153] The mechanism of autoregulation appears to be due to increased expression of *fos* and *jun* proteins which bind to the AP-1 site in the TGFβ promotor resulting in increased transcription of TGFβ.[172,173] (See chapter 2, section vi.)

Perhaps the most important tumoricidal (and bactericidal) activities of macrophages, in addition to the release of TNFα,[101] are mediated through the production of reactive oxygen intermediates (ROI) and reactive nitrogen intermediates (RNI).[101,105] TGFβ suppresses the production of both of these important classes of mediators of tumor cell killing.[157,158,174,175]

1) Effector Cells

TGFβ markedly inhibits the function of cytotoxic T cells, NK cells and LAK cells.[97,124,126,127,145,176-181] The inhibitory effect of TGFβ on these important surveillance cells can be blocked in vivo by anti-TGFβ antibody.[177,182] In addition, effector cell function was significantly improved in animals inoculated with 9L glioma cells modified to inhibit TGFβ expression via an antisense vector as compared to controls.[183] Immunotherapy regimens which have been shown to have some activity in humans, such as IL-2 plus IFNα for melanoma or renal cell carcinoma, may interfere with the expression of TGFβ. Recent evidence suggests that effector cell function may be more sensitive to the inhibitory effects of TGFβ than is cell growth.[126] Thus, endogenous production of TGFβ by tumors may, in part, account for the lack of a therapeutic response to immunotherapy in cancer patients.

e) Systemic vs Local TGFβ

Models to study the local effects of TGFβ have been widely utilized for years. The development of TGFβ knockout strains of mice have enabled researchers to study the systemic effects of TGFβ as well.[184,185] Interestingly, the effects on the immune response of the host differ depending upon whether TGFβ is acting locally or systemically.

Circulating TGFβ appears to act as a natural suppressor of autoimmunity in conditions such as experimental autoimmune encephalomyelitis (EAE) and multiple sclerosis (MS).[186] The systemic administration of anti-TGFβ antibody will exacerbate both EAE and MS.[187] In a mouse model of systemic lupus erythematosis the animals have elevated circulating levels of TGFβ, and their increased susceptibility to bacterial infections (due to a defect in PMN function) is reversed by anti-TGFβ antibody.[188] This immunosuppressive effect of circulating TGFβ appears to be due to the downregulation of leukocyte adhesion molecules, inhibition of leukocyte recruitment,[134,189] decreased proliferation of activated T cells[190] and deactivation of macrophages.[157]

In contrast, once outside the circulatory system, TGFβ acts locally to increase adhesion and infiltration of leukocytes via upregulation of integrin expression.[191,192] In an arthritis model, local administration of TGFβ has been shown to stimulate the inflammatory process, whereas systemic administration inhibits it.[191-193]

vi) Tumor Promotion/Progression

Malignant transformation is a complex multistage process. TGFβ inhibits the proliferation of normal epithelial and hematopoietic cells and promotes cell differentiation. However, many malignancies of epithelial and hematopoietic origin are resistant to the growth inhibitory effects of TGFβ.[194-201] Current evidence suggests that the acquisition of resistance to the TGFβ family of growth inhibitors represents potentially important property of malignant cells. The mechanisms behind this resistance of transformed cells to TGFβ are currently under investigation. Multiple pathways appear to be involved. For example, activation of oncogenes (e.g., Ras, myc, myb, E2F) or loss of tumor suppressor genes (e.g., Rb, p53) may contribute to decreased TGFβ responsiveness.[195] Other possible mechanisms include the inability to activate the latent TGFβ complex, loss of expression or function of transmembrane serine/threonine receptor kinases (TGFβ type I and II receptors) and defects in the postreceptor signal transduction pathway.[195] The evidence supporting the role of these mechanisms in acquired TGFβ resistance in tumors is discussed below.

As TGFβ is mainly produced and secreted in a latent form, bioactivation is required before it can bind to the signaling receptor. In order to be activated, TGFβ binds to the mannose 6-phosphate/insulin-like growth factor 2 receptor (M6P/IGF2r), which facilitates activation by proteolytic enzymes, such as plasmin. This receptor has been found to be lost in human liver and breast carcinoma,[201-203] suggesting that loss of the M6P/IGF2r may be responsible for resistance to TGFβ in some tumors. Recent evidence suggests that the M6P/IGF2r may, in fact, be a tumor suppressor gene.[201-203] Reduction or loss of TGFβ type I or II receptors is also observed in many rodent and human malignancies which have lost their growth inhibitory response to TGFβ.[204-211] Restoration of the type II receptor by stable transfection suppresses tumorigenicity in receptor negative cells.[212]

In contrast to inhibiting normal epithelial cell proliferation, TGFβ may stimulate the growth of transformed epithelial cells.[213-216] The mechanisms responsible for this paradox are not well understood. One means through which TGFβ may promote proliferation of malignant epithelial cells is via increased DNA synthesis. TGFβ induces expression of a rate-limiting enzyme of DNA synthesis, ribonucleotide reductase, in highly malignant cell lines.[217] Alternatively, TGFβ may work indirectly through stimulating angiogenesis, extracellular matrix production or via interactions with other growth factors, such as platelet derived growth factor (PDGF) or epidermal growth factor (EGF).[217]

The significance of the tumor stroma as an important determinant of tumor growth has also been demonstrated in many systems. It has been suggested that genetic lesions in stromal cells may promote tumor progression.[218] For example, a correlation has been noted between fibrotic stromal alterations and increased risk of cancer in the liver, skin,[219-221] breast and lung.[222,223] Experimentally induced areas of fibrosis express increased levels of TGFβ1 mRNA and were also shown to be preferred sites of tumor development in carcinogen-treated rats.[224,225] The exact nature of this TGFβ-stroma interaction in multistage carcinogenesis continues to be defined.

It has also been shown that tumor cells develop resistance to TGFβ induced growth inhibition without losing either their signaling or activation receptors. Alteration in the signal transduction pathways may convey resistance to TGFβ. For example, the retinoblastoma (Rb) gene product, a tumor suppressor gene, has been implicated in TGFβ signaling.[226] Phosphorylation of the Rb protein is required for progression through the cell cycle and TGFβ may inhibit growth by blocking this step. Recently, a protein upstream from Rb in the TGFβ signal transduction pathway, known as deleted in pancreatic cancer 4 (DPC4), has been found to be mutated or deleted in pancreatic cancer,[227] lending further support to this hypothesis.

The evidence supporting the role of TGFβ in tumor promotion and progression[177,228,229] have lead to efforts to develop cancer therapies directed against TGFβ.[177,183,230] For example, anti-TGFβ antibodies have recently been shown to inhibit breast cancer cell tumorigenicity,[177] and TGFβ antisense oligonucleotides can eradicate established intracranial gliomas in animals.[183] Therapeutic strategies are discussed further in chapter 7.

vii) Metastasis

Tumor metastasis involves a complex series of events including progression; invasion into the underlying stroma; the detachment of cells from the primary tumor; intravasation, embolization and survival in the circulatory system; as well as adhesion, extravasation and growth in a distant organ. TGFβ promotes many of these processes. Furthermore, many cancer patients demonstrate increased expression of TGFβ locally and/or systemically.[231-243]

Therefore, a tumor is growing in an environment of increased potential bioavailability of TGFβ. As previously noted, many tumors are resistant to the growth inhibitory effects of TGFβ.[195,196,237,239,241,242] In addition, highly metastatic clones not only secrete TGFβ, but also their growth is stimulated by it.[213-215] For example, TGFβ expressing tumor cell lines injected intravenously or subcutaneously produce more lung and lymph node metastases as compared to the parental cell lines which do not express TGFβ.[244,245] The mechanisms through which TGFβ is thought to promote the processes associated with metastases are discussed below.

Angiogenesis is a process of neovascular formation usually of capillary origin. It is an essential component of tumor invasion and metastasis.[63] TGFβ promotes angiogenesis, as previously noted, through its effects on endothelial cell migration, proliferation and matrix formation.[78,85,246] Specifically, TGFβ promotes proteolysis of the basement membrane; endothelial cell invasion, migration and proliferation, as well as capillary lumen formation (see preceding section in this chapter).[63,81,85,86,101,229,247-249]

Tumor cells use the process of proteolysis to invade the surrounding stroma. Highly malignant and invasive cells show increased protease activity when compared with normal and poorly invasive cells.[211,250,251] TGFβ stimulates plasminogen activator in the human lung carcinoma A549 cell line.[252] TGFβ1 stimulates collagenase type IV and procathepsin L transcription in H-ras-transformed fibrosarcomas, whereas it inhibits protease transcription in the parental line.[245] TGFβ1 modulates proteolytic activity of human prostate cancer cell lines by upregulating plasminogen activator.[253] TGFβ stimulates basement membrane lysis by increasing type IV collagenase in extramedullary tumor sites in leukemia,[254] and by inducing gelatinase production in metastatic renal cell carcinoma,[255] murine metastatic colon carcinoma cells,[256] and in mammary adenocarcinoma.[244] Many other tumor cell lines have also been shown to increase proteolysis in response to TGFβ.[244,257-261] This increased protease gene and protein expression promotes invasion and enhances tumor metastatic potential.

Motility is an essential property of cells that contributes to the spread of cancer either locally or at sites distant from the primary tumor. Active migration enhances metastatic spread and is a property of most metastatic tumor cells. It is obvious that tumor cell migration occurs in conditions where normal somatic cell locomotion is restrained. Tumor cells can up-regulate their locomotion either by producing motility-promoting factors themselves (autocrine mechanism) or inducing surrounding cells to produce proteins that enhance tumor cell chemokinesis and chemotaxis (paracrine mechanism).[262] TGFβ is an example of such a factor. TGFβ is not only a potent inducer of chemoattractants, such as collagen and fibronectin, but it is also directly promotes both chemotaxis and chemokinesis of many cells, including human dermal fibroblasts, neutrophils, human keratinocytes, and transformed fibroblast.[263-266] TGFβ1 enhances the migration behavior of mouse melanoma cells on collagen type I substrata by upregulating the expression of mouse melanoma cell CD44-chondroitin sulfate proteoglycan.[267] It has also been shown to promote the motility of transformed cells through a hyaluronin mediated pathway.[268,269] TGFβ's effect on cell motility is also cell type and concentration specific. It can stimulate transformed cell locomotion at a concentration which has no effect on the normal parental cells.

The majority of tumor cells which migrate into the circulation will be killed by host defenses.[270] As noted above, however, TGFβ is highly immunosuppressive. Among other mechanisms, TGFβ may enable tumor cells to escape immunosurveillance which increases their chance of survival in the circulation (see preceding section).

In order to escape from the circulation, tumor cells have to adhere to the endothelial surface of vessels, migrate through the vessel wall and attach to extracellular matrix in the distant organ. Many cancer cell lines expressing the metastatic phenotype demonstrate increased adhesiveness.[271,272] TGFβ regulates the adhesion of both normal and malignant cells by regulating expression of various adhesion molecules.[155,194,273-278] As noted above, TGFβ also promotes proteolysis, cell motility, angiogenesis and extracellular matrix deposition, all of which facilitate tumor cell growth and progression in distant organs.

viii) Conclusions and Future Directions

It is clear from this review that much progress has been made in unraveling the mechanisms behind the pleiotropic functions of TGFβ. Much work in this area, however, remains to be done. TGFβ affects all of the processes discussed above both directly and indirectly. Furthermore, it may affect all of them simultaneously. Many frontiers in TGFβ biology remain open to researchers. For instance, several steps in the signal transduction pathway remain to be defined. Undoubtedly, a number of new tumor suppressor genes will be discovered along the way. New therapies,[279] such as anti-angiogenesis agents, anti-TGFβ antibodies or TGFβ antisense oligonucleotides[280] are being introduced into clinical trials which represent radically different approaches to cancer treatment. Drugs which restore the normal growth phenotype in the cell, rather than kill it (differentiation inducing agents) are being tested as both antineoplastic therapies and chemoprevention agents. Thus, many new avenues continue to be explored. Ultimately, a better understanding of how normal cell growth control mechanisms have gone awry in cancer will lead to more effective therapies for many of these diseases.

References

1. Roberts AB, Sporn MB, Assoian RK et al. Transforming growth factor type β: Rapid induction of fibrosis and angiogenesis in vivo and stimulation of collagen formation in vitro. Proc Natl Acad Sci USA 1986: 83:4167-4171.
2. Ignotz RA, Massague J. Transforming growth factor-B stimulates the expression of fibronectin and collagen and their incorporation into the extracellular matrix. J Biol Chem 1986: 261:4337-4345.
3. Penttinen RP, Kobayashi S, Bornstein P. Transforming growth factor β increases mRNA for matrix proteins both in the presence and in the absence of changes in mRNA stability. Proc Natl Acad Sci USA 1988: 85:1105-1108.
4. Edwards DR, Murphy G, Reynolds JJ et al. Transforming growth factor beta modulates the expression of collagenase and metalloproteinase inhibitor. EMBO J 1987: 6:1899-1904.
5. Gronwald RGK, Seifert RA, Bowen-Pope DF. Differential regulation of expression of two platelet-derived growth factor receptor subunits by transforming growth factor-β. J Biol Chem 1989; 264:8120-8125.
6. Ishikawa O, Leroy EC, Trojanowska M. Mitogeneic effect of TGF-β1 on human fibroblasts involves induction of platelelt-derived growth factor a receptors. J Cell Physiol 1990; 145:181-186.
7. Janat MF, Liau G. TGF-β1 is a powerful modulator of platelet-derived growth factor action in vascular smooth muscle cells. J Cell Physiol 1992; 150:2323-242.
8. Frazier K, Williams S, Kothapalli D et al Stimulation of fibroblast cell growth, matrix production and granulation tissue formation by connective tissue growth factor. J Invest Dermatol 1996; 107:404-411.
9. Igarashi A, Ocochi H, Bradham DM et al. Regulation of connective tissue growth factor gene expression in human skin fibroblasts and during wound repair. Mol Biol Cell 1993; 4:637-645.
10. Kothapalli D, Frazier KS, Welply A et al. Transforming growth factor b induces anchorage-indpendent growth of NRK fibroblasts via a connective tissue growth factor-dependent signaling pathway. Cell Growth Diff 1997; 8:61-68.
11. Rifkin DB, Moscatelli D, Bizik J et al. Growth factor control of extracellular proteolysis. Cell Differentiation and Development 1990; 32:313-318.
12. Silberstein GB, Daniel CW. Reversible inhibition of mamry gland growth by transforming growth factor-beta. Science 1987; 237:291-293.

13. Liu S, Sanfilippo B, Perroteau I et al. Expression of transforming growth factor alpha in differentiated rat mammary tumors: Estrogen induction of transforming growth factor alpha production. Molec Endo 1987; 1:683.

14. Zwiebel JA, Davis M, Kohn E et al. Anchorage-independent growth-conferring factor production by rat mammary tumor cells. Cancer Res 1982; 42:5117.

15. Carr BI, Huang TH, Itakura K et al. TGFβ gene trascription in normal and neoplastic liver growth. J Cell Biochem 1989; 39:477-487.

16. Hirayama F, Shih JP, Awgulewitsch A et al. Clonal proliferation of murine lympho-hemopoietic progenitors in culture. Proc Natl Acad Sci USA 1992; 89:5907-5911.

17. Mohanam S, Salomon DS, Kidwell WR. Substratum modulation of epidermal growth factor receptor expression by normal mouse mammary cells. J Dairy Sci 1988; 71:1507-1514.

18. Salomon DS, Liotta LA, Kidwell WR. Differential response to growth factor by rat mammary epithelium plated on different collagen substrata in serum-free medium. Proc Natl Acad Sci USA 1981; 78:382-386.

19. Lee EH, Lee WH, Kaetzel CS et al. Interaction of mouse mammary epithelial cells with collagenous substrata: Regulation of casein gene expression and secretion. Proc Natl Acad Sci USA 1985; 82:1419-1423.

20. Miyazono K, Olofsson A, Colosetti P et al. A role of the latent TGF-β1-binding protein in the assembly and secretion of TGF-β1. EMBO J 1991; 10:1091-1101.

21. Dallas SL, Miyazono K, Skerry TM et al. Dual role for the latent transforming growth factor-β binding protein in storage of latent TGF-β in the extracellular matrix and as a structural matrix protein. J Cell Biol 1995;131:539-549.

22. Olofsson A, Ichijo H, Moren A et al. Efficient association of an amino-terminally extended form of human latent transforming growth factor-β binding protein with the extracellular matrix. J Biol Chem 1995; 52:31294-31297.

23. Nunes I, Gleizes PE, Metz CN et al. Latent transforming growth factor β binding protein domains involved in activation and transglutaminase -dependent cross-linking of latent transforming growth factor -β. J Cell Biol 1997; 136:1151-1163.

24. Roberts DD. Regulation of tumor growth and metastasis by thrombospondin-1. FASEB J 1996; 10:1183-1191.

25. Murphy-Ullrich JE, Schultz-Cherry S, Hook M. Transforming growth factor-β complexes with thrombospondin. Mol Biol Cell 1992; 3:181-188.

26. Schultz-Cherry S, Murphy-Ullrich JE. Thrombospondin causes activation of latent transforming growth factor-β secreted by endothelial cells by a novel mechanism. J Cell Biol 1993; 122:923-932.

27. Moses HL, Coffey Jr RL, Leof EB et al. Transforming growth factor β regulation of cell proliferation. J Cell Physiol (Suppl) 1987; 5:1-7.

28. Roberts AB, Anzano MA, Wakefield LM et al. Type β trnasforming growth factor: A bifunctional regulator of cellular growth. Proc Natl Acad Sci USA 1985; 82:119-123.

29. Davis BH. Transforming growth factor β responsiveness is modulated by the extracellular collagen matrix during hepatic Ito cell culture. J Cell Physiol 1988; 136:547-553.

30. Madri JA, Pratt BM, Tucker AM. Phenotypic modulation of endothelial cells by transforming growth factor-beta depends upon the composition and organizaion of the extracellular matrix. J Cell Biol 1988; 106:1375-1384.

31. Stampfer MR, Yaswen P, Alhadeff M et al. TGFβ induction of extracellular matrix associated proteins in normal and transformed human mammary epithelial cells in culture is independent of growth effects. J Cell Physiol 1993; 155:210-221.

32. Pepper MS. Transforming growth factor-beta: Vasculogenesis, angiogenesis, and vessel wall integrity. Cytokine & Growth Factor Rev 1997; 8:21-43.

33. Hosobuchi M, Stampfer MR. Effects of transforming growth factor β on growth of human mammary epithelial cells in culture. In Vitro 1989; 25:705-712.

34. Jhappan C, Geiser AG, Kordon EC et al. Targeting expression of a transforming growth factor β1 transgene to the pregnant mammary gland inhibits alveolar development and lactation. EMBO J 1993; 12:1835-1845.

35. Pierce DFJ, Johnson MD, Matsui Y et al. Inhibition of mammary duct development but not alveolar outgrowth during pregnancy in transgenic mice expressing active TGF-beta 1. Genes & Devel 1993; 7:2308-2317.

36. Arteaga CL, Tandon AK, Von Hoff DD et al. Transforming growth factor-β: Potential autocrine growth inhibitor of estrogen receptor-negative human breast cancer cells. Cancer Res 1988; 48:3898.

37. Herman MH, Katzenellenbogen BS. Alterations in transforming growth factor-α and -β production and cell responsiveness during the progression of MCF-7 human breast cancer cells to estrogen-autonomous growth. Cancer Res. 1994; 54:5867-5874.

38. Knabbe C, Lippman ME, Wakefield LM et al. Evidence that transforming growth factor-β is a hormonally regulated negative growth factor in human breast cancer cells. Cell 1987; 48:417-428.

39. Dalal BI, Keown PA, Greenberg AH. Immunocytochemical localization of secreted transforming growth factor-β1 to the advancing edges of primary tumors and to lymph node metastases of human mammary carcinoma. Am J Path 1993; 143:381-389.

40. Gorsch SM, Memoli VA, Stukel TA et al. Immunohistochemical staining for transforming growth factor β1 associates with disease progression in human breast cancer. Cancer Res 1992; 52:6949-6952.

41. McCune BK, Mullin BR, Flanders KC et al. Localization of tranforming growth factor-β isotypes in lesions of the human breast. Human Pathology 1992; 23:13-20.

42. Reiss M, Barcellos-Hoff MH. The role of transforming growth factor-β in breast cancer: A working hypothesis. Br Cancer Res Treat 1997; In press.

43. Kyprianou N, English HF, Davidson NE et al. Programmed cell death during regression of the MCF-7 human breast cancer following estrogen ablation. Cancer Res. 1991; 51:162-166.

44. Lin JK, Chou CK. In vitro apoptosis in the human hepatoma cell line induced by transforming growth factor β1. Cancer Res 1992; 52:385-388.

45. Martikainen P, Kyprianou N, Isaacs JT. Effect of transforming growth factor-β1 on proliferation and death of rat prostatic cells. Endocrinology 1990; 127:2963-2968.

46. Oberhammer FA, Pavelka M, Sharma S et al. Induction of apoptosis in cultured hepatocytes and in regressing liver by transforming growth factor β1. Proc Natl Acad Sci USA 1992; 89:5408-5412.

47. Rotello RJ, Lieberman RC, Purchio AF et al. Coordinated regulation of apoptosis and cell proliferation by transforming growth factor β1 in cultured uterine epithelial cells. Proc Natl Acad Sci USA 1991; 88:3412-3415.

48. Langer C, Jurgenmeier JM, Bauer G. Reactive oxygen species act at both TGF-β dependent and -independent steps during induction of apoptosis of transformed cells by normal cells. Expt Cell Res 1996; 222:117-124.

49. Ohba M, Shibanuma M, Kuroki T et al. Production of hydrogen peroxide by transforming growth factor-β1 and its involvement in induction of EGR-1 in mouse osteoblastic cells. J Cell Biol 1994; 126:1079-1088.

50. Sanchez A, Alvarez AM, Benito M et al. Apoptosis induced by transforming growth factor–β in fetal hepatocyte primary cultures: involvement of reactive oxygen intermediates. J Biol Chem 1996; 271:7416-7422.

51. Shibanuma M, Kuroki T, Nose K. Release of H2O2 and phorphorylation of 30 kilodalton proteins as early responses of cell cycle-dependent inhibition of DNA synthesis by transforming growth factor β1. Cell Growth & Diff 1991; 2:583-591.

52. Thannickal VJ, Fanburg BL. Activation of an H_2O_2-generating NADH oxidase in human lung fibroblasts by transforming growth factor β1. J Biol Chem 1995; 270:30334-30338.

53. Thannickal VJ, Hassoun PM, White AC et al. Enhanced rate of H2O2 release from bovine pulmonary artery endothelial cells induced by TGF-β1. Am J Physiol 1993; 265:L622-L626.

54. Jacobson MD. Reactive oxygen species and programmed cell death. TIBS 1996; 21:83-86.

55. Barcellos-Hoff MH, Dix TA. Redox-mediated activation of latent transforming growth factor-β1. Molec Endocrin 1996; 10:1077-1983.

56. Barcellos-Hoff MH. Radiation-induced transforming growth factor β and subsequent extracellular matrix reorganization in murine mammary gland. Cancer Res 1993; 53:3880-3886.

57. Barcellos-Hoff MH, Derynck R, Tsang MLS et al. Transforming growth factor-β activation in irradiated murine mammary gland. J Clin Invest 1994; 93:892-899.
58. Ehrhart EJ, Carroll A, Segarini P et al. Quantitative and functional *in situ* evidence of radiation-induced latent transforming growth factor-β activation. Submitted 1997.
59. Shenkar R, Coulson WF, Abraham E. Anti-transforming growth factor-β monoclonal antibodies prevent lung injury in hemorrhaged mice. Am J Respir CellMol Biol 1994; 11:351-357.
60. Bahadori L, Milder J, Gold L et al. Active macrophage-associated TGF-β colocalizes with type I procollagen gene expression in atherosclerotic human pulmonary arteries. Am J Path 1995; 146:1228-1237.
61. Anscher MS, Crocker IR, Jirtle RL. Transforming growth factor β1 expression in irradiated liver. Radiat Res 1990; 122:77-85.
62. Canney PA, Dean, S. Transforming growth factor beta: a promotor of late connective tissue injury following radiotherapy? Br J Radiology 1990; 63:620-623.
63. Szatrowski TP, Nathan CF. Production of large amounts of hydrogen peroxide by human tumor cells. Cancer Res 1991; 51:794-798.
64. Bikfalvi A. Significance of angiogenesis in tumour progression and metastasis. Eur J Cancer 1995; 31A(7-8):1101-1104.
65. Folkman J, Klagsbrun M. Angiogenic factors. Science 1995; 235:442-447.
66. Folkman J. Clinical applications of research on angiogenesis. N Eng J Med 1995; 333:1757-1763.
67. Saksela O, Moscatelli DM, Rifkin DB. The opposing effects of basic fibroblast growth factor and transforming growth factor beta on the regulation of plasminogen activator activity in capillary endothelial cells. J Cell Biol 1995; 105:957-963.
68. Mignatti P, Tsuboi R, Robbins E et al. In vitro angiogenesis on the human amniotic membrane: requirement for basic fibroblast growth factor-induced proteinases. J Cell Biol 1989; 108:671-682.
69. Muller G, Behrens J, Nussbaumer U et al. Inhibitory action of transforming growth factor β on endothelial cells. Proc Natl Acad Sci USA 1989; 85:5600-5604.
70. Frater-Schroder M, Muller G, Birchmeier W et al. Transforming growth factor-beta inhibits endothelial cell proliferation. Biochem Biophys Res Commun 1986; 137:295-302.
71. Baird A, Durkin T. Inhibition of endothelial cell proliferation by type β-transforming growth factor: Interactions with acidic and basic fibroblast growth factors. Biochem Biophys Res Commun 1986; 138:476-482.
72. RayChaudhury A, Frazier WA, D'Amore PA. Comparison of normal and tumorigenic endothelial cells: Differences in thrombospondin production and responses to transforming growth factor-beta. J Cell Sci 1994; 107:39-46.
73. Merwin JR, Anderson JM, Kocher O et al. Transforming growth factor beta 1 modulates extracellular matrix organization and cell-cell junctional complex formation during in vitro angiogenesis. J Cell Physiol 1990; 142.
74. Norgaard P, Hougaard S, Poulsen HS et al. Transforming growth factor β in cancer. Cancer Treatment Reviews 1995; 21:367-403.
75. Ueki N, Ohkawa T, Yokoyama Y et al. Potentiation of metastatic capacity by transforming growth factor-β1 gene transfection. Jpn J Cancer Res 1993; 84:589-593.
76. Yang EY, Moses HL. Transforming growth factor β1-induced changes in cell migration, proliferation, and angiogenesis in the chicken chorioallantoic membrane. J Cell Biol 1990; 111:731-741.
77. Brogi E, Wu T, Namiki A et al. Indirect angiogenic cytokines upregulate VEGF and bFGF gene expression in vascular smooth muscle cells, whereas hypoxia upregulates VEGF expression only. Circulation 1994; 90:649-652.
78. Pertovaara L, Kaipainen A, Mustonen T et al. Vascular endothelial growth factor is induced in response to transforming growth factor-β in fibroblastic and epithelial cells. J Biol Chem 1994; 269:6271-6274.

79. Mandriotta SJ, Menoud PA, Pepper MS. Transforming growth factor beta 1 down-regulates vascular endothelial growth factor receptor2/flk-1 expression in vascular endothelial cells. J Biol Chem 1996; 271:11500-11505.

80. Swerlick RA. Angiogenesis. J Dermatol 1995; 22:845-852.

81. Falcone DJ, McCaffrey TA Haimovitz-Friedman A et al. Transforming growth factor-β1 stimulates macrophage urokinase expression and release of matrix bound basic fibroblast growth factor. J Cell Physiol 1993; 155:595-605.

82. Pepper MS, Vassalli JD, Orci L et al. Biphasic effect of transforming growth factor-β1 on in vitro angiogenesis. Exper Cell Res 1993; 204:356-363.

83. Fajardo LF, Kwan HH, Kowalski J et al. Dual role of tumor necrosis factor-a in angiogenesis. Am J Pathol 1992; 140:539-544.

84. Fajardo LF, Prionas SD, Kwan HH et al. Transforming growth factor β1 induces angiogenesis in vivo with a threshold pattern. Lab Invest 1996; 74:600-608.

85. Chen JK, Hoshi H, McKeehan WL. Transforming growth factor type β specifically stimulates synthesis of proteoglycans in human adult arterial smooth muscle cells. Proc Natl Acad Sci USA 1987; 84:5287-5291.

86. Gajdusek CM, Luo Z, Mayberg MR. Basic fibroblast growth factor and transforming growth factor beta-1: synergistic mediators of angiogenesis in vitro. J Cell Physiol 1993; 157:133-144.

87. Iruela-Arispe M, Sage EH. Endothelial cells exhibiting angiogenesis in vitro proliferate in response to TGFβ1. J Cell Biochem 1993; 52:414-430.

88. Ingber DE, Folkman J. Mechanochemical switching between growth and differentiation during fibroblast growth factor stimulated angiogenesis. J Cell Biol 1989; 109:317-330.

89. Flaumenhaft R, Rifkin DB. Extracellular matrix regulation of growth factor and protease activity. Current Opinion Cell Biol 1991; 3:817-823.

90. Flaumenhaft R, Rifkin DB. The extracellular regulation of growth factor action. Mol Biol Cell 1992; 3:1057-1065.

91. Lyons RM, Gentry LE, Purchio AF et al. Mechanisms of activation of latent recombinant transforming growth factor β1 by plasmin. J Cell Biol 1990; 110:1361-1367.

92. Raines EW, Lane TF, Iruela-Arispe ML et al. The extracellular glycoproteinSPARC interacts with platelet-derived growth factor (PDGF)-AB and BB and inhibits binding of PDGF to its receptor. Proc Natl Acad Sci USA 1992; 89:1281-1285.

93. Saksela O, Moscatelli D, Sommer A et al. Endothelial cell derived heparin sulfate binds basic fibroblast growth factor and protects it from proteolytic degradation. J Cell Biol 1988; 107:743-751.

94. Sankar S, Mahooti-Brooks, Bensen L et al. Modulation of transforming growth factor β receptor levels on microvascular endothelial cells during in vitro angiogenesis. J Clin Invest 1996; 97:1436-1446.

95. Roberts AB, Sporn MB. The transforming growth factor β's. In: Peptide Growth Factors and Their Receptors. Berlin: Springer-Verlag. 1990:419-472.

96. Massague J. The transforming growth factor-β family. Annu Rev Cell Biol 1990; 6:597-641.

97. Miesher S, Whiteside TL, Carrel S et al. Functional properties of tumor infiltrating and blood lymphocytes in patients with solid tumors: Effects of tumor cells and their supernatants on proliferative responses of lymphocytes. J Immunol 1986; 136:1899-1907.

98. Sporn MB, Roberts AB. Transforming growth factor-β: Multiple actions and potential clinical applications. J Am Med Assoc 1989; 262:938-941.

99. Roszman T, Elliott L, Brooks W. Modulation of T-cell function by gliomas. Immunol Today 1991; 12:370-374.

100. Ebert EC, Roberts AJ, Devereux D et al. Selective immunosuppressive action of a factor produced by colon cancer cells. Cancer Res 1990; 50:6158-6161.

101. Roberts AB, Sporn MB. Physiological actions and clinical applications of transforming growth factor-β (TGF-β). Growth Factors 1993; 8:1-9.

102. Ruscetti F, Varesio L, Ochoa A et al. Pleiotropic effects of transforming growth factor-β on cells of the immne system. Ann NY Acad Sci 1993; 685:488-500.

103. Lawrence DA. Transforming growth factor-β: An overview. Kidney International 1995; 47(Suppl 49):S19-S23.

104. Lawrence DA. Transforming growth factor-β: A general review. Eur Cytokine Network 1996; 7:363-374.
105. Grande JP. Role of transforming growth factor-β in tissue injury and repair. PSEBM 1997; 214:27-40.
106. Wahl SM. Transforming growth factor β: The good, the bad, and the ugly. J Exp Med 1994; 180:1587-1590.
107. Lee G, Ellingsworth LR, Gillis S, Wall R, Kincade PW. β Transforming growth factors are potential regulators of of B lymphopoiesis. J Exp Med 1987; 166:1290-1299.
108. Cheifetz S, Weatherbee JA, Tsang L-S et al. The transforming growth factor-β system: a complex pattern of cross-reactive ligands and receptors. Cell 1987; 48:409-415.
109. Ottmann OG, Pelus LM. Differential proliferative effects of transforming growth factor-β on human hematopoietic progenitor cells. J Immunol 1988; 140:2661-2665.
110. Suda T, Zlotnik A. In vitro induction of CD8 expression on thymic pre-T cells. I. Transforming growth factor-beta and tumor necrosis factor-alpha induce CD8 expression on CD8- thymic subsets including the CD25+CD3-CD4-CD8- pre-T cell subset. J Immunol 1992; 148:1737-1745.
111. Inge TH, McCoy KM, Susskind BM et al. Immunomodulatory effects of transforming growth factor-β on T lymphocytes. Induction of CD8 expression in the CTLL-2 cell line and in normal thymocytes. J Immunol 1992; 148:3847-3856.
112. Harada M, Matsunaga K, Oguchi Y et al. The involvement of transforming growth factor β in the impaired antitumor T-cell rsponse at the gut-associated lymphoid tissue (GALT). Cancer Res 1995; 55:6146-6151.
113. Sitnicka E, Ruscetti FW, Priestley GV et al. Transforming growth factor beta 1 directly and reversibly inhibits the initial cell divisions of long-term repopulating hematopoietic stem cells. Blood 1996; 88:82-88.
114. Keller JR, Mantel C, Sing GK et al. Transforming growth factor beta 1 selectively regulates early murine hematopoietic progenitors and inhibits the growth of IL-3-dependent myeloid leukemia cell lines. J Exp Med 1988; 168:737-750.
115. Mossalayi MD, Mentz F, Ouaaz F et al. Early human thymocyte proliferation is regulated by an externally controlled autocrine transforming growth factor-beta 1 mechanism. Blood 1995; 85:3594-3601.
116. Keller JR, Jacobsen SE, Dubois CM et al. Transforming growth factor-beta: a bidirectional regulator of hematopoietic cell growth. Int J Cell Cloning 1992; 10:2-11.
117. Hestdal K, Jacobsen SE, Ruscetti FW et al. Increased granulopoiesis after sequential administration of transforming growth factor-beta 1 and granulocyte-macrophage colony-stimulating factor. Exp Hematol 1993; 21:799-805.
118. Jacobsen SE, Keller JR, Ruscetti FW et al. Bidirectional effects of transforming growth factor beta (TGF-beta) on colony-stimulating factor-induced human myelopoiesis in vitro: differential effects of distinct TGF-beta isoforms. Blood 1991; 78:2239-2247.
119. Keller JR, Jacobsen SE, Sill KT et al. Stimulation of granulopoiesis by transforming growth factor beta: synergy with granulocyte/macrophage-colony-stimulating factor. Proc Natl Acad Sci USA 1991; 88:7190-7194.
120. Celada A, Maki RA. Transforming growth factor-beta enhances the M-CSF and GM-CSF-stimulated proliferation of macrphages. J Immunol 1992; 148:1102-1105.
121. Ruegemer JJ, Ho SN, Augustine JA et al. Regulatory effects of transforming growth factor-β on IL-2 and IL-4 dependent T cell-cycle progression. J Immunol 1990; 144:1767-1776.
122. Gately M, Desai BB, Wolitzki AG et al. Regulation of human leukocyte proliferation by a heterodimeric cytokine, IL-12 (cytotoxic lymphocyte maturation factor). J Immunol 1992; 147:874-882.
123. Edwards DR, Heath JK. Regulation of transcription by Transforming growth factor-β. In: Cohen P, Foulkes JG, eds. The Hormonal Control Regulation of Gene Transcription. New York: Elsevier Sciences Publisher, 1991:333-347.
124. Ortaldo JL, Mason AT, O'Shea JJ et al. Mechanistic studes of transforming growth factor-β inhibition of IL-2 dependent activation of CD3- large granular lymphocyte functions. J Immunol 1991; 146:3791-3798.

125. Fox E, Ford HC, Douglas R et al. TGF-β can inhibit human T-lymphocyte proliferation through paracrine and auticrine mechanisms. Cell Immunol 1993; 150:45-58.

126. Geller RL, Smyth MJ, Strobl SL et al. Generation of lymphokine-activated killer activity in T cells. J Immunol 1991; 146:3280-3288.

127. Smyth MJ, Strobl SL, Young HA et al. Regulation of lymphokine-activated killer activity and pore-forming protein gene expression in human peripheral blood CD8+ T lymphocytes. Inhibition by transforming growth factor-beta. J Immunol 1991; 146:3289-3297.

128. Uhm J-R, Kettering JD, Gridley DS. Modulation of transforming growth factor-β1 effects by cytokines. Immunol Invest 1993; 22:375-388.

129. Lee HM, Rich S. Costimulation of T cell proliferation by transforming growth factor-beta 1. J Immunol 1991; 147:1127-1133.

130. Swain SL, Huston G, Tonkonogy S et al. Transforming growth factor-beta and IL-4 cause helper T cell precursors to develop into distinct effector helper cells that differ in lymphokine secretion pattern and cell surface phenotype. J Immunol 1991; 147:2991-3000.

131. Kehrl JH, Wakefield LM, Roberts AB et al. Production of transforming growth factor β by human T lymphocytes and its potential role in the regulation of T cell growth. J Exp Med 1986; 163:1037-1050.

132. Gamble JR, Vadas MA. Endothelial adhesiveness for blood neutrophils is inhibited by transforming growth factor-β. Science 1988; 242:97-99.

133. Gamble JR, Vadas MA. Endothelial adhesiveness for human T lymphocytes is inhibited by TGF-β. J Immunol 1991; 146:1149-1154.

134. Gamble JR, Khew-Goodall Y, Vadas MA. TGF-β inhibits E-selectin expression of human endothelial cells. J Immunol 1993; 150:4494-4503.

135. van Vlasselaer P, Punnonen J, deVries JE. Transforming growth factor-beta directs IgA switching in human B cells. J Immunol 1992; 148:2062-2067.

136. Kehrl JH, Roberts AB, Wakefield LM et al. Transforming growth factor beta is an important immunomodulatory protein for human B lymphocytes. J Immunol 1986; 137:3855-3860.

137. Kehrl JH, Taylor AS, Delsing GA et al. Further studies of the role of transforming growth factor β in human B cell function. J Immunol 1989; 143:1868-1874.

138. Flescher E, Fossum D, Ballester A et al. Characterization of B cell growth in systemic lupus erythematosus. Effects of recombinant 12-kDa B cell growth factor, interleukin 4 and transforming growth factor-beta. Eur J Immunol 1990; 20:2425-2430.

139. Lee G, Namen AE, Gillis S et al. Normal B cell precursors responsive to recombinant murine IL-7 and inhibition of IL-7 activity by transforming growth factor β. J Immunol 1989; 142:3875-3883.

140. Sing GK, Keller JR, Ellingsworth LR et al. Transforming growth factor β selectively inhibits normal and leukemic human bone marrow cell growth in vitro. Blood 1988; 72:1504-1511.

141. Kehrl JH. Transforming growth factor β: An important mediator of immunoregulation. Int J Cell Cloning 1991; 9:438-450.

142. Machold KP, Carson DA, Lotz M. Transforming growth factor-β (TGFβ) inhibition of Epstein-Barr virus (EBV)- and interleukin-4 (IL-4)-induced immunoglobulin production in human B lymphocytes. J Clin Immunol 1993; 13:219-227.

143. Boddan C, Nathan C. Modulation of macrophage function by transforming growth factor beta, interleukin-4 and interleukin-10. Ann NY Acad Sci. 1993; 685:713-739.

144. Fiorentino DF, Bond MW, Mosmann TR. Two types of mouse T helper cells. IV. Th2 clones secrete a factor that inhibits cytokine production by Th1 clones. J Exp Med 1989; 170:2081-2095.

145. Espevik T, Figari IS, Ranges GE et al. Transforming growth factor β1 and recombinant human tumor necrosis factor α reciprocally regulate the generation of lymphokine-activated killer cell activity. Comparison between natural porcine platelet-derived TGF-β1 and TGF-β2 and recombinant human TGF-β1. J Immunol 1988; 140:2312-2316.

146. Espevik T, Figari IS, Shalaby MR et al. Inhibition of cytokine production by cyclosporine A and transforming growth factor β. J Exp Med 1987; 166:571-576.

147. Fargeas C, Wu CY, Nakajima T et al. Differential effect of transforming growth factor β on the synthesis of Th1- and Th2-like lymphokines by human T lymphocytes. Eur J Immunol. 1992; 22:2173-2176.

148. Turner M, Chantry D, Katsikis P et al. Induction of interleukin 1 receptor antagonist protein by transforming growth factor-β. Eur J Immunol 1991; 21:1635-1639.

149. Hatzfeld J, Li ML, Brown EL et al. Release of early human hematopoietic progenitors from quiescence by antisense transforming growth factor-β1 or Rb oligonucleotides. J Exp Med 1991; 174:925-929.

150. Wahl SM, Hunt DA, Wakefield LM et al. Transforming growth factor type β induces monocyte chemotaxis and growth factor production. Proc Natl Acad Sci USA 1987; 84:5788-5792.

151. Wiseman DM, Polverini PJ, Kamp DW, et a. Transforming growth factor beta (TGFβ) is chemotactic for human monocytes and induces their expression of angiogenic activity. Biochem Biophys Res Comm 1988; 157:793-800.

152. Reibman J, Meixler S, Lee TC et al. Transforming growth factor β1, a potent chemoattractant for human neutrophils, bypasses classic signal-transduction pathways. Proc Natl Acad Sci USA 1991; 88:6805-6809.

153. McCartney-Francis N, Maizel D, Wong H et al. TGF-β regulates production of growth factors and TGF-β by human peripheral blood monocytes. Growth Factors 1990; 4:27-35.

154. Bauvois B, Rouillard D, Sanceau J et al. IFNγ and transforming growth factor-β1 differently regulate fibronectin and laminin receptors of human differentiating monocyte cells. J Immunol 1992; 148:3912-3919.

155. Wahl SM, Allen JB, Weeks BS et al. Transforming growth factor beta enhances integrin expression and type IV collagenase secretion in human monocytes. Proc Natl Acad Sci USA 1993; 90:4577-4581.

156. Chin YH, Cai JP, Xu XM. Transforming growth factor-β1 and IL-4 regulate the adhesiveness of Peyer's patch high endothelial venule cells for lymphocytes. J Immunol 1992; 148:1106-1112.

157. Tsunawaki S, Sporn M, Ding A et al. Deactivation of macrophages by transforming growth factor-β. Nature 1988; 334:260-262.

158. Nelson BJ, Ralph P, Green SJ et al. Differential succeptibility of activated macrophage cytotoxic effector reactions to the suppressive effects of transforming growth factor β. J Immunol 1991; 146:1849-1857.

159. Wahl SM, McCartney-Francis N, Allen JB et al. Macrophage production of TGF-β and regulation by TGF-β. Ann NY Acad Sci 1990; 593:188-196.

160. Wahl SM, Allen JB, Welch GR et al. Transforming growth factor-β in synovial fluids modulates FcγRIII (CD16) expression on mononuclear phagocytes. J Immunol 1992; 148:485-490.

161. Bottalico LA, Wager RE, Agellon LB et al. Transforming growth factor-β1 inhibits scavenger receptor activity in THP-1 human macrophages. J Biol Chem 1991; 266:22866-22871.

162. Tanaka M, Lee K, Yodoi J et al. Regulation of Fcε receptor 2 (CD23) expression on a human eosinophilic cell line Eol 3 and a human monocytic cell line U937 by transforming growth factor β. Cell Immunol 1989; 122:96-107.

163. Unanue E. Macrophages, antigen-presenting cells, and the phenomenon of antigen handling and presentation. In: Paul, WE, ed. Fundamental Immunology. New York: Raven Press, 1989:95-115.

164. Springer TA. Adhesion receptors of the immune system. Nature 1990; 346:425-433.

165. Siepl C, Bodmer S, Frei K et al. The glioblastoma-derived T cell suppressor factor/transforming growth factor-β2 inhibits T cell growth without affecting the interaction of interleukin 2 with its receptor. Eur J Immunol 1988; 18:593-600.

166. Darley R, Morris A, Passas J et al. Interactions between interferonγ and retinoic acid with transforming growth factor β in the induction of immune recognition molecules. Cancer Immunol Immunother 1993; 37:112-118.

167. Fidler IJ, Schroit AJ. Recognition and destruction of neoplastic cells by activated macrophages: Discrimination of altered self. Biochem Biophys Acta 1988; 948:151-173.

168. Nathan CF. Coordinate actions of growth factors in monocyte/macrophages. In: Sporn MB, Roberts AB, eds. Handbook of Experimental Pharmacology, Vol 95/II. Berlin: Springer Verlag, 1990:427-462.
169. Chantry D, Turner M, Abney E et al. Modulation of cytokine production by transforming growth factor-β. J Immunol. 1989; 142:4295-4300.
170. Turner M, Chantry D, Feldmann M. Transforming growth factor β induces the production of interleukin 6 by human peripheral blood mononuclear cells. Cytokine 1990; 2:211-216.
171. Musso T, Espinoza-Delgado I, Pulkii K et al. Transforming growth factor β downregulates IL-1 induced IL-6 production by human monocytes. Blood 1990; 76:2466-2469.
172. Kim SJ, Jeang KT, Glick A et al. Promotor sequences of the human transforming growth factor-β1 gene responsive to transforming growth factor-β1 autoinduction. J Biol Chem 1989; 264:7041-7045.
173. Kim SJ, Angel P, Lafyatis R et al. Autoinduction of transforming growth factor β1 is mediated by the AP-1 complex. Mol Cell Biol 1990; 10:1492-1497.
174. Ding A, Nathan CF, Graycar J et al. Macrophage deactivating factor and transforming growth factors-β1, -β2 and -β3 inhibit induction of macrophage nitrogen oxide synthesis by IFNγ. J Immunol 1990; 145:940-944.
175. Gazzinelli RT, Oswald IP, Hieny S et al. The microbicidal activity of IFNγ-treated macrophages against *Trypanosoma cruzi* involves an L-arginine-dependent, nitrogen oxide-mediated mechanism inhibitable by interleukin 10 and transforming growth factor-β. Eur J Immunol 1992; 22:2501-2506.
176. Torre-Amione G, Beauchamp RD, Koeppen H et al. A highly immunogenic tumor transfected with a murine transforming growth factor type β1 cDNA escapes immune surveillence. Proc Natl Acad Sci USA 1990; 87:1486-1490.
177. Arteaga CL, Hurd SD, Winnier AR et al. Anti-transforming growth factor (TGF)-β antibodies inhibit breast cancer cell tumorigenicity and increase mouse spleen natural killer cell activity. Implications for a possible role of tumor cell/host TGF-β interactions in human breast cancer progression. J Clin Invest 1993; 92:2569-2576.
178. Grimm EA, Crump WL III, Durett A et al. TGFβ inhibits the in vitro induction of lymphokine-activated killing activity. Cancer Immunol Immunother. 1988; 27:53-58.
179. Hirte H, Clark DA. Generation of lymphokine-activated killer cells in human ovarian carcinoma ascitic fluid: Identification of transforming growth factor β as a suppressive factor. Cancer Immunol Immunother. 1991; 32:296-302.
180. Kuppner MC, Hamou MF, Bodmer S et al. The glioblastoma-derived T-cell suppressor factor/transforming growth factor beta 2 inhibits the generation of lymphokine-activated killer (LAK) cells. Int J Cancer 1988; 42:562-567.
181. Wrann M, Bodmer MS, Martin R de et al. T cell suppressor factor from human glioblastoma cells in a 12.5-kd protein closely related to transforming growth factor beta. EMBO J 1987; 6:1633-1636.
182. Tada T, Ohzeki S, Utsumi K et al. Transforming growth factor-beta-induced inhibition of T cell function. Susceptibility difference in T cells of various phenotypes and functions and its relevance to immunosuppression in the tumor-bearing state. J Immunol 1991; 146:1077-1082.
183. Fakhrai H, Dorigo O, Shawler DL et al. Eradication of established intracranial rat gliomas by transforming growth factor β antisense gene therapy. Proc Natl Acad Sci USA 1996; 93:2909-2914.
184. McCartney-Francis NL, Wahl SM. Transforming growth factor β: A matter of life and death. J Leuk Biol 1994; 55:401-409.
185. Letterio JJ, Roberts AB. Transforming growth factor-β1-deficient mice: identification of isoform-specific activities in vivo. J Leuk Biol 1996; 59:769-774.
186. Racke MK, Dhib-Jallbut S, Cannella B et al. Prevention and treatment of chronic relapsing experimental allergic encephalomyelitis by transforming growth factor-β1. J Immunol 1991; 146:3012-3017.

187. Racke MK, Cannella B, Albert P et al. Evidence of endogenous regulatory function of trans-forming growth factor-β1 in experimental allergic encephalomyelitis. Int Immunol 1992; 4:615-620.
188. Lowrance JH, O'Sullivan FX, Caver TE et al. Spontaneous elaboration of transforming growth factor β suppresses host defense against bacterial infections in autoimmune MRL/lpr mice. J Exp Med 1994; 180:1693-1703.
189. Santambrogio L, Hochwald GM, Saxena B et al. Studies on the mechanism by which trans-forming growth factor-β (TGF-β) protects against allergic encephalomyelitis. J Immunol 1993; 151:1116-1127.
190. Wahl SM, Hunt DA, Wong HL et al. Tramsforming growth factor beta is a potent immu-nosuppressive agent which inhibits interleukin-1 dependent lymphocyte proliferation. J Immunol 1988; 140:3026-3032.
191. Wahl SM, Allen JB, Costa GL et al. Reversal of acute and chronic synovial inflammation by anti-transforming rowth factor β. J Exp Med 1993; 177:225-230.
192. Allen JB, Manthey CL, Hand AR et al. Rapid onset synovial inflammation and hyperplasia induced by transforming growth factor β. J Exp Med 1990; 171:231-247.
193. Brandes ME, Allen JB, Ogawa Y et al. Transforming growth factor β1 suppresses acute and chronic arthritis in experimental animals. J Clin Invest 1991; 87:1108-1113.
194. Filmus J, Kerbel RS. Development of resistance mechanisms to the growth-inhibitory ef-fects of transforming growth factor-beta during tumor progression. Curr Op Oncology 1993; 5:123-129.
195. Fynan TM, Reiss M. Resistance to inhibition of cell growth by transforming growth factor-beta and its role in oncogenesis. Crit Rev Onc 1993; 4:493-540.
196. Kerbel RS. Expression of multi-cytokine resistance and multi-growth factor independence in advanced stage metastatic cancer. Malignant melanoma as a paradigm. Am J Path 1992; 141:519-524.
197. Fearon ER, Vogelstein B. A genetic model for colorectal tumorigenesis. Cell 1990; 61:7757-7767.
198. Polyak K. Negative regulation of cell growth by TGF beta. Biochem Biophys Acta 1996; 1242:185-199.
199. Kaiser U, Schardt C, Brandscheidt D et al. Expression of insulin-like growth factor recep-tors I and II in normal human lung and in lung cancer. J Cancer Res Clin Oncol 1993; 119(11):665-668.
200. Levy LS, Bost KL. Mechanisms that contribute to the development of lymphoid malignan-cies: roles for genetic alterations and cytokine production. Crit Rev Immunol 1996; 16:31-57.
201. De Souza AT, Hankins GR, Washington MK et al. Frequent loss of heterozygosity on 6q at the mannose 6-phosphate/insulin-like growth factor II receptor locus in human hepatocel-lular tumors. Oncogene 1995; 10:1725-1729.
202. Rodeck U, Bossler A, Graeven U et al. Transforming growth factor β production and re-sponsiveness in normal human melanocytes and melanoma cells. Cancer Res 1994; 54:575-581.
203. De Souza AT, Hankins GR, Washington MK et al. M6P/IGF2r gene is mutated in human hepatocellular carcinomas with LOH. Nature Genet 1995; 11:447-449.
204. Hankins GR, De Souza AT, Bentley RC et al. M6P/IGF2 receptor: A candidate breast tu-mor suppressor gene. Oncogene 1996; 12:2003-2009.
205. Sue SR, Chari RS, Kong F-M et al. Transforming growth factor beta receptors and man-nose 6-phosphate/insulin-like growth factor II receptor expression in human hepatocellu-lar carcinomas. Ann Surg 1995; 222:171-178.
206. Kimchi A, Wang XF, Weinberg RA et al. Absence of TGF-β receptors and growth inhibi-tory responses in retinoblastoma cells. Science 1988; 240:196-198.
207. Markowitz S, Wang J, Myeroff L et al. Inactivation of the type II TGF-β receptor in colon cancer cells with microsatellite instability. Science 1995; 268:1336-1338.
208. Kaufmann AM, Stoeck M, Schirrmacher V et al. Transforming growth factor-beta produc-tion and induction of cellular responses in 13762NF rat mammary adenocarcinoma cell clones. Invasion & Metastasis 1993; 13:244-252.

209. Mansbach JM, Mills JJ Boyer IJ et al. Phenobarbital selectively promotes initiated cells with reduced TGFβ receptor levels. Carcinogenesis 1996; 17:171-174.

210. Factor VM, Kao CY, Santoni-Rugui E et al. Constituive expression of mature transforming growth factor b1 in the liver accelerates hepatocarcinogenesis in transgenic mice. Cancer Res 1997; 57:2089-2095.

211. Yingling JM, Wang XF, Bassing CH. Signaling by the transforming growth factor-beta receptors. Biochem Biophys Acta 1995; 1242:115-136.

212. Sloane BF, Rozhin J, Johnson K, Taylor H, Crissman JD, Honn KV. Cathepsin B. Associations with plasma membrane in metastatic tumors. Proc Natl Acad Sci USA 1986; 83:2483.

213. Serra R, Moses HL. Tumor suppressor genes in the TGFβ pathway? Nature Med 1996; 2:390-391.

214. Jennings MT, Maciunas RJ, Carver R et al. TGF beta 1 and TGF beta 2 are potential growth regulators for low-grade and malignant gliomas in vitro: evidence in support of an autocrine hypothesis. Int J Cancer 1991; 49:129-139.

215. Mulder KM, Ramey MR, Hoosein NM et al. Characterization of transforming growth factor-beta-resistant subclones isolated from a transforming growth factor-beta-sensitive human colon carcinoma cell line. Cancer Res 1988; 48:7120-7125.

216. Perrotti D, Cimino L, Ferrari S et al. Differential expression of transforming growth factor-beta 1 gene in 3LL metastatic variants. Cancer Res 1991; 51:5491-5494.

217. Sehgal I, Baley PA, Thompson TC. Transforming growth factor beta 1 stimulates contrasting responses in metastatic versus primary mouse prostate cancer-derived cell lines in vitro. Cancer Res 1996; 56:3359-3365.

218. Wright JA, Turley EA, Greenberg AH. Transforming growth factor beta and fibroblast growth factor as promoters of tumor progression to malignancy. Crit Rev Oncogen 1993; 4:473-492.

219. Schor SL. Fibroblast subpopulations as accelerators of tumor progression: The role of migration stimulating factor. EXS 1995; 74:273-296.

220. Lieber CS, Garro A, Leo MA et al. Alcohol and cancer. Hepatology 1986; 6:1005-1009.

221. Alter HJ. Transfusion-associated non-A, non-B hepatitis: the first decade. New York: Alan R. Liss, 1988.

222. van Vloten WA, Hermans J, van Daal WAJ. Radiation induced skin cancer and radiodermatitis of head and neck. Cancer 1987; 59:411-414.

223. Vorherr H. Fibrocystic breast disease: Pathophysiology, pathomorphology, clinical picture, and management. Am J Ostet Gynecol 1986; 154:836-838.

224. Kawai TK, Yakumaru M, Suski K et al. Diffuse interstitial pulmonary fibrosis and lung cancer. Acta Pathologica Japonica 1987; 37:11-19.

225. Ohwada H, Hayashi Y, Seki M. An experimental study on carcinogenesis related to localized fibrosis in the lung. Gann 1980; 71:285-291.

226. Phan SH, Kunkel SL. Lung cytokine production in bleomycin-induced pulmonary fibrosis. Exp Lung Res 1992; 18:29-43.

227. Alexandrow MG, Moses HL. Transforming growth factor β and cell cycle regulation. Cancer Res 1995; 55:1452-1457.

228. Hahn SA, Schutte M, Hoque AT et al. DPC4, a candidate tumor suppressor gene at human chromosome 18q21.1. Science 1996; 271:350-353.

229. Arteaga CL, Dugger TC, Winnier AR, Forbes JT. Evidence for a positive role of transforming growth factor-beta in human breast cancer cell tumorigenesis. J Cell Biochem (Suppl) 1993; 17G:187-193.

230. Ueki N, Nakazato M, Ohkawa T et al. Excessive production of transforming growth factor-β1 can play an important role in the development of tumorigenesis by its action for angiogenesis: Validity of neutralizing antibodies to block tumor growth. Biochem Biophys Acta 1992; 1137:189-196.

231. Spearman M, Taylor WR, Greenberg AH et al. Antisense oligodeoxyribonucleotide inhibition of TGF-beta 1 gene expression and alterations in the growth and malignant properties of mouse fibrosarcoma cells. Gene 1994; 149:25-29.

232. Shirai Y, Kawata S, Ito N et al. Elevated levels of plasma transforming growth factor-β in patients with hepatocellular carcinoma. Jpn J Cancer Res 1992; 83:676-679.

233. Shirai Y, Kawata S, Tamura S et al. Plasma transforming growth factor-β1 in patients with hepatocellular carcinoma: Comparison with chronic liver diseases. Cancer 1994; 73:2275-2279.

234. Ivanovic V, Melman A, Davis-Joseph B et al. Elevated plasma levels of TGFb1 in patients with invasive prostate cancer. Nature Med 1995; 1:282-283.

235. Kong F-M, Anscher MS, Abbot BD et al. Elevated plasma transforming growth factor-β1 levels in breast cancer patients decrease after surgical removal of the tumor. Ann Surg 1995; 222:155-162.

236. Wakefield LM, Letterio JJ, Chen T et al. Transforming growth factor-β1 circulates in normal human plasma and is unchanged in advanced metastatic breast cancer. Clin Cancer Res 1995; 1:129-136.

237. Kong FM, Washington MK, Jirtle RL et al. Plasma transforming growth factor-β1 reflects disease status in patients with lung cancer after radiotherapy: A possible tumor marker. Lung Cancer 1996; 16:47-59.

238. Derynck R, Goeddel DV, Ullrich A et al. Synthesis of messenger RNAs for transforming growth factors α & β and the epidermal growth factor receptor by human tumors. Cancer Res 1987; 47:707-712.

239. Kim S-J, Kehrl JH, Burton J et al. Transactivation of the transforming growth factor β1 (TGF-b1) gene by human T lymphotrophic virus type 1 tax: A potential mechanism for increased production of TGF-β1 in adult T cell leukemia. J Exp Med 1990; 172:121-129.

240. Jasani B, Wyllie FS, Wright PA et al. Immunocytochemically detectable TGF-β associated with malignancy in thyroid epithelial neoplasia. Growth Factor 1990; 2:149-155.

241. Ito N, Kawata S, Tamura S et al. Elevated levels of transforming growth factor β messenger RNA and its polypeptide in human hepatocellular carcinoma. Cancer Res 1991; 51:4080-4083.

242. Kremer JP, Reisbach G, Nerl C et al. B-cell chronic lymphocytic leukemia cells express and release transforming growth factor-beta. Br J Haematol 1992; 80:480.

243. Lotz M, Ranheim E, Kipps TJ. Transforming growth factor beta as endogenous growth inhibitor of chronic lymphocytic leukemia B cells. J Exp Med 1994; 179:99.

244. Blanckaert VD, Schelling ME, Elstad CA et al. Differential growth factor production, secretion, and response by high and low metastatic variants of B16BL6 melanoma. Cancer Res 1993; 53:4075-4081.

245. Welch DR, Fabra A, Nakajima M. Transforming growth factor β stimulates mammary adenocarcinoma cell invasion and metastatic potential. Proc Natl Acad Sci USA 1990; 87:7678-7682.

246. Samuel SK, Hurta RAR, Kondaiah P et al. Autocrine induction of tumor protease production and invasion by a metallothionein-regulated TGF-β1(Ser-223,225). EMBO J 1992; 11:1599.

247. Haralson MA. Extracellular matrix and growth factors: An integrated interplay controlling tissue repair and progression to disease. Lab Invest 1993; 69:369-372.

248. Koh GY, Kim SJ, Klug MG et al. Targeted expression of transforming growth factor-beta 1 in intracardiac grafts promotes vascular endothelial cell DNA synthesis. J Clin Invest 1995; 95:114-121.

249. Agrotis A, Bobit A. Vascular remodelling and molecular biology: new concepts and therapeutic possibilities. Clin Exper Pharmacol Physiol 1996; 23:363-368.

250. Phillips GD, Whitehead RA, Stone AM et al. Transforming growth factor beta (TGF-β) stimulation of angiogenesis: an electron microscopic study. J Submicroscopic Cytol Pathol 1993; 25:149-155.

251. Matrisian LM, Bowden GT, Krieg P et al. The mRNA coding for secreted protease transin is expressed more abundantly in malignant than in benign tumors. Proc Natl Acad Sci USA 1986; 83:9413.

252. Stetler-Stevenson WG. Type IV collagenases in tumor invasion and metastasis. Cancer Metast Rev 1990; 9:289.

253. Keski-Oja J, Blasi F, Leof E et al. Regulation of the synthesis and activity of urokinase plasminogen activator in A549 human lung carcinoma cells by transforming growth factor-β. J Cell Biol 1988; 106:451.
254. Desruisseau S, Ghazarossian-Ragni E, Chinot O et al. Divergent effect of TGFbeta1 on growth and proteolytic modulation of human prostatic-cancer cell lines. Int J Cancer 1996; 66:796-801.
255. Kobayashi M, Hamada J, Li YQ et al. A possible role of 92 kDa type IV collagenase in the extramedullary tumor formation in leukemia. Jpn J Cancer Res 1995; 86:298-303.
256. Gohji K, Nakajima M, Fabra A et al. Regulation of gelatinase production in metastatic renal cell carcinoma by organ-specific fibroblasts. Jpn J Cancer Res 1994; 85:152-160.
257. Shimizu S, Nishikawa Y, Kuroda K et al. Involvement of transforming growth factor beta 1 in autocrine enhancement of gelatinase B secretion by murine metastatic colon carcinoma cells. Cancer Res 1996; 56:3366-3370.
258. Kawamata H, Kameyama S, Nan L et al. Response to epidermal growth factor (EGF) and transforming growth factor β1 (TGF-β1) of newly established rat bladder carcinoma cell lines. Proc 84th Annual Meeting of the AACR 1993:171.
259. Hsu S, Huang F, Hafez M et al. Colon carcinoma cells switch their response to transforming growth factor β1 with tumor progression. Cell Growth Diff 1994; 5:267-275.
260. Merzak A, McCrea S, Koocheckpour S et al. Control of human glioma cell growth, migration and invasion in vitro by transforming growth factor β1. Br J Cancer 1994; 70:199-203.
261. Mooradian DL, McCarthy JB, Komanduri KV et al. Effects of transforming growth factor-β1 on human pulmonary adenocarcinoma cell adhesion motility and invasion in vitro. J Natl Cancer Inst 1992; 84:523-527.
262. Reed JA, McNutt S, Prieto VG et al. Expression of transforming growth factor-β2 in malignant melanoma correlates with the depth of tumor invasion. Am J Pathol 1994; 145:97-104.
263. Rosen EM, Goldberg ID. Protein factors that regulate cell motility. In Vitro Cell Dev Biol 1989; 25:1079.
264. Postlethwaite AE, Keski-Oja J, Moses HL et al. Stimulation of the chemotactic migration of human fibroblasts by transforming growth factor beta. J Exp Med 1987; 165:251.
265. Brandes ME, Mai WEH, Ohura K et al. Type I transforming growth factor-β receptors on neutrophils mediate chemotaxis to transforming growth factor-b. J Immunol 1991; 147:1600.
266. Riebman J, Meixler S, Lee TC et al. Transforming growth factor β-1, a potent chemoattractant for human neutrophils,by passes classic signal-transduction pathways. Proc Natl Acad Sci USA 1991; 88:6805.
267. Nickoloff BJ, Mitra RS, Riser BS et al. Modulation of keratinocyte motility. Correlation with production of extracellular matrix molecules in response to growth promoting and antiproliferative factors. Am J Pathol 1988; 132:543.
268. Faassen AE, Mooradian DL, Tranquillo RT et al. Cell surface CD44-related chondroitin sulfate proteoglycan is required for transforming growth factor-beta-stimulated mouse melanoma cell motility and invasive behavior on type I collagen. J Cell Sci 1993; 105:501-511.
269. Turley EA, Austen L, Vandelight K et al. Hyaluronan and a cell-associated hyaluronan binding protein regulate the locomotion of ras-transformed cells. J Cell Biol 1991; 112:1041.
270. Hardwick C, Hoare K, Owens R et al. Molecular cloning of a novel hyaluronan receptor that mediates tumor cell motility. J Cell Biol 1992; 117:1343.
271. Fidler IJ. In: Vincent TD Jr, Samuel H, Steven AR, eds. Molecular Biology of Cancer: Invasion and Metastasis. Philadelphia: Lippincott-Raven Publishers, 1997:135-152.
272. Saiki I, Naito S, Yoneda J et al. Chracterization of the invasive and metastatic phenotype in human renal cell carcinoma. Clin Exp Metast 1991; 9:551-566.
273. Updyke TV, Nicolson GL. Malignant melanoma cell line selected in vitro for increased homotypic adhesion properties have increased experimental metastasis potential. Clin Exp Metast 1986; 4:237-284.
274. Ignotz RA, Heino J, Massague J. Regulation of cell adhesion receptors by transforming growth factor-β. J Biol Chem 1989; 264:389-392.

275. Kahari V, Peltonen J, Chen YQ et al. Differential modulation of basement membrane gene expression in human fibrosarcoma HT-1080 cells by transforming growth factor-β1. Lab Invest 1991; 64:807-818.

276. Arrick BA, Lopez AR, Elfman F et al. Altered metabolic and adhesive properties and increased tumorigenesis associated with increased expression of transforming growth factor β1. J Cell Biol 1992; 118:715-726.

277. Couffinhal T, Duplaa C, Moreau C et al. Regulation of vascular cell adhesion molecule-1 and intercellular adhesion molecule-1 in human vascular smooth muscle cells. Circulation Res 1994; 74:225-234.

278. Norgaard P, Damstrup L, Rygaard K et al. Growth suppression by transforming growth factor b_1 of human small-cell lung cancer cell lines is associated with expression of the type II receptor. Br J Cancer 1994; 69:802-808.

279. Tsonis PA, Del Rio-Tsonis K, Millian JL et al. Expression of N-cadherin and alkaline phosphatase in chick limb bud mesenchymal cells: Regulation by 1,25-dihydroxy-vitamin D3 or TGF-β1. Exp Cell Res 1994; 213:433-437.

280. Lagadec P, Reveneau S, Lejune P et al. Immunomodulator OM 163-induced reversal of tumor-mediated immunosuppression and downregulation of TGF-β1 in vivo. J Pharmacol Exp Ther 1996; 278:926-933.

281. Hoefer M, Anderer FA. Anti-(transforming growth factor beta) antibodies with predefined specificity inhibit metastasis of highly tumorigenic human xenotransplants in nu/nu mice. Cancer Immunol Immunother 1995; 41:302-308.

CHAPTER 4

Stromal-Epithelial Interactions

J.R. Benson

i) Introduction

Many of the studies mentioned in the preceding chapter have involved breast epithelial cells in isolation. However, a tumor is composed of several cell types in addition to neoplastic epithelium. These include various mesenchymal derivatives such as fibroblasts and endothelial cells, which in vivo have important interactions with epithelial cells in both topographical and functional contexts. The nature of these stromal-epithelial interactions remain ill-defined and poorly understood. Experimental data substantiates a role for such interactions in morphogenesis and other developmental processes.[1,2] In particular, these have confirmed the importance of mesenchymal elements as key determinants in fundamental mechanisms of cell proliferation and differentiation, even in the adult organism once morphological and functional maturity have occurred.

Mesenchymal-epithelial interactions during embryogenesis and their continuance throughout an organism's life span raise questions about possible involvement in carcinogenesis. Firstly, does any derangement of epithelial proliferation and differentiation represent a regressive state in which features of the embryonic/fetal phenotype are re-expressed by transformed cells? Secondly, if mesenchymal-epithelial interactions in the adult organism serve to keep in check any abnormal epithelial proliferation, then how are these interactions perturbed in cancer? Finally, should specific abnormalities in stromal-epithelial interactions be identified, therapy may be directed at rectifying these. For example, any deficiency of growth factors might be corrected, or expression of others either augmented or suppressed such that any imbalance of opposing influences on epithelial proliferation are amended and a steady state re-attained. Stromal-epithelial interactions are especially pertinent to hormone dependent tumors where endocrine effects may be mediated indirectly upon epithelium by its associated mesenchyme.

ii) Stromal-Epithelial Interactions During Development

Hormonally sensitive tissues in the developing genital tract have provided a model for investigating the role of mesenchymal elements during development. In the genital tract of developing male rodents, androgen receptors are initially expressed exclusively within mesenchymal tissue, at a time when neighboring epithelium is undergoing hormone dependent morphogenesis.[1] This suggests that any hormonal influence may be exerted indirectly via the mesenchyme (which alone possesses androgen receptors), this in turn acting in a paracrine manner upon neighboring epithelial cells. ER are likewise expressed in mesenchyme at a time when they are absent within neighboring epithelium. Neonatal mouse epithelium can respond to estrogen despite lacking ER which are present on contiguous mesenchymal cells.[3]

TGFβ and Cancer, edited by J.R. Benson. ©1998 R.G. Landes Company.

Therefore stromal-epithelial interactions are not merely modulating endocrine effects in some subtle way, but are a principle pathway for mediation of hormonal action in these developing systems.

Elegant recombination experiments have demonstrated that epithelial differentiation and hormonal responsiveness are determined by mesenchymal characteristics. Using androgen insensitive tissues from animals with the testicular feminization syndrome (Tfm), a combination of wild-type mesenchyme with either wild-type or Tfm epithelium leads to prostatic (i.e., male pattern) differentiation. Mesenchyme from Tfm tissue is unable to direct male pattern differentiation in either type of epithelium. These recombination experiments suggest that mesenchyme may act not just in a permissive manner to facilitate development of a 'determined' epithelium, but can also direct or instruct pluripotential epithelial cells to differentiate along a particular phenotypic pathway. In some circumstances, this instructive influence may be incomplete; when mammary epithelium is recombined with salivary gland mesenchyme, the resultant epithelium morphologically resembles that of a salivary gland, yet functionally secretes a milk protein characteristic of mammary differentiation.[4]

iii) Stromal-Epithelial Interactions in Adult Tissues

In adult tissues, epithelia and stroma constitute an integrated, functional unit which is often responsible for regular epithelial renewal. In those tissues where epithelial turnover is high, such as the gut and skin, these stromal-epithelial interactions are likely to be especially important. In effect, these tissues resemble systems in a continuous state of development. The above evidence suggests an inductive capacity of mesenchyme upon epithelium during development. If this inductive ability is maintained in the fully mature, differentiated counterparts of developing mesenchyme, then mesenchymal determinants may serve to keep in check abnormal epithelial proliferation. Derangement of stromal-epithelial interactions are more likely to affect tumor progression than initiation, and could initially lead to immortalization of epithelium as a prelude to complete malignant transformation.

Recombination experiments using renal subcapsular grafts further confirm that stromal elements can influence epithelial proliferation in adult tissues.[1] Tissue recombinants of wild-type urogenital mesenchyme (UGM) and a single adult prostatic duct result in marked epithelial proliferation which does not occur with UGM from the Tfm variant. When wild-type fetal urogenital mesenchyme is combined with either wild-type or Tfm adult bladder epithelium, mature prostatic tissue results. Moreover, castration of the host in which the recombinants are grown results in prostatic atrophy which may be restored by administration of testosterone. The Tfm bladder epithelium has no functional androgen receptors,[5] these being confined exclusively to the wild-type stromal cells. Thus androgens appear to mediate both morphogenesis and regeneration of prostatic tissue via a direct effect upon stromal cells and in turn an indirect action upon neighboring epithelial cells. This evidence for a role of stroma in mediating androgenic effects in mature prostatic tissue is partially indirect, for experiments with adult prostatic stroma are lacking. However, UGM in recombinants differentiates and matures into prostatic stroma and isolated prostatic epithelium in culture is unresponsive to androgens. Moreover, in contrast to recombinants, prostatic ducts implanted alone without mesenchyme fail to grow.[6]

Further evidence for involvement of stromal elements in epithelial behavior and hormonal responsiveness comes from reconstitution experiments with primary cultures of mammary epithelial cells and fibroblasts. In contrast to organ cultures, epithelial differentiation and functional responsiveness are usually absent in isolated epithelial cells in vitro. Haslam found the presence of fibroblasts to be necessary for a proliferative response of epithelial cells to estrogen and in the absence of which fibroblasts may be inhibitory to epithelial cell proliferation.[7] Fibroblasts not only permitted a proliferative response of mammary epithelial cells to estrogen, but also resulted in increased levels of progesterone receptors within these cells, together with distinct morphological changes. Of interest, conditioned media derived from fibroblasts could mimic this response, whilst irradiated, metabolically inactive cells were incapable of inducing a proliferative response. Many workers have confirmed that isolated normal mammary epithelium is not directly responsive to estrogens and this emphasizes the limitations of studies on individual isolated elements, and reinforces the importance of stromal elements not only for morphogenesis but also expression of differentiated function.[8] In support of this notion, adult mammary stroma can support fetal mammary epithelial development, and conversely fetal mammary mesenchyme can induce ductal morphogenesis in adult mammary tissue.[9]

iv) Stromal-Epithelial Interactions and Malignancy

If stromal-epithelial interactions are important in regulation of epithelial proliferation in mature tissues, then derangements thereof may be involved in carcinogenesis. The neoplastic process can be conceptually divided into two phases. Firstly, the initiation and early reversible promotional phase, and secondly, the later autonomous phase of tumor development. The first phase probably involves an epithelial initiating event acting in conjunction with a subtle change in stromal-epithelial interactions which together promote excessive epithelial proliferation and immortalization. One manifestation of deranged stromal-epithelial interactions may be a mesenchymal defect which could either be an inherited, systemic abnormality, or an acquired locally induced effect resulting from epigenetic phenomena secondary to primary events within epithelial cells. Skin fibroblasts display fetal-like characteristics in approximately 90% of breast cancer patients with a strong family history, and this phenotype is found in 50% of their relatives.[10,11] Moreover, approximately half of all cases of sporadic breast cancers have fibroblasts with similar features. This implies the existence of a systemic abnormality of fibroblasts and retention of a fetal-like phenotype has been suggested to predispose to cancer development by disturbance of stromal-epithelial interactions.[12] The mechanism by which this disturbance is manifest is unknown, but a primary deficiency in secretion of a paracrine inhibitory growth factor such as TGFβ by stromal cells is plausible.[13] Alternatively, deranged stomal-epithelial interactions could result from a mesenchymal abnormality which is locally induced in stromal cells by transformed epithelial cells. Growth of colonies of malignant epithelial cell lines is stimulated by conditioned media of fibroblasts derived from the same tumor tissue, but other fibroblast types have lesser effects.[14] This alludes to heterogeneity of fibroblasts between different tissues, suggesting local inductive effects of epithelium upon stromal cells via paracrine interactions. Furthermore, the precise nature of these may differ between normal and neoplastic tissues. In sporadic cases of breast cancer, a stromal defect is likely to be acquired secondarily. The occurrence of fetal-like fibroblasts in these patients is thought to result from clonal expansion of a population of fibroblasts induced by epigenetic phenomena.[15]

Experimental evidence from a number of different systems supports a role for stromal-epithelial interactions in carcinogenesis, but with some inconsistencies. These probably reflect the complexity of any such interactions, and perhaps the changing role of stroma as a tumor evolves. Following tumor initiation, fibroblasts may change from being inhibitory for epithelial cells to stimulatory, this being associated with general stromal expansion to provide support for emerging neoplastic cells. Moreover, the role of stromal factors differs between organ systems, and this is likely to be reflected in the varying significance to carcinogenesis of deranged stromal-epithelial interactions between different tissues. Horgan and co-workers demonstrated that MCF-7 tumor cell growth was enhanced in vivo in the presence of fibroblasts derived from benign and malignant breast tissue and skin,[16] and have recently confirmed that the conditioned media of fibroblasts derived from malignant or benign breast tissue together with skin is invariably stimulatory to growth of MCF-7 cells.[17] No particular fibroblast type excelled in stimulating tumor growth. Conditioned media of fibroblasts derived from benign and malignant breast tumors were found by Adams and co-workers to have a stimulatory effect upon growth of MCF-7 cells in vitro, whilst media from normal skin fibroblasts was inhibitory to these cells.[18] Similar results were obtained by Mukaida and colleagues who reported that conditioned media of primary fibroblasts from a variety of human malignancies was generally stimulatory to growth of epithelial cells derived from the same tumor type. Skin fibroblasts were inhibitory to colony growth, but interestingly breast tumor fibroblasts were invariably stimulatory.[14] Enami and co-workers also found that conditioned medium from mouse mammary fibroblasts stimulated cell proliferation in monolayer cultures of neoplastic and normal mouse mammary epithelial cells.[19] A differential response has been found between ER positive and negative cells to conditioned media from breast tumor fibroblasts by Van Roozendaal.[20] Thus conditioned media of fibroblasts derived from malignant tumors and skin were markedly stimulatory to ER positive cells (MCF-7 and ZR-75) whilst minimal effects were observed on ER negative cells (BT-20, MB MDA 231). Curiously, conditioned media of benign breast tissue fibroblasts (reduction mammoplasty or breast tissue adjacent to tumor) was only slightly stimulatory and this response was confined to ER positive cells. Therefore fibroblasts derived from malignant breast tumors appears to be generally stimulatory to ER positive cells or xenografts, whereas those derived from skin or benign breast tissue have a variable influence. This may in part reflect the problems of obtaining 'normal' breast fibroblasts as opposed to those from a benign tumor. Moreover, genetic abnormalities may exist in fibroblasts of some patients with breast cancer or a positive family history, thereby further complicating the issue of fibroblast normality.

The inhibitory effects of normal skin fibroblasts upon malignant epithelial cells observed by Adams is consistent with observations demonstrating that when carcinoma cells are combined with 'nontumorous' mesenchyme, they tend to acquire a more normal phenotype. De Cossa and co-workers showed that mammary carcinoma cells grown with mesenchyme exhibited a reduced proliferative rate and a more organized morphology.[21] Colon carcinoma cells undergo attempts at glandular formation when combined with fetal mesenchyme in organ culture.[22]

Further insight into the influence of mesenchyme on its associated epithelium comes from experiments in which basal-cell carcinomas were induced in rat skin and then transplanted heterotopically into the uterus. These tumors subsequently underwent a reconversion from malignant to a more benign appearing epithelium. This suggests that dermal mesenchyme may induce a state of immortalization in overlying epidermal cells and prevent terminal differentiation in these cells which can revert to benign behavior once free of this specific 'adverse' stromal influence.[23]

v) Mechanisms of Stromal-Epithelial Interaction in Carcinogenesis

The above evidence suggests that putative soluble factors are secreted by mesenchymal cells which can diffuse through the extra-cellular matrix (ECM) and act upon epithelial cells via a paracrine mechanism.[7,18,19] Stromal cells may also influence epithelial cells more directly via modification of composition and rate of deposition of ECM which it lays down,[24] or by direct cell-to-cell contact.

Epithelial differentiation can be induced and maintained on and within a variety of biomatrices derived from ECM components. Both normal and neoplastic mouse mammary epithelium grows at a higher rate and displays some morphogenesis when grown on and within collagen gels;[25-27] though attempts at tubule formation never approximate to normal morphology. The much greater rates of growth suggest that the gels may not simply be acting as a scaffolding, but are facilitating both 2- and 3-dimensional interaction of epithelial cells. Of interest, killed fibroblasts can increase incidence but not growth of tumors in vivo,[16] suggesting a passive substratum effect. Others have found that lethally irradiated fibroblasts can accelerate xenograft tumor growth when coimplanted with epithelial cells, suggesting that components of the ECM can promote epithelial proliferation once a tumor is initiated. However, the presence of metabolically active cells is essential for maximal rates of proliferation.[28]

None of the above studies involving conditioned media have identified any specific soluble factors. Not all of these studies were carried out in serum-free media, and therefore serum components could interact with those in conditioned media to produce the observed responses of epithelial cells. A mitogenic factor has been isolated from serum-free conditioned media with a molecular weight of 8000, which is similar to that of TGF alpha and insulin-like growth factor (IGF).[17] Implanted pellets of EGF can induce epithelial cell proliferation and formation of duct structures in the mammary gland of ovariectomized mice.[29]

Experiments with mammary epithelial cells in culture indicate that morphological and functional differentiation are greatly encouraged by growth of cells either in 3-dimensional systems or a 2-dimensional substrate composed of ECM components.[27,30] ECM may modulate epithelial morphology and function by a 3-dimensional effect in which cell shape is determined by multi-directional forces established within a 3-dimensional system.[31] In vivo, epithelial cells possess various types of cell surface receptors collectively termed integrins, which bind to components of the ECM.[32] The density of these receptors partly determines the nature of the interaction between ECM and epithelial cells. The ECM may indirectly affect epithelial cells by controlling the bioavailability and rate of transmission of paracrine growth factors secreted by fibroblasts and other cell types. For example, TGFβ binds to components of the ECM via the latent TGFβ binding protein (LTBP) and both fibroblast growth factor (FGF) and platelet-derived growth factor (PDGF) are specifically bound to ECM.[33] The glycoprotein tenascin is normally only present in embryonic tissue and doesn't occur normally in mature mammary tissue. However, it is found in adult stroma in pathological states, including malignancy, where carcinoma cells may stimulate the stroma to produce this substance.[34] Immunohistochemical studies reveal the presence of tenascin in malignant but not benign tissue sections.[35] In particular, the association of this substance with tumors of poor prognosis points to a role in cell invasion and metastases, whereby tenascin may promote cell detachment and migration. TGFβ secreted by MCF-7 cells can stimulate production of the ECM glycoprotein tenascin by fibroblasts, thus interfering with cell-cell adhesion and promoting tumor spread.[36] The versatility of stromal behavior and function may be largely attributable to modulators such as TGFβ. This may not only interact with other growth factors, but also secretory products such as stromelysin-3, a metalloproteinase secreted by stromal cells of invasive breast tumors which may be central to transition from in situ to invasive disease.[37] TGFβ can also stimulate hyaluronate production by fibroblasts, thereby modifying properties of the ECM and indirectly influencing cell-cell interactions.[38] The concept of 'dynamic reciprocity' invokes changes in gene expression as a direct result of the extracellular matrix interacting with transmembrane proteins which communicate with the nuclear matrix via a cell's cytoskeleton. This modified gene expression may involve alterations in the profile of secreted growth factors and hence lead indirectly to changes in paracrine interactions and hence intercellular communication.[39]

Direct cell-to-cell contact may be relatively less important in parenchymal organs where epithelium is often formally separated from stromal cells by a basal lamina, and the latter are usually outnumbered by epithelial cells, thus precluding extensive cell-to-cell contact. Confrontation experiments between mammary epithelial cells and fibroblasts grown in

2-dimensional monolayer systems permitting exchange of media, have shown direct contact between the two cell types to be essential for an epithelial response to estrogen.[40]

A mesenchymal defect involving a primary deficiency of TGFβ has been proposed as a possible mechanism for development of gastro-intestinal polyps and desmoid tumors in patients with Gardner's syndrome who possess both ectodermal and mesodermal tumors.[13] This hypothesis was formulated to account for certain disparate clinical observations, including the effects of adjuvant tamoxifen in early breast cancer and the association between GI polyps and desmoid tumors. Stromal-epithelial interactions and in particular the potential role of mesenchymal determinants are invoked as central elements of this hypothesis, which is elaborated upon in the following section.

Breast Cancer, Desmoid Tumors and Familial Polyposis Coli— A Unifying Hypothesis

The results of adjuvant trials[41-43] revealing that the efficacy of tamoxifen in early breast cancer was partially independent of estrogen receptor (ER) status were counter-intuitive as the anti-estrogen tamoxifen is precluded from acting as a competitive antagonist for the conventional ER. A negative paracrine hypothesis was proposed[44] and later corroborated by experimental[44,45] and clinical data,[46] in which tamoxifen directly stimulates fibroblasts to produce and secrete inhibitory growth factors for neighboring epithelial cells, be they ER positive or ER negative.

Desmoid tumors are benign proliferative lesions of fibroblasts and may occur in association with Familial adenomatous polyposis coli in the condition known as Gardner's syndrome, in which affected individuals develop both ectodermal and mesodermal tumors.[47] In contrast to desmoids, gastro-intestinal polyps are composed of a mixture of epithelial and mesenchymal elements. So could fibroblasts within the stroma of polyps share some abnormality with those of desmoids, this contributing both to desmoid formation and epithelial proliferation within polyps?

Mesenchymal elements such as fibroblasts and endothelial cells have important interactions in vivo with epithelial cells both in topographical and functional contexts. As discussed above, there is experimental data to substantiate a role for such interactions in morphogenesis and other developmental processes with ongoing stromal-epithelial interactions in the adult organism once morphological and functional maturity have been attained.

To suggest that a mesenchymal abnormality might underly development of polyps and desmoid tumors in patients with Gardner's syndrome implies some systemic abnormality of stromal tissue. Not only do fibroblasts from patients with a family history of breast cancer display fetal-like characteristics with abnormal migration patterns on collagen gels,[48] but skin fibroblasts from patients with FAP show abnormal growth characteristics in vitro with a reduced requirement for serum and a morphology similar to embryonal fibroblasts with overgrowth and loss of contact inhibition.[49]

These observations allude to a possible systemic abnormality of fibroblasts in cancer patients and it was proposed that an intrinsic systemic abnormality of fibroblasts in FAP patients predisposes to both desmoid tumors and GI polyps with local factors initiating tumor formation. Based on evidence for stromal induction of TGFβ both in vitro and in vivo by anti-estrogens, it was proposed that this intrinsic mesenchymal defect might be a primary deficiency of TGFβ. This would produce a local imbalance of growth factors within tissues which in conjunction with putative fetal-like characteristics would lead to: (a) the promotion of fibroblast activity encouraging desmoid formation. The clinical response of desmoid tumors to anti-estrogens is presumed to be secondary to induction of TGFβ to which these tumors display an inhibitory, though aberrant response. (b) disturbance of stromal-epithelial interactions with reduction of negative stromal paracrine influences resulting in excessive epithelial proliferative activity of gastro-intestinal mucosa.

This intrinsic mesenchymal defect could be a phenotypic manifestation of a genetic abnormality at the 5q21 locus. Lesions at this locus have been demonstrated in polyps of FAP patients and desmoid tissue of patients with Gardner's syndrome.[50,51] Any inherited germline mutation would be present in all cells including fibroblasts. In accordance with Knudson's theory,[52] heterozygosity at this locus in epithelial cells predisposes to polyps with a further somatic mutation in the homologous allele resulting in malignant change. This heterozygosity at the 5q locus might confer an abnormal phenotype characterized in fibroblasts by defective secretion of TGFβ. Such a fault would predispose to both polyps and desmoids. A further somatic mutation of the homologous allele on the cognate chromosome of colonic epithelial cells would trigger actual malignant transformation with development of colorectal carcinoma. The elements of this hypothesis are assimilated schematically in Figure 4.1.

Though abnormalities at the 5q locus are not implicated in breast cancer, certain familial forms could be associated with derangement of stromal-epithelial interactions based on a local imbalance of growth factors. TGFβ is a preeminent growth inhibitory signal, upon which several different pathways may ultimately converge. Defective function could result from abnormalities at more than one locus which involve synthesis, secretion or activation of TGFβ. Of interest, there is an association between breast cancer and nonfamilial GI polyps;[53] this is most likely a consequence of environmental factors, but could involve a common mechanistic, if not inherited defect, based on deranged stromal-epithelial interactions. Fibroblasts from a subset of breast cancer patients with a strong family history may have significantly lower levels of TGFβ1 secretion which could be implicated in defective paracrine mechanisms leading to excessive proliferation of breast epithelium.

This intrinsic, inherited mesenchymal defect which would be present in all fibroblasts and is manifest as a primary deficiency of TGFβ production/secretion represents a breakdown of a systemic growth restraint. TGFβ is a central component of one of the principal negative signaling pathways between cells.[54] The formation of GI polyps, desmoid tumors and perhaps some forms of familial breast cancer may be viewed as local manifestations of this systemic disorder. According to the above hypothesis, an epithelial tumor would be initiated by local factors, but a stromal defect would promote epithelial proliferation and immortalization. Though the proposed mesenchymal defect is considered neither to initiate GI polyps nor indeed malignant transformation, it nonetheless has a crucial role in the early promotional phases of neoplasia where subtle changes in the balance of growth factors in the local tissue milieu can influence rogue proliferative activity. The differential expression of IGF-I and II mRNA by fibroblasts derived from breast tumor tissue, with benign tumor fibroblasts over-expressing IGF-I, and those from malignant tumors over-expressing IGF-II mRNA (see insulin-like growth factors in chapter 1) may reflect a preexisting, intrinsic difference between such fibroblasts. Therefore specific stromal characteristics may precede and predispose to malignant transformation. Similarly, benign and malignant breast tumor fibroblasts have been shown to display differential rates of secretion of the TGFβ2 isoform.[45] Though there is no statistically significant difference in levels of TGFβ1 secretion between malignant and benign breast tumor fibroblasts, absolute levels of TGFβ2 secretion are significantly higher for benign breast tumor fibroblasts compared to fibroblasts from malignant tumors. Furthermore, levels of secretion of secretion of TGFβ1 appear to be generally higher for breast tumor fibroblasts than normal skin fibroblasts.[45] These data suggest that differential quantitative expression of TGFβ isoforms may be important during neoplastic development, with alterations in the expression profile of TGFβ as a tumor evolves. Immunohistochemical studies reveal no difference in the qualitative expression of TGFβ1,

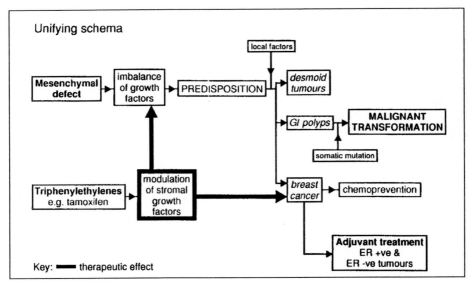

Fig. 4.1. Schema for Unifying Hypothesis. Predisposition to desmoid tumors, gastrointestinal polyps and breast cancer is determined by a basic mesenchymal defect manifest as a deficiency of the negative growth modulator, TGFβ. This results in an imbalance of growth factors which could be corrected by modulation of stromal synthetic capacity by agents such as tamoxifen which have been shown to enhance expression of TGFβ both in vivo and in vitro. Any pre-existing imbalance of growth factors could also be compensated for by pharmacological intervention, thus suggesting a role for such a strategy in both treatment and prevention of early breast cancer and possibly GI polyp formation. Reprinted with permission from: Benson JR, Baum M. Lancet 1993; 342:848-850 © The Lancet Limited.

TGFβ2 or TGFβ3 between malignant and nonmalignant human breast tumor tissue.[55] However, once again, such studies do not reveal the dynamic aspects of protein expression within tissues. The relatively higher levels of secretion by breast tumor fibroblasts compared with 'normal' skin fibroblasts is consistent with immunohistochemical studies indicating a slightly higher overall expression of TGFβ1 in tumor tissue.[56] This may represent a homeostatic response of stromal cells to enhanced epithelial proliferation, be this in a benign tumor or an early stage breast cancer. Conditioned media from benign and malignant breast tumor fibroblasts is stimulatory to MCF-7 cells in vitro,[17] whilst media from normal skin fibroblasts is inhibitory to these cells.[14,18] Furthermore, stromal cells from malignant breast tissue express high levels of smooth muscle actin, unlike fibroblasts from normal breast tissue.[57] These findings suggest that fibroblasts from both benign and malignant tumors may display phenotypic features which are not shared by other somatic fibroblasts, and which may be acquired during neoplastic development. Aberrant stromal phenotypes in breast tumors may lead to deranged stromal-epithelial interactions and promote neoplastic progression. Moreover, the acquired expression of this aberrant phenotype may permit pharmacological induction of TGFβ within these fibroblasts. Whether this be a fortuitous and incidental manifestation of an abnormal stromal phenotype, it can potentially be exploited therapeutically (Fig. 4.2.). This aspect of a putative stromal phenotype will be further discussed in chapter 7. Should such a phenotype appear in premalignant and/or benign breast lesions, this could have important implications for chemoprevention where subtle changes

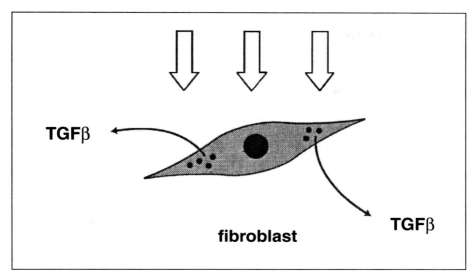

Fig. 4.2. Fibroblasts within the peritumoral stroma constitute a potential target for pharmacological induction of TGFβ by anti-estrogens and other agents. The therapeutic implications of such a phenomenon are discussed in chapter 7.

in the balance of growth factors determine behavior of cells. A crucial question is at what stage in the development of a neoplastic lesion is this phenotype acquired? Moreover, what are the other features of this phenotype which relate to neoplastic development per se?

References
1. Cunha GR, Donjacour A. Stromal-epithelial interactions in normal and abnormal prostatic development. Prog Clin Biol Res 1987; 239:251-272.
2. Cunha GR, Bigsby RM, Cooke PS, Sugimura Y. Stromal-epithelial interactions in adult organs. Cell Differentiation 1985; 17:137-148.
3. Bigsby RM, Cunha GR. Estrogen stimulation of DNA synthesis in uterine epithelial cells which lack oestrogen receptors. Endocrinology 1986; 119:390-396.
4. Sakakura T, Nishizuka Y. Mesenchymal dependent morphogenesis and epithelium specific cyto-differentiation in mouse mammary gland. Science 1976; 194:1439-1441.
5. Shannon JM, Cunha GR. Characterisation of androgen binding sites and DNA synthesis in prostate like structures induced in testicular feminised mice. Biol Reprod 1984; 31:175-183.
6. Norman JT, Cunha GR, Sugimura Y. The induction of new ductal growth in adult prostatic epithelium in response to an embryonic prostatic inductor. Prostate 1986; 8:209-220.
7. Haslam SZ. Mammary fibroblast influence on normal mouse mammary epithelial cell responses to oestrogen in vitro. Cancer Res 1986; 46:310-316.
8. Nandi S, Imagawa W, Tomooka Y et al. Collagen gel culture system and analysis of estrogen effects on mammary carcinogenesis Arch Toxicol 1984; 55:91-96.
9. Sakakura T, Sakagami I, Nishizuka Y. Persistence of responsiveness of adult mouse mammary gland to induction by embryonic mesenchyme. Dev Biol 1979; 72:201-210.
10. Schor SL, Haggie JA, Durning P et al. Occurrence of a fetal fibroblast phenotype in familial breast cancer. Int J Cancer 1986; 37:831-836.
11. Haggie JA, Sellwood RA, Howel A et al. Fibroblasts from relatives of patients with hereditary breast cancer show fetal-like behaviour in vitro. Lancet 1987; (i):1455-1457.

12. Schor SL, Schor AM, Howell A, Crowther D. Hypothesis: Persistent expression of fetal phenotypic characteristics by fibroblasts is associated with an increased susceptibility to neoplastic disease. Exp Cell Biol 1987 (b); 55:11-17.
13. Benson JR, Baum M. Breast cancer, desmoid tumors and familial adenomatous polyposis-a unifying hypothesis. Lancet 1993; 342:848-850 and 1560.
14. Mukaida H, Hirabayashi N, Hirai T et al. Significance of freshly cultured fibroblasts from different tissues in promoting cancer cell growth. Int J Cancer 1991; 48:423-427.
15. Schor SL, Schor AM. Clonal heterogeneity in fibroblast phenotype: Implications for the control of epithelial-stromal interactions. BioEssays 1987 (a); 7:200-204.
16. Horgan K, Jones DL, Mansel RE. Mitogenicity of human fibroblasts in vivo for human breast cancer cells Br J Cancer 1987; 74:227-229.
17. Ryan MC, Orr DJA, Horgan K. Fibroblast stimulation of breast cancer cell growth in a serum-free system. Br J Cancer 1994; 67:1268-1273.
18. Adams EF, Newton CJ, Braunsberg H et al. Effects of human breast fibroblasts on growth and 17β estradiol dehydrogenase activity of MCF-7 cells in culture. Breast Cancer Res Treat 1988; 11:165-172.
19. Enami J, Enami S, Koga M. Growth of normal and neoplastic mouse mammary epithelial cells in primary culture: Stimulation by conditioned medium from mouse mammary fibroblasts. Gann 1983; 74:845-853.
20. von Roozendaal CEP, van Ooijen B, Klijn JGM et al. Stromal influences on breast cancer cell growth. Br J Cancer 1992; 65:77-81.
21. De Cosse JJ, Gossens CL, Kuzma JF et al Breast cancer: Induction of differentiation by embryonic tissue. Science 1973; 181:1057 -1058.
22. Fukamachi I, Mizuno T, Kim YS. Gland formation of human colon cancer cells combined with fetal rat mesenchyme in organ culture: An ultra-structural study. J Cell Sci 1987; 87:615-621.
23. Cooper M, Pinkus H. Intrauterine transplantation of rat basal cell carcinoma: A model for reconversion of malignant to benign growth. Cancer Res 1977; 37:2544-2552.
24. Bissell MJ, Glenn Hall H, Parry G. How does the extracellular matrix direct gene expression? J Theor Biol 1982; 99:31-38.
25. Emerman JT, Pitelka DR. Maintenance and induction of morphological differentiation in dissociated mammary epithelium on floating collagen membranes. In Vitro 1977; 13:316-328.
26. Foster CS, Smith CA, Dinsdale EA et al. Human mammary gland morphogenesis in vitro : The growth and differentiation of normal breast epithelium in collagen gel cultures defined by electron microscopy, monoclonal Ab and autoradiography. Develop Biol 1983; 96:197-216.
27. Yang J, Richards J, Bowman P et al. Sustained growth and three dimensional organisation of primary mammary tumor epithelial cells embedded in collagen gels. PNAS (USA) 1979; 76:No.7 3401-3405.
28. Camps JL, Chang S-M, Hsu TC et al. Fibroblast-mediated acceleration of human epithelial tumour growth in vivo. Proc Natl Aca Sci (USA) 1990; 87:75-79.
29. Coleman S, Silberstein GB, Daniel CW. Ductal morphogenesis in the mouse mammary gland: Evidence supporting a role for epidermal growth factor Develop Biol 1988; 127:304-315.
30. Lee EY-H, Parry G, Bissel MJ. Modulation of secreted proteins of mouse mammary epithelial cells by the extracellular matrix. J Cell Biol 1991; 98:146-155.
31. Streuli CH, Bissell MJ. Mammary epithelial cells, extracellular matrix and gene expression. In: Lippman ME, Dickson RB, eds. Breast Cancer-Cellular and Molecular Biology. Boston: Kluwer Academic Publishers, 1991:365-381.
32. Hynes RO. Integrins: A family of cell surface receptors. Cell 1987; 48:549-554.
33. Gospodarowicz D. Molecular and developmental biology aspects of fibroblast growth factor. Adv Exp Med Biol 1988; 234:23-39.

34. Inaguma Y, Kusakabe M, Mackie EJ et al. Epithelial induction of stromal tenascin in the mouse mammary gland: From embryogenesis to carcinogenesis. Develop Biol 1988; 128:245-255.

35. Mackie EJ, Chiquet-Ehrismann R, Pearson CA et al. Tenascin is a stromal marker for epithelial malignancy in the mammary gland. Proc Natl Aca Sci (USA) 1987; 84:4621-4625.

36. Chiquet-Ehrismann R, Kalla P, Pearson CA. Participation of Tenascin and transforming growth factor beta in reciprocal epithelial-mesenchymal interactions of MCF-7 cells and fibroblasts. Cancer Res 1989; 49:4322-4325.

37. Basset P, Bellocq JP, Wolf C et al. A novel metallo-proteinase gene specifically expressed in stromal cells of breast carcinoma. Nature 1990; 348:699-704.

38. Heldin C-H, Westermark B, Wasteson A. Chemical and biological properties of a growth factor from human-cultured osteosarcoma cells: Resemblance with platelet-derived growth factor. J Cell Physiol 1980; 105:235-246.

39. Bissel MJ. Extracellular matrix influence on gene expression: Is structure the message? B J Cancer 1988; 58:223 (abstract).

40. McGrath CM. Augmentation of response of normal mammary epithelial cells to estradiol by mammary stroma. Cancer Res 1983; 43:1355-1357.

41. Early Breast Cancer Trialists Collaborative Group. Systemic treatment of early breast cancer by hormonal, cytotoxic or immune therapy. 133 randomised trials involving 31,000 recurrences and 24,000 deaths among 75,000 women. Lancet 1992; 339:1-15 and 71-75.

42. Nolvadex Adjuvant Trial Organisation. Controlled trial of tamoxifen as a single adjuvant agent in the management of early breast cancer. Br J Cancer 1988; 57:608-611.

43. Medical Research Council Scottish Trials Office. Adjuvant tamoxifen in the management of operable breast cancer. Lancet 1987; 11:171-175.

44. Colletta AA, Wakefield LM, Howell FV et al. Anti-estrogens induce the secretion of active transforming growth factor beta from human fetal fibroblasts. Br J Cancer 1990; 62:405-409.

45. Benson JR, Wakefield LM, Colletta AA et al. Synthesis and secretion of TGFβ isoforms by primary cultures of human breast tumour fibroblasts in vitro and their modulation by tamoxifen. Br J Cancer 1996; 74:352-358.

46. Butta A, Maclennan K, Flanders KC et al. Induction of transforming growth factor beta 1 in human breast cancer in vivo following tamoxifen treatment. Cancer Res 1992; 52:4261-4264.

47. MacAdam WAF, Goligher JC. The occurrence of desmoids in patients with familial polyposis coli. Br J Surg 1970; 57:618-631.

48. Grey AM, Shor AM, Rushton G et al. Purification of the migration stimulatory factor produced by foetal and breast cancer patient fibroblasts. PNAS 1989; 86:2438-2442.

49. Pfeffer L, Lipkin M, Stutman O et al. Growth characteristics of cultured human skin fibroblasts derived from individuals with hereditary adenomatosis of the colon and rectum. J Cell Physiol. 1976; 89:29-37.

50. Okamoto M, Sato Ch, Kohno Y et al. Molecular nature of chromosome 5q loss in colorectal tumours and desmoids from patients with familial adenomatous polposis. Hum Genet 1990; 85:595-599.

51. Nishisho I, Nakamura Y, Miyoshi Y et al. Mutations of chromosome 5q21 genes in FAP and colorectal cancer patients. Science 1991; 253:665-669.

52. Knudson A.G. Jr Genetics of human cancer. Ann Rev Genetics 1986; 20:231-251.

53. Jouin H, Baumann R, Derlon A, et al. Is there an increased incidence of adenomatous polyps in breast cancer patients? Cancer 1989; 63:599-603.

54. Benson JR, Wells K. Microsatellite instability and a TGFβ receptor-clues to a growth control pathway. BioEssays 1995; 17 (12):1009-1012.

55. McCune BK, Mullin BR, Flanders KC et al. Localisation of transforming growth factor β isotypes in lesions of the human breast. Human Pathol 1991; 23:13-20.

56. Wakefield LM, Colletta AA, McCune BK, Sporn MB. Roles for transforming growth factors β in the genesis, prevention and treatment of breast cancer. In: Dickson RB, Lippman ME, eds. Genes, Oncogenes and Hormones: Advances in Cellular and Molecular Biology Breast Cancer. Boston: Kluwer Academic Publishers, 1991:97-136.
57. Sappino A-P, Skalli O, Jackson B et al. Smooth muscle differentiation in stromal cells of malignant and nonmalignant breast tissues. Int J Cancer 1988; 41:707-712.

CHAPTER 5

TGFβ in the Developing Organism

J. MacCallum

i) Introduction

As is discussed in previous chapters, transforming growth factor (TGFβ) belongs to a large family of distinct and diverse proteins sharing a similar structure based on the seven conserved cysteine residues of the monomeric unit[1] (Fig. 5.1). As such there is conservation of the peptides between species,[2] and members of the family are known to be involved in various important developmental processes such as pattern formation in both fly[3] and toad[4,5] (Table 5.1). In this chapter, the presence and distribution of TGFβ in developing organisms will be discussed. This will include evidence for the importance of TGFβ in embryogenesis, and specifically with development of the mammary gland. Roles for TGFβ in relation to the events occurring throughout embryogenesis and development will be discussed.

TGFβ isoforms are expressed by many normal cell types.[1,6] Most transformed and nontransformed fibroblasts and epithelial cells in culture express the three mammalian TGFβ mRNAs and secrete the corresponding protein in latent form into conditioned medium.[7,8] They characteristically oppose or antagonize the action of other mitogenic growth factors and act to inhibit cell growth.[1] For example, proliferation of normal mammary epithelial cells is generally suppressed and production of differentiated proteins modified,[9] whilst stromal cells are stimulated to proliferate and lay down extracellular matrix (ECM).[10]

Production of TGFβ by both epithelial and stromal cells can influence growth directly or indirectly,[11,12] during development.[13] Being contextual, responses to TGFβ are complicated. Functional consequences depend on numerous cell and tissue-specific parameters and include: target cell type; state of cellular differentiation and activation, receptor expression;[14] presence of binding proteins; ECM composition;[15] presence and concentration of other cytokines growth factors and antagonists in the pericellular environment;[16] and the state of latency and isoform expression profile.[17]

ii) Evidence for a Role in Embryogenesis

Members of the TGFβ superfamily are known to regulate a variety of developmental and homeostatic processes such as hematopoiesis, angiogenesis, immune function, inflammation, myogenesis, osteogenesis, tissue repair, remodeling and steroidogenesis[1,6,18,19] (Fig. 5.2). Evidence suggests that TGFβ isoforms play an important role in the regulation of mammary development and function,[20] and affect vital functions in many cell types.[1,21] Therefore it is not inconceivable that TGFβs may have a wider role during developmental processes in general. Suggestive evidence for this is detailed below.

TGFβ and Cancer, edited by J.R. Benson. ©1998 R.G. Landes Company.

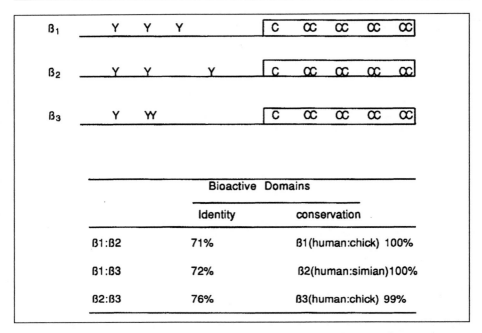

Fig. 5.1. Precursor structure and homology of TGFβs. Reprinted with permission from: Massague J, Cheifetz S, Laiho M et al. Transforming growth factor-β. 1992; 12:81-103. © Cancer Surveys published for the Imperial Cancer Research Fund by Cold Springs Harbor Laboratory Press.

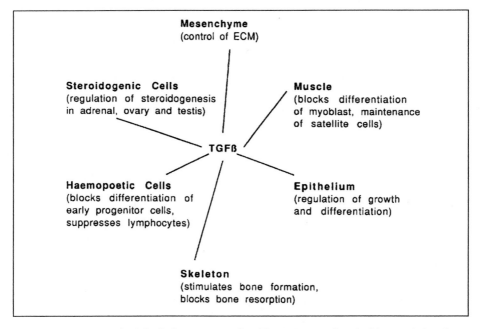

Fig. 5.2. Some major physiological systems regulated by TGFβ. Reprinted with permission from: Roberts AB, Flanders KC, Heine UI et al. Transforming growth factor-β: multifunctional regulator of differentiation and development. Phil Trans 1990; 327:145-154. © Royal Society London.

Table 5.1. Properties of the members of the TGFβ gene family

Peptide	Precursor number of amino acids	Processed number of amino acids (cys)	M.W.	mRNA (Kb)	Homology[a] (%)	Function	Reference
TGFβ1	390	112(9)	25,000	2.4	100	Multifunctional regulators of growth, differentiation and function	Derynck et al, 1985; de Martin et al, 1987
TGFβ2	414	112(9)	25,000	4.1, 6.5	71		
Inhibins [b]	364( )	134(7)	32,000	1.5	28	Inhibition of secretion of FSH by pituitary cells	Mason et al,1985
	424(βA)	116(9)		4.5, 7.2	38		
	423(βB)	115(9)		4.5	33		
Activins [c]			28,000			simulation of secretion of FSH by pituitary gland	Ling et al,1986; Vale et al,1986; Cate et al,1986
MIS	560	(7)	140,000	2.0	32	Induces regulation of mullerian ducts in male embryos	
DPP-C	588	100(7)	?	4.5	36	Establishment of dorsal-ventral specification in Drosophila embryos	Padgett et al,1987
Vgl	360	114(7)	?	4.5	38	Function as an inducer of mesoderm during frog development	Wechs and Melton, 1987

a based on homology of porcine inhibin and activin subunits, human MIS and drosophila DPP-C to human TGFβ1.

b Inhibins are heterodimers—alpha crosslinks to either βA or βB subunit.

c Activins are heterodimers or homodimeric combinations of βA or βB subunits of inhibin.

Reprinted with permission from: Roberts AB, Flanders KC, Kondaiah P et al. Transforming growth factor beta: Biochemistry and role in embryogenesis, tissue repair and remodelling, and carcinogenesis. Recent Prog Horm Res 1988; 44:157–197. © Academic Press, Inc.

TGFβs can influence the expression of many genes,[22] and by acting as a cellular switch, they can dictate patterns of gene expression, depending on the environment and state of differentiation of any target cell.[23] Thus they have the ability to modulate cell proliferation[24-27] differentiation[28-33] and physiology.[10] They can also elicit phenotypic transformation under certain conditions, such as mesenchymal-like transformation of epithelial cells,[34] and the development of myofibroblast characteristics in chronically exposed stromal cells.[35]

In addition, TGFβs they have specific effects on matrix formation[36] encouraging mesenchymal deposition of ECM in vitro by increasing biosynthesis of ECM proteins,[10,28] decreasing rates of degradation[37,38] and augmenting cellular receptors for proteins such as fibronectin.[28] These effects collectivey serve to alter the architecture of the extracellular matrix (Fig. 5.3, Table 5.2). TGFβs specifically modulate the capacity of cells to adhere to the ECM, ultimately leading to a change in the pattern of target cell gene transcription. Thus the composition and organization of ECM is an important determinant of cellular behavior.

TGFβs have a chemotactic role within tissues of mesenchymal origin.[24,27,39] Immunocompetent function is also under TGFβ control through potent immunosuppression of T and B cell populations.[40] Furthermore, as a chemotactic factor for macrophages, TGFβs might also mediate granulation responses in macrophages and other phagocytic cells.[41]

The remarkable conservation of TGFβs, and their ability to modulate cellular differentiation and function, their effects on ECM and chemotaxis,[39,41] angiogenesis[10,42] and immune function suggest a fundamental role in development, with these various factors contributing an important role in the remodeling of embryonic and adult tissues.

Extensive studies have been carried out to determine the expression and distribution of TGFβ isoforms at the level of both mRNA and protein within various mammalian tissues. Although it is difficult to unequivocally confirm that TGFβ is causally related to these events, its expression early in embryogenesis in a tissue specific and developmentally-dependent manner strongly suggests that TGFβ has a pivotal role in morphogenic and histogenic events.[23] This is discussed in the next section with emphasis on the role of TGFβ in mammary development.

iii) Expression of TGFβ Isoforms in Embryonic and Developing Tissues

Investigation of the expression of TGFβs during murine, bovine and chick embryogenesis, in addition to studies of human development, have shown that TGFβ expression occurs at the earliest stages of development, appearing initially after fertilization,[43-46] with levels remaining high during development[47-50] and throughout neonatal and adult life.[51] Since all three TGFβ isoforms are produced and expressed in the pre and post implantation mouse uterus, they are thought to influence embryogenesis and embryo-uterine interactions, and may regulate preimplantation differentiation events, including morula to blastocyst transformation and blastocyst maturation.[45,52]

TGFβ production at the fetal-maternal interface has a significant regulatory role in the proliferation and differentiation of the trophoblast,[53] together with control of trophoblast invasion in situ.[54] In the *Xenopus* blastula, cells in the animal hemisphere are induced to form mesoderm by proteins homologousto TGFb in conjuction with FGF from the vegetal hemisphere,[55] and there is prominent in situ expression in the haemopoetic cells of early mouse embryos.[56] In the following sections, expression of the three mammalian TGFβ isoforms is discussed. It should be emphasized that the majority of investigations have examined TGFβ1 expression as the predominant isoform. Expression at levels of messenger RNA and protein is discussed.

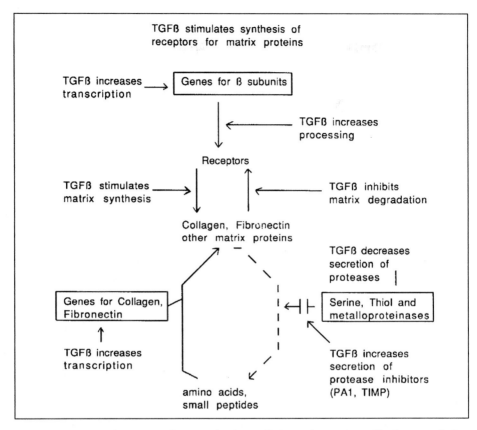

Fig. 5.3. Properties of TGFβ members. Mechanisms of TGFβ enhancement of both accumulation of ECM proteins and their interactions with cells, including enhancement of synthesis of matrix proteins inhibition of the degradation of matrix proteins and enhanced synthesis of receptors for matrix proteins. Reprinted with permission from: Roberts AB, Flanders KC, Kondaiah P et al. Transforming growth factor beta: Biochemistry and role in embryogenesis, tissue repair and remodelling, and carcinogenesis. Recent Prog Horm Res 1988; 44:157-197. © Academic Press, Inc.

In contrast to mammalian systems, in the developing chick embryo no TGFβ1, or homologus thereof are found although a TGFβ4 isoform is detectable. Expression of TGFβ2 and β3 mRNA is detected 1.5 days after incubation and increases with developmental age.[57] Although expressed in all embryonic tissue, particularly high levels are found in brain and muscle, compared with much lower levels in kidney and liver. TGFβ2 is down-regulated during development in the heart and a role in epithelial-mesenchymal cell transformation to yield valve progenitor cells in early chicken heart[58] has been suggested.

TGFβ expression in the developing mouse has been extensively studied (Table 5.3). Each isoform shows a different mRNA expression pattern in mice 9.5-16.5 days post coitum. In the murine lung, where all three isoforms are found from birth to adulthood, levels vary throughout the first 2 weeks post partum only.[59] TGFβ1 mRNA predominates in the mesenchymal component of lung[60] 14.5 days post coitum with no protein product

Table 5.2. Effects on extracellular matiex

Increased synthesis of ECM components
Collagen
Fibronectin
Proteoglycan
Tenascin
Decreased synthesis of proteinases
Collagenase
Transin
Cathepsin L
Increased synthesis of protinase inhibitor
Plasminogen Activator Inhibitor
Tissue Specific Metalloproteinase Inhibitor
Urokinase
Increased synthesis of adhesion receptors
Vitronectin Receptor
LFA-1
Fibronectin Receptor
Other integrins

Reprinted with permission from: Barnard JA, Lyons RM, Moses HL. The cell biology of transforming growth factor β. Biochem Biophys Acta 1990; 1032:79-87. © Elsevier Science-NL.

being detectable,[47] and at 16.5 days, TGFβ2 mRNA expression is high within, conducting airways and large blood vessels of the lung (63-748). TGFβ1 mRNA is also found in the submucosa of the developing intestine, in cushion tissue of developing heart valves, and in fetal bone and liver megakaryocytes.[61,62]

Heine et al[47] found the distribution of TGFβ protein in 11-18 day mouse embryos to be associated with mesenchyme or mesenchyme-derived tissues (Table 5.3) (e.g., connective tissue, cartilage, bone). Strong TGFβ1 staining was observed in tissues derived from neural crest mesenchyme such as palate, larynx, facial mesenchyme, nasal sinuses, meninges and teeth. Staining was most intense during morphogenesis, with high levels of TGFβ1 expression in mesenchyme within the vicinity of critical sites of interactions with adjacent epithelium (e.g., hair follicles, teeth and submandibular gland). High levels have also been detected where there is remodeling of the mesenchyme or mesoderm, such as formation of digits from limb buds or formation of palate and heart valves,[60,63] and often correlate angiogenic activity.[47] Intense staining is seen in the myocardium of the developing and mature heart,[51] where TGFβ is thought to mediate cardioprotection[64] (Fig. 5.4). TGFβ is identified in embryonic murine CNS, and may regulate proliferation and differentiation of meningeal and neuroepithelial cells during development.[66] There is also localization in the developing skeletal system, TGFβ being implicated in various effects on osteoclasts and Schwann cells.[47,60-62] Exogenous TGFβ injected subperiosteally into the femur of a newborn rat can induce formation of localized masses of new bone.[65]

Thus a major role for TGFβ in developmental processes involving tissues of different lineage and diverse mechanisms of action is postulated.[60] In general, TGFβ expression has a unique pattern of distribution both spatially and temporally, this correlating with morphogenetic and histogenetic events, involving mesoderm or mesenchymal elements. It would therefore appear fundamental to much of the basic architecture and organization of the developing embryo.[36]

Table 5.3. Differential localization of RNA's encoding TGFβ₁, β₂ and β₃ during murine embryogenesis

	TGFβ$_1$	TGFβ$_2$	TGFβ$_3$
Hemopoetic Tissue	+		–
Endothelia	+	–	–
Thyroid	+	–	–
Parathyroid	+	–	–
Thymus	+	–	–
Epithelia			
whisker follicles	+	+	+
salivary glands	+	+	–
tooth bud	+	+	–
secondary palate	+	–	+
bronchial epithelia	–	+(s)	+(c)
optic epithelia	–	+	–
olifactory epithelia	–	+	–
lens epithelia	–	+	–
retina	–	+	–
hyperplastic nodularity	–	+	–
suprabasal keratinocytes	–	+	–
Cartilage and bone			
precartilaginous blastema	–	+(limb)	+(iv)
growth zone of long bone	–	+	–
perichondria	–	–	+
hypertrophic cartilage	–	–	–
osteoblasts, osteoclasts	+	–	–
Cardiac tissue			
prevalvular endothelia	+	–	–
prevalvular myocardium	–	+	–
Neuronal tissue			
ventral spinal cord	–	+	–
ventral forebrain	–	+	–
Muscle	–	(+)	(+)
Mesothelia	–	–	+
Mesenchyme	–	+	+

s squamos
c cuboidal
iv intervertebral disc analgen

In some murine tissues TGFβ1, β2 and β3 are expressed in the same cell types (e.g., pericardium and bone) whilst in others distinct distribution patterns are seen (e.g., lung, tooth bud, liver, whisker follicle[70] and secondary palate). Such distinctive expression patterns in micehave been documented in many studies, and are also observed during human embryogenesis.[71] Immunohistochemical localization of TGFβ protein in the large proximal conducting airways of murine lungs[59] show coincident patterns with mRNA expression, although individual isoforms show differing temporal and spatial localization.[67-69,72] In fact, TGFβ1 mRNA expression is often abundant within epithelial cells when staining for the

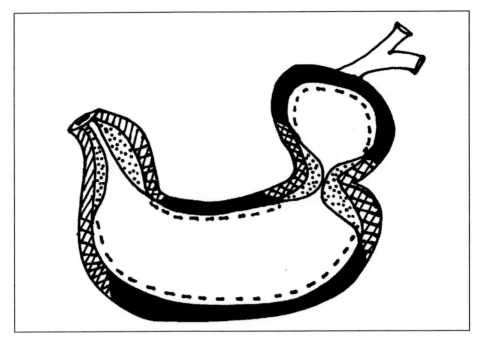

Fig. 5.4. Expression of TGFβ isoforms in early murine cardiogenesis. The diagram summarizes the localization of TGFβ$_1$ and β$_2$ RNA and protein distribution at around 8.5-9 days gestation: Note that, at this stage and earlier, the surrounding mesenchyme also expresses high levels of TGFβ$_2$ RNA, but not protein. ▬▬▬ TGFβ$_1$ RNA, ▦ TGFβ$_1$ protein, ▨ TGFb2 protein and RNA, ■ TGFβ$_2$ protein, ▨ TGFβ$_2$ RNA. Ackhurst RJ, Fitzpatrick DR, Fowlis DJ et al. The role of TGF-βs in mammalian development and neoplasia. Mol Repr Dev 1992; 32:127-135. © Wiley-Liss, Inc.

protein is localized to the underlying mesenchyme.[47,60,73] If TGFβ1 is synthesized within the epithelia overlying mesenchymal tissues known to contain the corresponding protein, then involvement of autocrine and paracine mechanisms of action can be postulated.[23,47,60,74] TGFβ2 has amore widespread distribution, being associated with epithelium underlying areas of growth and differentiation.[75]

Differentiating components tend to be a rich source of both the β1 and β2 isoforms,[49,76] with involvement in neovascularization and late paracrine interactions between endothelial and mesenchymal cells in developing embryos. TGFβ1 also has a role in establishment of the primitive vascular system and later on in the morphogenesis of cardiac valves and septae. In contrast, TGFβ2 could be thought of as an endogenous regulator of growth and differentiation of cardiomyocytes exerting influence on the formation of cushion tissue within the heart. Therefore, TGFβ1 and possibly β3 may be associated with morphogenesis, whilst TGFβ2 may regulate growth and/or differentiation of the epithelium per se.

iv) Role in Mammary Development

With the onset of ovarian function, between three and four weeks after birth, the terminal end buds of the developing murine mammary gland drive growth and dichotomous branching of mammary epithelium, filling the adipose-rich stroma with a tree-like network.[77] The mammary gland retains embryonic potential well into postnatal life, such that static ducts can reinitiate ductal growth and morphogenesis when implanted into paren-chyma-free mammary fat pads. Epithelial-mesenchymal interactions,[78] hormones[79] and lo-cal regulation by growth factors[80] are all involved in this response.

Patterns of ductal growth in the mammalian mammary gland may be regulated at least in part by TGFβ, with operation of autocrine feedback and paracrine circuits associated with epithelial-stromal interactions.[13] Ductal patterning is a function of hormonal status, and generation of form and pattern is determined by locally acting negative regulators such as TGFβ, that modulate the action of mitogens which are under systemic control (Fig. 5.5). Thus, as a large terminal end bud penetrates the surrounding stroma, the subtending mam-mary duct is formed as the bud narrows and stromal fibroblasts synthesize the fibrous periductal matrix under the influence of TGFβ. Exogenous TGFβ1 has been shown to in-hibit epithelial cell division and to strongly stimulate ECM synthesis. Thereafter, lateral branches form in regions of the periductal stroma low in TGFβ and elongate until they reach an area of high TGFβ, when their growth is terminated (Fig. 5.5).[13]

Once the mammary ductal tree is established, ductal spacing must be maintained by active suppression of lateral buds so that alveolar development and secretory differentiation can occur at pregnancy.[77,81,82] This ability of the mammary gland to undergo repeated rounds of alveolar development and involution implies ongoing maintenance of the alveolar stem cell population. Lobular-alveolar structures persist until the end of lactation, after which massive apoptosis characteristic of involution occurs.[83] Individual TGFβ isoforms are ex-pressed differentially throughout mammary gland development (Table 5.4), are distributed in unique patterns, and they are thought to have roles determined by specific spatial and temporal localization.[77]

v) TGFβ in the Developing Mammalian Mammary Gland

In early bovine mammary gland development, TGFβ1 inhibits ductal elongation, but has little effect on cellular proliferation of lobuloalveolar structures in later development.[82] TGFβ mRNAs are only transiently expressed during development and key regulatory steps are posttranslational, with release of TGFβ precursors from storage granules and subse-quent activation[1] being prerequisites for autocrine and paracrine effects.

All three isoforms are present in lactating and nonlactating bovine adult mammary gland,[84] although they show different spatial distributions. TGFβ1 predominates in epithe-lial cells of the lobules and within intralobular stromal cells lining the epithelium, whilst TGFβ2 localizes to epithelial cells TGFβ3 is the most abundant isoform, and is present in most cells.[84] During pregnancy TGFβ2 and β3 expression increases, whilst all three isoforms are drastically reduced in the lactating gland.[77]

TGFβ1 and β3 mRNA are expressed in the intralobular stroma cells, and secretion and activation of the respective proteins, may influence the secretion of ECM components or induce final differentiation of epithelial cells in the infant as well as modulate milk expres-sion in the adult.[84] TGFβ1 and β2 proteins have been isolated from milk[85,86] and it has been proposed that the function of these isoforms may be dependent on lactational secretion. Indeed TGFβ1 has been shown to induce terminal differentiation of intestinal epithelial cells in vitro,[87] suggesting that TGFβs may induce terminal differentiation of the gastrointes-tinal epithelia in the neonate. TGFβ1 also induces IgA synthesis in gut-associated lymph node cells,[88] and a similar process may occur in the neonate to protect against infection by microorganisms at the gut mucosal interface.

In the mouse, comparative analysis of TGFβ gene expression and localization again shows overlapping patterns within the epithelium of actively growing mammary end buds during branching morphogenesis and in the epithelium of growth quiescent ducts.[77] TGFβ1

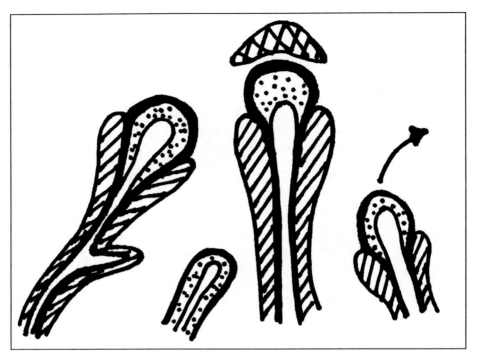

Fig. 5.5. Possible roles for TGFβ1 in reegulation of branching morphogenesis. Intracellular TGFβ1 is found in all mammary epithelial cells. On the left is depicted a laarge, rapidly growing terminal end duct. The basal lamina of the bud tip is in direct contact with the stroma, whereas the end bud and the subtrending duct is encased by fibrous ECM. A small adventitious lateral bud has begun to grow in resonse to high levels of TGFβ in the stroma. Center, a terminal end bud is capped with ectopic ECM in response to exogenous TGFβ. Right, a growing duct turns to the right as it encounters high levels of TGFβ around the adjacent duct. ▨ TGFβ, ◪ fibrous ECM, ■ basal lamina, ⊠ cap cells (located basally in large end buds), ▦ lumenal epithelium, ☐ lumen. Reprinted with permission from: Daniel CW, Robinson S, Silbertstein GB. The role of TGF-β in patterning and growth of the mammary ductal tree. J Mamm Gland Biol Neop 1996; 1(4):331-341. © Plenum Publishing Corporation.

inhibits mammary development of prepubertal mice, although once the gland is committed to differentiation, TGFβ no longer affects mammary morphology.[89] TGFβ may also help to regulate ductal penetration of the fatty stromal tissue in juvenile mice.[77,90] In the virgin gland TGFβ mRNA is present at low levels, but increases rapidly in mid-pregnancy.

Since milk protein secretion by the mammary epithelium is controlled by the composition of ECM,[91,92] it is proposed that TGFβ plays an important role in regulating functional changes which precede milk protein secretion. One model proposes the following; DNA synthesis is increased as a result of estrogen and progesterone induction of TGFα, EGF and EGF receptor, whilst decreased levels of TGFβ removes the normal inhibition of mammary development, thereby allowing the tissue to respond to different hormones and other growth factors. During lobuloalveolar development, continued proliferation leads to active secretion of milk proteins, at which point the gland becomes sensitized to TGFβ1, which may inhibit any lactational response. Withdrawal of all hormones, except insulin, subsequently causes the gland to involute, milk protein secretion ceases and the gland regresses to a morphologically inactive form[89] (Table 5.5).

Table 5.4. Expression of TGFβ genes determined by molecular hybridization in situ and by northern analysis

	Virgin			Pregnant			Lactating	
	End buds	Ducts	Fat pad	Alveoli	Ducts	Fat pad	Alveoli	Fat pad
TGFβ₁	+++	+++	++	++	++	+	−	+/−
TGFβ₂	+	+	+/−	+++	+++	+	−	+/−
TGFβ₃	+++	+++	++	+++	+++	+	+/−	+

Results representative of composite of northern analysis and in situ hybridisation. Fat pad includes, but is not limited to adipocytes and fibroblasts. Reprinted with permission from: Robinson SD, Silberstein GB, Roberts AB et al. Regulated expression and growth inhibitory effects of transforming growth factor-β isoforms in mouse mammary gland development. Dev 1991; 113:867-878. © Company of Biologists, Ltd.

Table 5.5. TGFβ₁ and TGFβ₂ concentrations in rat milk at various times after birth

days post partum[b]	pM TGFβ₁[a]	pM TGFβ₂[a]
1	74 ± 6 (68-80)	842 ± 174 (300-1070)
2	17.5 ± (3-32)	626 ± 201 (340-1350)
3	16.7 ± (6-29)	763 ± 207 (394-1350)
8	<3	206 ± 132 (74-338)
15	<3	159 ± 18 (134-195)

[a] mean TGFβ₂ concentration ± S.E. (range)
[b] day of parturition is day 1 (3-24 hours post partum) Reprinted with permission from: Scneider SL, Gollnick SO, Grande C et al. Differential regulation of TGF-b2 hormones in rat uterus and mammary gland. J Repr Biol 1996; 32:125-144. © Elsevier Science-NL.

TGFβs may have a role in conjuction with several hormones in the delicately balanced process of mammary development.[93] Normal mammary epithelial cells can be induced to produce milk fat globule antigen by TGFβ[94] which itself is a component of human milk.[95] Whilst TGFβ can suppress the onset of lactation and subsequent production of β-caesin, it does not inhibit protein synthesis nor secretion from acini.[96]

vi) Role in Reproductive Function and Embryogenic Development

TGFβ1 may mediate migration of primordial germ cells to genital ridges in vivo.[97] In the testes, paracrine and autocrine actions of growth factors appear to mediate interactions between sertoli, peritubular, and leydig cells as well as between sertoli and germinal cells,[98] though TGFβ₁ does not appear to be an absolute requirement for testicular function. In the ovary, TGFβs show cell specific patterns of distribution during different reproductive stages, with differential responsiveness to hormonal stimulation.[99,100] Expression and secretion of ovarian origin cell types suggests that TGFβ may function as an autocrine/paracrine regulator of function, influencing not only follicular growth and differentiation, but also oocyte development and luteal function.[101] TGFβ has additional roles in implantation, decidualization and placentalization[72,102-104] and in establishing maternal tolerance to the allogenic conceptus.[105]

Expression patterns of TGFβs during embryogenesis and in the adult organism, together with activities in ex vivo assays of biological processes, suggest a role for TGFβ in reproductive function and embryogenic development.[106] These functions have been investigated in detail with the use of knockout mice where the low number of homozygous mutants produced from a heterozygote cross is indicative of some embryolethality (Table 5.6).[107] This is consistent with a role for TGFβ1 in embryonic development and implantation. The frequency of heterozygotes produced is also reduced, which may reflect losses in utero and in turn suggest a role for TGFβ1 in haploid germ cell function.[106] Thus, disruption of the TGFβ gene results in abnormalities of both reproductive function and embryonic development.

The homozygous mutants produced have no detectable TGFβ mRNA or protein, product and after normal growth for approximately 3-5 weeks succumb to a rapid wasting syndrome and die. This is a consequence of an excessive inflammatory response, with massive lymphocytic infiltration in many organs, particularly in the heart and lungs, and suggesting a role for TGFβ1 in the homeostatic regulation of immune cell production and extravasation into tissues.[107] Absence of TGFβ1 in these mice may facilitate generalized activation of the immune system by stimuli that are unable to provoke disease in normal mice. Thus, absence of TGFβ1 does not preclude implantation, but it does affect the immune, amongst other systems. Functional redundancy may exist with TGFβ2 and β3 substituting for TGFβ1 in some cases.[1,43]

Perhaps surprisingly, these mice show no adverse effects of either specification or determination of mammary epithelial cells during embryonic and perinatal development.[107] Therefore, neither paracrine nor autocrine TGFβ1 may be essential for modeling and construction of the primitive mammary epithelial architecture.[108] However, glands of transgenic mice show more ductal branching and precocious lobuloalveolar development. This increases with age, and the females are infact unable to feed their litters.[109] TGFβ1 is thought to suppress the production of milk proteins in differentiated mammary epithelium, and, although it may contribute essential signals for secretory maturation of the mammary epithelium,[110-112] is not thought to play an active role in the synthesis or secretion of milk within fully differentiated lactating mammary epithelium.[108] In contrast, overexpression of the TGFβ transgene during puberty reduces the rate of growth of the ductal tree resulting in a simplified pattern of arborization, and failure of lactation.[13]

vii) Implications and Conclusions

In accordance with the interchangeable binding patterns and functional redundancies between the TGFβ family members, it is anticipated that targeted disruption of a single isoform in a gene knockout mouse might be compensated for by one or other of the two remaining isoforms.[113] However, evidence cited above suggests that synthesis and expression cannot be compensated for by the β2 and β3 isoforms. Nonetheless, TGFβ1 knockout mice can survive for up to 3-5 weeks, and this may be due either to compensatory activities of TGFβ2 and β3, or, possibly the presence of maternal TGFβ1as death coincides with weaning.[114]

Differences in biological activity have been detected between TGFβ1 and β2[115,116] although in general all three isoforms of TGFβ show qualitatively similar activities when added to cells in culture[117-119] and competition studies indicate interaction with the same binding sites. The isoforms show striking differences in gene expression and distribution, suggesting that they may have distinct roles not only in mammary growth

Table 5.6. TGFβ₁ knockout mice

Gene Target	Mouse Strain	Pathology	Target Organs	Lethality
Exon 6 (mature peptide)	129/svJ[a] x C57Bl/6J[b] x CF₁	infiltration, necrosis, wasting.	Heart, stomach liver, lung, pancreas salivary gland, striated muscle	*in utero* >50% 2-3 weeks 100%
Exon 1 (entire peptide)	129/svJ[a] x C57Bl/6J[b] x C57Bl/6J	infiltration, necrosis, wasting	heart, lung, pancreas salivary gland, colon, lymph nodes	*in utero* >50% 2-3 weeks 100%

[a] embryonic stem cells
[b] blastocysts
Reprinted with pe rmission from: McCartney-Francais Taken from McCartney-Francis *et al*, 1994 [113]

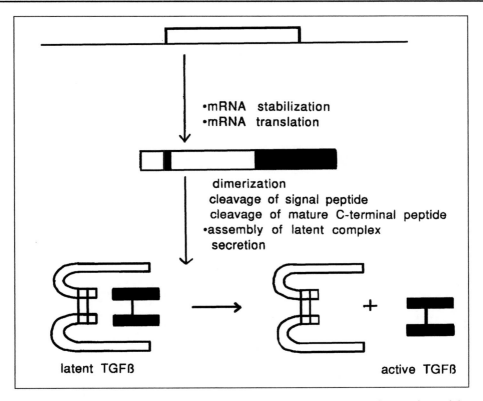

Fig. 5.6. Possible sites of post-transcriptional regulation of TGFβ secretion by members of the steriod/retinoid family of receptors. Candidate sites of action include steps regulating the stability or translatability of the TGFβ mRNAs as well as those controlling either intracellular assembly or extracellular activation of the latent complex of TGFβ. Reprinted with permission from: Roberts AB, Sporn MB. Differential expression of the TGF-b isoforms in embryogenesis suggests specific roles in developing and adult tissues. Mol Repr Dev 1992; 32:91-98. © Wiley-Liss, Inc.

and differentiation,[77] but also in morphogenesis and embryogenic development in general. Indeed, specific and unique activities have been assigned to individual TGFβ isoforms.[5,116,120]

It is known that the promoter region of each gene has distinct regulatory elements, such that each isoform can be independently regulated.[121] In addition to this, where mRNA is detected, it is often assumed to be translated to active protein. However, posttranslational mechanisms are known to control the production of biologically active TGFβs (Fig. 5.6), and in certain situations not only secretion of protein but also activation of latent forms may be subject to regulation.[1] Thus, differences in TGFβ1 activity may relate not only to mRNA expression, but also to the efficiency of translational, posttranslational processing, secretion and activation of mechanisms.[60,89]

In summary, TGFβ influences the developing organism through effects on gene expression; proliferation, differentiation and function; matrix protein formation; chemotaxis; tissue repair and remodeling; and immunosuppression. Extensive studies have shown TGFβ to be abundantly expressed during embryogenesis and at all stages of development of the adult organism. TGFβ isoforms are widely distributed, often in association with critical sites of mesenchyme-epithelial interactions and areas of remodeling of mesenchyme or mesoderm. Such studies suggest a substantial role for TGFβ in embryogenesis. TGFβ appears to be intimately involved in the regulation of branching morphogenesis, within the mammary gland during development and throughout pregnancy and lactation. Furthermore, TGFβ is secreted into breast milk, and into the placental circulation, which may help the neonate to survive in it's first weeks of life, by offering protection against infection. This is consistent with studies of knockout mice, in which homozygotes survive to weaning. These studies have highlighted the importance of TGFβ1 in embryonic development, and reproductive function and milk production.

References

1. Roberts AB, Sporn MB. The transforming growth factor-β. In: Sporn MB, Roberts AB, eds. Handbook of experimental pharmacology. Peptide growth factors and their receptors. 95th Edition. Berlin: Springer-Verlag, 1990:419-472.
2. Sporn MB, Roberts AB, Wakefield LM et al. Some recent advances in the chemistry and biology of TGF beta. J Cell biol 1987; 105:1039-1045.
3. Padgett RW, Johnston DSt, Gerhart WM. A transcript from a drosophila pattern gene predicts a protein homologous to the transforming growth factor β family. Nature Lond 1987; 325:81-84.
4. Weeks DL, Melton DA. A maternal mRNA localised to the vegetal hemisphere in xenopus eggs codes for a growth factor related to TGFβ. Cell 1987; 51:861-867.
5. Rosa F, Roberts AB, Danielpour D et al. Mesoderm induction in amphibians: The role of TGFβ₂-like factors. Science 1988; 239:783-785.
6. Massague J. The transforming growth factor-β family. Ann Rev Cell Biol 1990; 6:597-641.
7. Derynck R, Linquist PB, Lee A et al. A new type of transforming growth factor-beta, TGF-beta 3. EMBO J 1988; 7:3737-3743.
8. Lawrence DA, Pircher R, Kryceve-Martinerie C et al. Normal embryo fibroblasts release transforming growth factors in a latent form. J Cell Physiol 1984; 121:184-188.
9. Wakefield L, Colletta AA, McCune BK et al. Roles for transforming growth factors-β in the genesis, prevention and treatment of breast cancer. In: Dickson RB, Lippman ME, eds. Genes, Oncogenes and Hormones: Advances in Cellular and Molecular Biology of Breast Cancer. Boston: Kluwer Academic Publishers, 1991:97-136.
10. Roberts AB, Sporn MB, Assoian RK et al. Transforming growth factor type β: Rapid induction of fibrosis and angiogenesis in vivo and stimulation of collagen formation in vitro. Proc Natl Acad Sci USA 1986; 83:4167-4171.

11. Leof EB, Proper JA, Goustin AS et al. Induction of c-sis mRNA and activity similar to PDGF by TGF-β. A proposed model for indirect mitogenesis involving autocrine activity. Proc Natl Acad Sci USA 1986; 83:2453-2457.
12. Massague J, Cheifetz S, Laiho M et al. Transforming growth factor-β. Cancer Surveys 1992; 12:81-103.
13. Daniel CW, Robinson S, Silbertstein GB. The role of TGF-β in patterning and growth of the mammary ductal tree. J Mamm Gland Biol Neop 1996; 1(4):331-341.
14. Arrick BA. Therapeutic implications of the TGF-β system. J Mamm Gland Biol Neop 1996; 1(4):391-397.
15. Arteaga CL, Dugger TC, Hurd SD. The multifunctional role of (TGF)-βs on mammary epithelial cell biology. Breast Cancer Res Treat 1996; 38:49-56.
16. Pepper MS, Vassalli J-D, Orci L et al. Biphasic effect of transforming growth factor-$β_1$ on in vitro angiogenesis. Exp Cell Res 1993; 204:356-363.
17. Wahl SM. Transforming growth factor beta (TGF-β) in inflammation: a cause and a cure. J Clin Immunol 1992; 12:1-14.
18. Rizzino A. Transforming growth factor-β: Multiple effects on cell differentiation and extracellular matrices. Dev Biol 1988; 130:411-422.
19. Barnard JA, Lyons RM, Moses HL. The cell biology of transforming growth factor β. Biochem Biophys Acta 1990; 1032:79-87.
20. Barcellos-Hoff MH. Latency and activation in the control of TGF-β. J Mamm Gland Biol Neop 1996; 1(4):353-363.
21. Moses HL. The biological action of transforming growth factor β. In: Sara V, Hall K, Low H, eds. Growth factors from genes to clinical applications. New York: Raven Press, 1990:141-155.
22. Van Obbergehen-Schilling E, Roche NS, Flanders KC et al. Transforming growth factor β1 positively regulates its own expression in normal and transformed cells. J Biol Chem 1988; 263:7741-7746.
23. Roberts AB, Flanders KC, Heine UI et al. Transforming growth factor-β: multifunctional regulator of differentiation and development. Phil Trans R Soc Lond B 1990; 327:145-154.
24. Moses HL, Tucker RF, Leof EB et al. Type beta transforming growth factor is a growth stimulator and a growth inhibitor. In: Feramisco J, Ozanne B, Stiles C, eds. Cancer Cells. Vol 3. Cold Spring Harbour, NY: Cold Spring Harbour Laboratory, 1985:65-71.
25. Centrella M, McCarthy TL, Canalis E. Transforming growth factor-beta system, a complex pattern of cross-reactive ligands and receptors. Cell 1987; 48:409-415.
26. Hill DJ, Strain AJ, Milner RDG. Presence of transforming growth factor-beta-like activity in multiple fetal rat tissues. Cell Biol Int Rep 1986; 10:915-922.
27. Robey PG, Young MF, Flanders KC et al. Osteoblasts synthesize and respond to TGF-beta in vitro. J Cell Biol 1987; 105:457-463.
28. Ignotz R, Massague J. Transforming growth factor-beta stimulates the expression of fibronectin and collagen and their incorporation into the extracellular matrix. J Biol Chem 1986; 261:4337-4345.
29. Seyedin SM, Thomas TC, Thompson AY et al. Purification and characterization of two cartilage-inducing factors from bovine demineralized bone. Proc Natl Acad Sci USA 1985; 82:2267-2271.
30. Seyedin SM, Thompson AY, Bentz H et al. Cartilage-inducing factor-A. J Biol Chem 1986; 261:5693-5695.
31. Florini JR, Roberts AB, Ewton DZ et al. Transforming growth factor-beta: A very potent inhibitor of myoblast differentiation, identical to the differentiation inhibitor secreted by buffalo rat liver cells. J Biol Chem 1986; 261:16509-16513.
32. Massague J, Cheifetz S, Endo T et al. Type beta transforming growth factor is an inhibitor of myogenic differentiation. Proc Natl Acad Sci USA 1986; 83:8206-8210.
33. Olson EN, Sternberg E, Hu JS et al. Regulation of myogenic differentiation by type beta transforming growth factor. J Cell Biol 1986; 103:1799-1805.

34. Miettinen PJ, Ebner R, Lopez AR et al. TGF-β induced transdifferentiation of mammary epithelial cells to mesenchymal cells: involvement of type I receptors. J Cell Biol 1994; 127:2021-2036.

35. Desmouliere A, Geinoz A, Gabbiani F et al. Transforming growth factor-β1 induces alpha-smooth muscle actin expression in granulation tissue myofibroblasts and in quiescent and growing cultured fibroblasts. J Cell Biol 1993; 122:103-111.

36. Roberts AB, Flanders KC, Kondaiah P et al. Transforming growth factor beta: Biochemistry and role in embryogenesis, tissue repair and remodelling, and carcinogenesis. Recent Prog Horm Res 1988; 44:157-197.

37. Lund LR, Riccio A, Andreasen PA et al. Transforming growth factor-β is a strong and fast acting positive regulator of the level of type-1 plasminogen activator inhibitor mRNA in WI-38 human lung fibroblasts. EMBO J 1987; 6:1281-1286.

38. Edwards DR, Murphy G, Reynolds JJ et al. TGF-β modulates the expression of collagenase and TIMP. EMBO J 1987; 6:1899-1904.

39. Postlethwaite AE, Keski-Oja J, Moses HL et al. Stimulation of the chemotactic migration of human fibroblasts by transforming growth factor beta. J Exp Med 1987; 165:251-256.

40. Huchet R, Bruley-Rosset M, Mathiot C et al. Involvement of the IFN- and transforming growth factor-β in graft-vs-host reaction-associated immunosuppression. J Immunol 1993; 6:2517-2524.

41. Wahl SM, Hunt DA, Wakefield LM et al. TGF-β induces monocyte chemotaxis and growth factor production. Proc Natl Acad Sci USA 1987; 84:5788-5792.

42. Madri JA, Pratt BM, Joseph LB et al. Phenotypic modulation of microvascular endothelial cells by transforming growth factor-β depends upon the composition and organization of the extracellular matrix. J Cell Biol 1988; 106:1375-1384.

43. Rappolee DA, Brenner CA, Schultz R et al. Developmental expression of PDGF, TGF-alpha, and TGF-β genes in preimplantation mouse embryos. Science Wash; 242:1823-1825.

44. Slager HG, Lawson KA, van den Eijnden-van Raaij AJM et al. Differential localisation of TGF-β2 in mouse preimplantation and early postimplantation development. Dev Biol 1991; 145:205-218.

45. Paria BC, Jones KL, Flanders KC et al. Localization and binding of transforming growth factor-β isoforms in mouse preimplantation embryos and in delayed and activated blastocysts. Dev Biol 1992; 151:91-104.

46. Tamada H, McMaster MT, Flanders KC et al. Cell type-specific expression of the transforming growth factor-β1 in the mouse uterus during the preimplantation period. Mol Endocrinol 1990; 4:965-972.

47. Heine UI, Munoz EF, Flanders KC et al. Role of transforming growth factor-β in the development of the mouse embryo. J Cell Biol 1987; 105:2861-2876.

48. Fitzpatrick DR, Denhez F, Kondaiah P et al. Differential expression of TGF-beta isoforms in murine palatogenesis. Dev 1990; 109:653-660.

49. Pelton RW, Nomura S, Moses HL et al. Expression of transforming growth factor-β2 during murine embryogenesis. Dev 1989; 106:759-767.

50. Pelton RW, Saxena B, Jones M et al. TGF-beta 2 and TGF-beta 3 in mouse embryo expression patterns suggest multiple roles during embryonic development. J Cell Biol 1991; 115:1091-1105.

51. Thompson NL, Flanders, KC, Smith M et al. Expression of transforming growth factor-β1 in specific cells and tissues of adult and neonatal mice. J Cell Biol 1989; 108:661-669.

52. Paria BC, Dey SK. Preimplantation embryo development in vitro: Cooperative interactions amongst embryos and role of growth factors. Proc Natl Acad Sci USA 1990; 87:4756-4760.

53. Graham CH, Lysiak JJ, McCrae KR et al. Localization of transforming growth factor-β at the human fetal-maternal interface: role in trophoblast growth and differentiation. Biol Rep 1992; 46:561-571.

54. Graham CH, Lala PK. Mechanism of control of trophoblast invasion in situ. J Cell Physiol 1991; 148:228-234.

55. Hsuan JJ. Transforming growth factor β. Br Med Bull 1989;45:425-437.

56. Wilcox JN, Derynk R. Developmental expression of transforming growth factors alpha and beta in mouse fetus. Molec Cell Biol 1988; 8:3415-3422.

57. Jakowlew SB, Ciment G, Tuan RS et al. Expression of transforming growth factor-β2 and β3 mRNAs and proteins in the developing chick embryo. Diff 1994; 55:105-118.

58. Potts JD, Runyan RB. Epithelial-mesenchymal cells transformation in the embryonic heart can be mediated, in part, by transforming growth factor-β. Devel Biol 1989; 134:392-401.

59. Pelton RW, Johnson MD, Perkett EA et al. Expression of transforming growth factor-β1, β2 and β3 mRNA and protein in the murine lung. Am J Respir Cell Mol Biol 1991; 5:522-530.

60. Lenhert SA, Ackhurst RJ. Embryonic expression pattern of TGF beta type-1 RNA suggest both paracrine and autocrine mechanisms of action. Dev 1988; 104:263-273.

61. Ellingsworth LR, Braman JE, Fok K et al. Antibodies to the n-terminal portion of cartilage-inducing factor A and TGF-β (Immunohistochemical localisation and association with differentiating cells). J Biol Chem 1986; 261:12362-12367.

62. Sandberg M, Vurion T, Hirrovan H et al. Enhanced expression of TGF-β and c-fos mRNAs in the growth plates of developing human long bones. Dev 1988; 102:461-470.

63. Hay ED. In: Hay ED, ed. Cell biology of extracellular matrix. New York: Plenum, 1981:379-409.

64. Lefer AM, Tsao P, Aoki N et al. Mediation of cardioprotection by transforming growth factor-beta. Science 1990; 249:61-64.

65. Joyce ME, Roberts AB, Sporn AB et al. Transforming growth factor-beta and the initiation of chondrogenesis and osteogenesis in the rat femur. J Cell Biol 1990; 110:2195-2207.

66. Johnson MD, Jennings MT, Gold LI et al. Transforming growth factor-β in neural embryogenesis and neoplasia. Human Pathol 1993; 24:457-462.

67. Yamauchi K, Martinet Y, Basset P et al. High levels of transforming growth factor-beta are present in the epithelial lining fluid of the normal human lower respiratory tract. Am Rev Respir Dis 1988; 137:1360-1463.

68. Perkett EA, Lyons RM, Moses HL et al. Transforming growth factor-β activity in sheep lung lymph during the development of pulmonary hypertension. J Clin Invest 1990; 86:1459-1564.

69. Khalil N, Bereznay O, Sporn M et al. Macrophage production of transforming growth factor β and fibroblast collagen synthesis in chronic inflammation. J Exp Med 1989; 170:727-737.

70. Lyons KM, Pelton RW, Hogan BLM. Organogenesis and pattern formation in the mouse: RNA distribution patterns suggest a role for Bone morphogenic protein-2A (BMP-2A). Dev 1990; 109:833-844.

71. Gatherer D, ten Dijke P, Baird DT et al. Expression of TGFβ isoforms during first trimester human embryogenesis. Dev 1990; 110:445-460.

72. MacCallum J, Poulsom R, Hanby AM, Miller WR. Expression and distribution of TGFβ mRNA isoforms in a small group of human breast cancers examined by in situ hybridization. The Breast 1995; 4:289-296.

73. Flanders KC, Thompson NL, Cissel DS et al. Transforming growth factor-beta 1:histochemical localization with antibodies to different epitopes. J Cell Biol 1989; 108:653-660.

74. Akhurst RJ, Lenhert SA, Faissner AJ et al. TGF β in murine morphogenetic processes: the early embryo and cardiogenesis. Dev 1990; 108:645-656.

75. Millan FA, Kondaiah P, Denhez F et al. Embryonic gene expression patterns of TGF betas 1, 2 and 3 suggest different developmental functions in vivo. Dev 1991; 111:131-144.

76. Glick AB, Flanders KC, Danielpour D et al. Retinoic acid induces transforming growth factor-beta2 in cultured keratinocytes and mouse epidermis. Cell Regul 1989; 1:87-97.

77. Robinson SD, Silberstein GB, Roberts AB et al. Regulated expression and growth inhibitory effects of transforming growth factor-β isoforms in mouse mammary gland development. Dev 1991; 113:867-878.

78. Bernfield MR, Cohn RG, Banerjee SD. Glycosaminoglycans and epithelial organ formation. Am Zool 1973; 13:1067-1083.

79. Topper YJ, Freeman CS. Multiple hormone interactions in the developmental biology of the mammary gland. Physiol Rev 1980; 60:1049-1106.
80. Daniel CW, Silberstein GB. Postnatal development of the rodent mammary gland. In: Neville MC, Daniel CW, eds. The mammary gland: development, regulation and function. New York: Plenum Press, 1987:3-36.
81. Faulkin LJ, DeOme KB. Regulation of growth and spacing of gland elements in the mammary fat pad of the C3H mouse. J Natl Cancer Inst 1960; 24:953-963.
82. Daniel CW, Silberstein GB, Van Horn K et al. TGF-β1 induced inhibition of mouse mammary ductal growth: developmental specificity and characterization. Dev Biol 1989; 135:20-30.
83. Strange R, Li F, Saurer S et al. Apoptotic cell death and tissue remodelling during mouse mammary gland involution. Dev 1992; 115:49-58.
84. Maier R, Schmid P, Cox D et al. Localization of transforming growth factor-β1, -β2 and -β3 gene expression in bovine mammary gland. Mol Cell Endocr 1991; 82:191-198.
85. Cox DA, Burk RR. Isolation and characterization of milk growth factor, a transforming growth factor-beta 2-related polypeptide, from bovine milk. Eur J Biochem 1991; 197:353-358.
86. Jin Y, Cox D, Cerletti N. Separation, purification, and sequence identification of TGF-beta 1 and TGF-beta 2 from bovine milk. J Protein Chem 1991;
87. Kurokowa M, Lynch K, Podolosky DK. Effects of growth factors on an intestinal epithelial cell line: transforming growth factor beta inhibits proliferation and stimulates differentiation. Biochem Biophys Res Commun 1987; 142:775-782.
88. Chen S-S, Li Q. Transforming growth factor-beta 1 (TGF-beta 1) is a bifunctional immunoregulator for mucosal IgA responses. Cell Immunol 1990; 128:353-361.
89. Plaut K. Role of epidermal growth factor and transforming growth factors in mammary development and lactation. J Dairy Sci 1993; 76:1536-1538.
90. Silberstein G, Daniel CW. Reversible inhibition of mammary gland growth by transforming growth factor-beta. Science 1987; 237:291-293.
91. Li HY, Aggeler J, Farson DA et al. Influence of a reconstituted basement membrane and its components on caesin gene expression and secretion in mouse mammary epithelial cells. Proc Natl Acad Sci USA 1987; 84:136-140.
92. Bisell MJ, Hall HG. In: Neville MC, Daniel CW, eds. The mammary gland. New York: Plenum Press, 1987:97-146.
93. Vonderhaar BK. Regulation of development of the normal mammary gland by hormones and growth factors. In: Lippman ME, Dickson RB, eds. Breast cancer: Cellular and molecular biology. Boston: Kulwer, 1988:251-266.
94. Lippman ME, Dickson RB. Growth control of normal and malignant breast epithelium. Proc Royal Soc Edin 1989; 95B: 89-106.
95. Noda K, Umeda M, Ono T. Transforming growth factor activity in human colostrum. Gann 1984; 75:109-112.
96. Sudlow AW, Wilde CJ, Burgoyne RD. Transforming growth factor-β1 inhibits casein secretion from differentiating mammary-gland explants but not from lactating mammary cells. Biochem J 1994; 304:333-336.
97. Godin I, Wylie CC. TGF-β1 inhibits proliferation and has a chemotrophic effect on mouse primordial germ cells in culture. Dev 1991; 113:1451-1457.
98. Skinner ML. Cell-cell interactions in the testis. Endocr Rev 1991; 12:45-77.
99. Mulheron GW, Schomberg DW. Rat granulosa cells express transforming growth factor-β type 2 messenger ribonucleic acid which is regulatable by follicle-stimulating hormone in vitro. Endocrinol 1990; 126:1777-1779.
100. Teerds KJ, Dorrington JH. Immunohistochemical localization of transforming growth factor-β1 and -β2 during follicular development in the adult rat ovary. Mol Cell Endocrinol 1992; 84:R7-R13.
101. Feng P, Catt KJ, Knecht M. Transforming growth factor-β stimulates meiotic maturation of the rat oocyte. Endocrinol 1988; 122:181-186.

102. Altman DJ, Schneider SL, Thompson DA et al. A transforming growth factor β1 (TGF-β2)-like immunosuppressive factor in amniotic fluid and localization of TGF-β2 mRNA in the pregnant uterus. J Exp Med 1990; 172:1391-1401.
103. Dungy LJ, Siddiqi TA, Kahn S. Transforming growth factor-β1 expression during placental development. Am J Obstet Gynecol 1991; 165:853-857.
104. Manova K, Paynton BV, Bachvarova RF. Expression of activins and TGFβ1 and β2 RNAs in early postimplantation mouse embryos and uterine decidua. Mech Dev 1992; 36:141-152.
105. Clark DA, Falbo M, Rowley RB et al. Active suppression of host-vs graft reaction in pregnant mice. J Immunol 1988; 141:3833-3840.
106. Shull MM, Doetschman T. Transforming growth factor-β1 in reproduction and development. Mol Rep Dev 1994; 39:239-246.
107. Kulkarni AB, Huh C-G, Becker D. et al. Transforming growth factor β1 null mutation in mice causes excessive inflammatory response and early death. Proc Natl Acad Sci USA 1993; 90:770-774.
108. Smith GH. TGF-β and functional differentiation. J Mamm Gland Biol Neopl 1996; 1:343-352.
109. Gorska AE, Serra R, Chen R-H et al. Mammary gland development in transgenic mice expressing a dominant-negative transforming growth factor-beta type II receptor under the control of the mouse mammary tumour virus promoter/enhancer. Proc Am Assoc Cancer Res 1995; 36:188.
110. Vassalli A, Matzuk MM, Gardner L et al. Activin/inhibin βB subunit gene disruption leads to defects in eyelid development and female reproduction. Genes Dev 1994; 8:414-427.
111. Schrewe H, Gendron-Maguire M, Harbison ML et al. Mice homozygous for a null mutation of activin βB are viable and fertile. Mech Dev 1994; 47:43-51.
112. Russo IH, Russo J. Role of hCG and inhibin in breast cancer. Int J Oncol 1994; 4:296-306.
113. McCartney-Francis NL, Wahl SM. Transforming growth factor β: A matter of life and death. J Leuk Biol 1994; 55:401-409.
114. Letterio JJ, Geiser AG, Kulkarni AB et al. Maternal rescue of transforming growth factor-β1 null mice. Science 1994; 264:1936-1938.
115. Ohta M, Greenberger JS, Anklesaria P et al. Two forms of transforming growth factor-beta distinguished by multipotential haemopoetic progenitor cells. Nature 1987; 329:539-541.
116. Jennings JC, Mohan S, Likhart TA et al. Comparison of the biological actions of TGF beta-1 and TGF beta-2:differential activity in endothelial cells. J Cell Physiol 1988; 137:167-172.
117. Graycar JL, Miller DA, Arrick BA et al. Human transforming growth factor-β3:recombinant expression, purification and biological activities in comparison with transforming growth factors-β1 ad -β2. Mol Endo 1989; 7:1977-1986.
118. Roberts AB, Rosa F, Roche NS et al. Isolation and characterization of TGF β2 and TGFβ5 from medium conditioned by *Xenopus* XTC cells. Growth Factors 1990; 2:135-147.
119. ten Dijke P, Hansen P, Iwata KK et al. Identification of another member of the transforming growth factor β gene family. Proc Natl Acad Sci USA 1988; 85:4715-4719.
120. Kimelman D, Kirschner M. Synergistic induction of mesoderm by FGF and TGF-β in the identification of an mRNA coding for FGF in the early *Xenopus* embryo. Cell 1987; 51:869-877.
121. Lafyatis R, Lechleider R, Kim SJ et al. Structural and functional characterization of the transforming growth factor β3 promoter: A cAMP response element regulates basal and induced transcription. J Biol Chem 1990; 265:19128-19136.
122. Scneider SL, Gollnick SO, Grande C et al. Differential regulation of TGF-β2 hormones in rat uterus and mammary gland. J Repr Biol 1996; 32:125-144.
123. Ackhurst RJ, Fitzpatrick DR, Fowlis DJ et al. The role of TGF-βs in mammalian development and neoplasia. Mol Repr Dev 1992; 32:127-135.
124. Roberts AB, Sporn MB. Differential expression of the TGF-β isoforms in embryogenesis suggests specific roles in developing and adult tissues. Mol Repr Dev 1992; 32:91-98.

CHAPTER 6

TGFβ and Colonic Neoplasia

A.M. Manning, A. Hague, C. Pareskeva

The complex multistep nature of cancer is now accepted to refer to an accumulation of definable genetic alterations that provide the cell with a growth advantage and allow it to become the predominant cell type in the tumor by clonal expansion.[1] The colon is a tightly controlled self renewing population where the management of proliferation, differentiation and cell death are heavily interdependent. It represents an excellent example of this complex multistage pathway to neoplasia due to the existence of clearly defined stages of progression. Consequently the cellular and molecular analysis of this cancer has allowed remarkable progress in the identification of the nature and role of some of the genetic alterations involved in human tumor progression.

i) Introduction to Colorectal Neoplasia

Colorectal cancer accounts for about 14% of all cancers and remains one of the major sites of malignant disease in Westernized countries. The majority of colorectal cancers are thought to arise from preexisting premalignant tumors or adenomas, (sometimes referred to as polyps), in what is referred to as the adenoma-carcinoma sequence.[2] Adenomas themselves arise from cellular hyperproliferations of the intestinal epithelium, that in turn originate from the normal colonic mucosa. Grades of atypical epithelia in adenomas suggest a gradual transition from the benign to a malignant phenotype which may take decades to produce a malignant tumor.[2]

a) Genetic Alterations in Colorectal Cancers

Unlike many other common human cancers, the availability of biopsy material representative of these early stages of colonic neoplasia has made it possible to develop a chronicle of somatic mutations that accompany these conversions. Vogelstein and colleagues[3-5] have elegantly demonstrated a median of 4/5 chromosomal losses per tumor and have further suggested that full malignant transformation of normal colonic epithelium may require 8 independent events, with patients having more than the median percentages of allelic losses acquiring a worse prognosis.[6] Common genetic alterations that occur during the development of colorectal cancer are deletions on chromosomes 5p, 17p, 18q and 22q.[7-9] Other less well characterized chromosome losses include 1p, 4p, 6p, 8p, 9q and 18p.[6,10-13] The increased incidence of cancer with age is consistent with the theory that successive events on independent genetic loci must accumulate with time to eventually reach a critical threshold.[14] Multiple loci are targets for genetic alterations during colorectal carcinogenesis including Ki-ras, APC, and p53.[3,9,15-17] It is probable that it is the accumulation of and not the sequence of these genetic changes that is responsible for the increasingly aggressive properties that eventually evolve into the malignant phenotype.[4]

Whilst in the majority of cases no obvious inherited genetic component can be identified,[18] inheritance of a single gene can result in a marked predisposition to the development of colorectal cancer in two distinct autosomal dominant syndromes.[18,19] These are familial adenomatous polyposis coli (FAP) and hereditary nonpolyposis coli (HNPCC). In FAP the "gatekeeper" function of the APC gene is mutated, altering the rate of tumor initiation such that the affected individual typically develops hundreds to thousands of polyps in the rectum and colon during the second and third decades of life.[5,16,20-22] Due to the large number of polyps, the patient is at grave risk that some will inevitably progress to invasive cancer. The APC gene is also thought to be involved as the initiating somatic mutation in sporadic colorectal cancers. Although in HNPCC much lower numbers of polyps are observed the early onset of colorectal cancer is again seen indicating that the feature of this syndrome is the high malignant potential of these adenomatous polyps.[23] Indeed the hereditary defect in HNPCC is now thought to accelerate tumor progression by targeting the integrity of the genome and its propensity for mutation through DNA mismatch repair genes.[5,24-29] Two types of hereditary nonpolyposis colorectal cancer have been distinguished on the basis of inheritance of colorectal cancer solely (Lynch syndrome type I), or inheritance with other types of cancer, e.g., endometrial, ovarian or stomach (Lynch syndrome type II). Interestingly it would appear that a cancer requires only one type of instability whether it be gross chromosomal changes or mismatch repair deficiency. Either is sufficient to produce the prerequisite multiple genetic alterations that ultimately lead to neoplasia.[5]

b) Cellular Models of Colorectal Neoplasia

In order to study these genetic alterations and understand how they give rise to benign and malignant phenotypes, it is important to develop in vitro model systems to attempt to correlate genetic lesions with observed biological characteristics. The scarcity of studies describing the neoplastic transformation of human colonic epithelium is probably due at least in part to the relative difficulty in developing long term cultures of adult normal colonic epithelium. Short term primary cultures of adult and fetal colonic epithelium have been reported as has the long term culture of fetal colonic epithelium.[30-32] Nonetheless, a number of colorectal carcinoma cell lines and cell lines of both hereditary and sporadic adenomas at different stages of tumor progression from early adenoma (< 1 cm in size) to late adenoma (> 2 cm in size) have been isolated.[33-36] In addition a human premalignant adenoma cell line has been transformed in vitro to develop a complete sequential model of malignant progression exhibiting the specific mutations determined during in vivo carcinogenesis.[37] This in vitro progression provided the first experimental evidence for the adenoma-carcinoma sequence and has allowed cells at different stages of malignancy but with a common genetic background to be studied in detail. Hence this panel of premalignant adenoma cell lines and in some cases their transformed counterparts have afforded a unique opportunity to observe colorectal tumor progression from the premalignant stage to invasive cancer. The investigation of these cell lines and others has increased our understanding of the genetic alterations involved and their consequent effect on tumor progression.[15,35,38-46]

ii) Growth Regulation in the Colorectum

The epithelial lining of the colonic mucosa consists of a sheet of single cell thickness organized into tubular invaginations or crypts amid narrow cuffs of surface epithelium between the crypt orifices. Epithelial cells along the colonic crypt axis represent a dynamic continuum of structure and function, such that the cells at the base of the crypt represent the rapidly proliferating less differentiated cells, whilst those towards the top represent differentiated cells with specialized absorptive and digestive functions such as columnar absorptive cells, mucus containing goblet cells and endocrine cells. Continuous exfoliations into the colonic lumen are counterbalanced by ongoing proliferation so that the net epithelial mass remains relatively constant and the sizes of the proliferating and differentiating compartments are maintained within precise topographical boundaries (see Fig. 6.1).

In the normal colorectum, this balance is influenced by both positive and negative growth factors, to provide a fine interactive tuning mechanism for growth control.[47,48] Requirements for more than one positive growth factor for autonomous growth have been demonstrated.[49] Other investigators have illustrated that overproduction or even independence of a positive growth regulator may contribute to unregulated proliferation and increasingly aggressive behaviour.[50,51] In contrast, TGF β1 has been well established as a negative growth regulator for a variety of epithelial cells.[52-59] Hence the detection of biologically relevant amounts of TGFβ1 like activities in the conditioned medium of several colon cell lines in vitro,[50,60] plus experiments using the rat jejunum,[61,62] suggested that it may also be important in the negative regulation of intestinal epithelial cell growth.

a) *TGFβ1 Regulation of Colonic Cell Growth*

TGFβ1 inhibition of colonic epithelial cell growth has now been amply demonstrated in the literature.[38,40-45,63,64] It has also been shown to inhibit the growth of normal intestinal epithelial cells in vivo by injection—where it decreases both villus and crypt heights.[65] Finally, immunohistochemical studies have confirmed that TGFβ1 is expressed in human colorectal carcinoma, adenoma, and normal colorectal mucosa.[66] A gradient of differential expression along the crypt epithelium was observed in normal mucosa. Cells in the upper part of the crypt towards the luminal surface showed enhanced immunoreactivity compared to cells in the lower proliferative compartment, similar to that observed in the rodent large bowel.[67] Furthermore, in the colon this differential staining was lost in dysplastic mucosa, indicating a possible deregulation of expression in neoplastic cells.[66] Indeed increased cloning efficiencies and tumor incidence in FET colon carcinoma cells transfected with antisense TGFβ1 to repress endogenous TGFβ expression suggest that loss of inhibition to TGFβ1 may contribute to the generation of significantly more aggressive growth characteristics.[44]

The observation that the transformed counterparts of some cell lines may be less sensitive or acquire partial or full resistance to growth inhibition by TGFβ1[53,57,68-71] support the idea that an escape from or loss of response to a negative growth control mechanism may be important in tumor development and progression.[72-74] Whilst most colon carcinoma cell lines have been shown to be resistant to growth inhibition by TGFβ1[42,50,75] several reports have shown that some human colorectal cancer cell lines retain some degree of sensitivity to the growth inhibitory effect of TGFβ1[38,76,77]—possibly due to the high ratio of heterogeneity in colorectal carcinomas. Even modest resistance may play a role in the formation of adenomas, resulting in a slow but steady accumulation of cells over years.[78] In fact, human premalignant colorectal adenoma cell lines have been demonstrated to be significantly more sensitive to the inhibitory effects of TGFβ1 than tumorigenic colorectal carcinoma cell lines.[42] Recent studies have demonstrated that a G1 growth arrest is induced in these colonic adenoma cells.[79] (Hague et al manuscript in preparation.) The fact that relatively late stage adenomas, i.e., adenomas with a relatively high malignant potential[34,37] were shown to remain sensitive to the inhibitory effect of TGFβ1 would argue that loss of responsiveness to TGFβ1 occurs at a relatively late stage in colorectal carcinogenesis.[42] Similar conclusions are implicit in other examples of multistage carcinogenesis such as the mouse skin[80] and the rat tracheal epithelium.[81,82] In addition, the conversion of the premalignant adenoma cell line PC/AA/C1 to a tumorigenic phenotype was also accompanied by a reduced response to the inhibitory effect of TGFβ1.[42] An analogous loss in TGFβ1 sensitivity was reported to accompany in vitro progression in the colorectal carcinogenesis model described by Markowitz et al.[46]

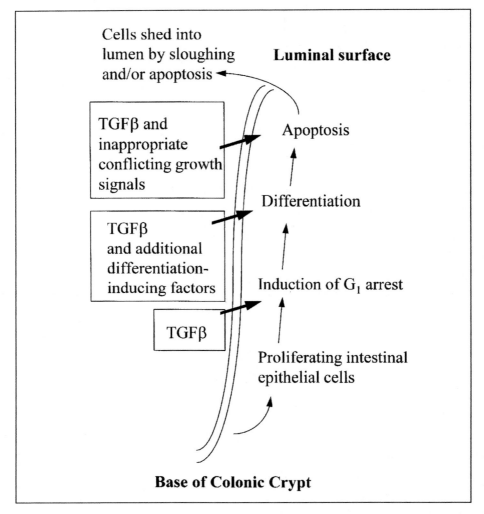

Fig. 6.1. TGFβ in the control of tissue homeostasis in the colonic epithelium. Cells proliferate in the lower 60% of the crypt and undergo growth arrest on encountering TGFβ. Bcl-2 levels may decrease in response to TGFβ, resulting in a delayed apoptotic response. Alternatively, TGFβ may produce a stable non-proliferative state for subsequent induction of differentiation, further signals for apoptosis being required higher up the colonic crypt.

iii) Mechanisms of TGFβ1 Growth Regulation in the Colon

At present, the mechanism for the escape from TGFβ mediated growth arrest is unclear. However genetic alterations strongly implicated in colorectal tumor progression are *Ki-ras* and *p53* mutations. Hence the possible involvement of these alterations in the mechanism of TGFβ mediated growth arrest in the colon has been addressed.

a) Ki-ras

The commonest oncogene alteration associated with colorectal cancer concerns members of the c-*ras* family. *Ki-ras* mutations have been reported in only a small proportion of adenomas less than 1cm[83] and are generally related to late stage adenomas with relatively high malignant potential.[6,84,85] Activation of a member of the *ras* gene family has been reported to be a crucial step in the acquisition of TGFβ1 resistance in other cell types.[86] However the presence of an activated *ras* gene in several human adenoma cell lines tested did not confer resistance to high levels of TGFβ1.[42] This is consistent with studies in the keratinocyte system concerning Ha-*ras*.[80] Conversely Ha-*ras* transfected CCL64 cells were shown to lose sensitivity to TGFβ1,[87] whilst experimental data using rat intestinal cells has suggested a relationship between loss of sensitivity to TGFβ1 and the degree of morphological transformation elicited by Ha-*ras*.[88] Possible differences in the acquisition of a Ha-*ras* or Ki-*ras* mutation with respect to response to TGFβ1, plus variations between different cell systems complicate the issue but clearly mutant *ras* cannot directly block the action of TGFβ1.[89]

b) p53

Deletions/mutations of the *p53* gene have also been demonstrated to be one of the most common genetic alterations in colorectal cancer occurring as a late event in progression.[4,7,15,90] Evidence for a tumor suppressor role has been provided by *p53* transfection experiments and chromosome 17 transfer experiments[91,92] although the precise role of *p53* in carcinogenesis is unclear. Studies in a variety of cell systems have suggested a direct correlation between the acquisition of mutant *p53* and the loss of response to the inhibitory effect of TGFβ1.[59,93,94] However in the colon, this does not appear to be the case: the premalignant adenoma cell line S/RG/C2, known to contain a *p53* mutation[15] has been shown to be sensitive to TGFβ1.[42] In addition some colonic cell lines have been shown to progress towards TGFβ1 resistance whether harboring a *p53* mutation or not.[42,46] There remains the possibility as with mutant *ras* that normal colon may be significantly more sensitive to the inhibitory effect of TGFβ1 and that the acquisition of a mutant *p53* may confer some degree of resistance.[59,93,94] However the transfection of a *p53* gene bearing one of up to 4 of the most common *p53* mutations detected in human cancer did not abrogate the TGFβ1 sensitivity of the colonic adenoma cell line PC/AA/C1, previously demonstrated to retain the wild type protein.[15,95,96] Further investigations suggest that 3 of the 4 mutations do not have a fully dominant mode of action over the wild type *p53* protein in vivo,[96] whilst it has also been reported that the ability of mutant *p53* to inhibit the transactivation function of the coexpressed wild type protein is cell type specific.[97] These studies serve to highlight the importance of studying a variety of cell systems to examine the specific biological consequences of both *p53* and TGFβ and also indicate the intricacy of any signaling pathway involving growth control.

In support of this it is well established that growth factors may activate multiple pathways, increasing the amount of information that can be transmitted, whilst some redundancy in the system could increase the likelihood of error free transmission.[98] It is also clear that the mechanisms involved in TGFβ mediated G1 growth arrest are both numerous, complex and cell specific.[99] The manipulations of multiple proteins such as the down regulation of c-*myc*,[40,100] the inhibition of expression and phosphorylation of the retinoblastoma protein,[40,100] and the inhibition/induction/activation of various cyclins, cyclin dependent kinases and cyclin dependent kinase inhibitors[99] all appear to be involved to some extent in the colon as elsewhere and will not be discussed here. Furthermore it is possible that mutational inactivation/alteration of any component of these intracellular signaling pathways could underly the acquisition of TGFβ resistance in a given situation. Continual research in this area will ultimately lead to meaningful advances in the understanding of the molecular events associated with loss of sensitivity to TGFβ in the colon and other epithelial cell systems.

iv) TGFβ Receptors and HNPCC

To this end, another more obvious possibility to explain a loss of response to the inhibitory effect of TGFβ would be the loss or inactivation of some part of the TGFβ cell surface receptor complex.[101] Loss or inactivation of either of the two receptors involved in the signaling of TGFβ has been observed in a few cases such as retinoblastoma cell lines,[102] many small-cell lung cancers[103,104] and some gastric cancer cell lines.[64] Reduced expression of TGFβ receptors has also been implicated in some cases to be sufficient to confer TGFβ resistance and a more malignant phenotype.[105] Nevertheless in many other cases no link between receptor levels and loss of response was detected. However, the discovery that certain human colon cancers bear somatic mutations that selectively inactivate TGFβ receptor II provided conclusive proof that a direct consequence of receptor mutation is TGFβ resistance.[106]

Briefly, all TGFβ isoforms signal by binding to a heteromeric receptor complex consisting of two distantly related transmembrane serine/threonine kinases designated receptors type I and II. TGFβ binds directly to the type II receptor, a constitutively active kinase. The bound factor is then recognized by the type I receptor which is accordingly recruited into the complex, then phosphorylated by the type II receptor. Phosphorylation allows the type I receptor to propogate the signal to downstream substrates. In this elegant model, the specificity of response may be defined by the particular type I receptor engaged in the complex, providing a succinct explanation for the achievement of many responses from the same factor.[107,108]

Examination of the TGFβ types I and II receptor (RI and RII) transcripts in a panel of 38 human colon cancer cell lines revealed a reduction in the expression of both transcripts.[106] In particular frameshift mutations were demonstrated to occur, consisting of the insertion/deletion of 1 or 2 adenine bases clustered within a 10 base pair polyadenine repeat of exon 3 (nucleotides 709-718) of the coding sequence of RII.[99,106,109] These mutations resulted in the introduction of early stop codons and the subsequent encoding of a severely truncated receptor almost certainly functionally inactive.[106] Significantly, these RII mutations were also discovered in the primary colon tumors from which some of the cell lines had been established, whilst they were not seen in normal cells from the same individual.[106] This would indicate that RII was inactivated by active selection during tumor progression.[99]

a) RII and Microsatellite Instability

This reduction in TGFβ receptor II transcript correlated with separate unrelated studies on the same panel of cell lines looking at microsatellite instability (MI).[106] DNA microsatellites are composed of repetitive runs of mono, di or trinucleotide repeats that are generally noncoding. In microsatellite cancers these repetitive sequences are prone to an accumulation of somatic mutations by the addition/subtraction of additional DNA sequence repeat units.[99] TGFβ RII frameshift mutations were identified exclusively in a subgroup of colon cancers that demonstrated MI.[110] MI is common in many sporadic human cancers and in particular is found in a significant proportion of the sporadic colon cancers occurring in the proximal or right hand side of the colon—as well as in many sporadic gastric and endometrial cancers.[110-117] The MI phenotype is also characteristic of HNPCC tumors, mutations in DNA repair factors resulting in a reduced fidelity for correcting mistakes.[24-29] Frameshift mutations in the type II TGFβ receptor have been shown to be common in inherited and sporadic colorectal cancers exhibiting extensive MI.[118-121] In contrast only a minority of cell lines without MI have demonstrated an inactivation of the TGFβ type II receptor thus demonstrating a close and specific association with a subset of colon cancer cell lines exhibiting replication errors. Bringing these two observations together makes a momentous and potentially extremely significant link between DNA repair defects and a specific pathway of tumor progression.[106]

Mutational inactivation of the TGFβ type II receptor has now been detected in certain other human cancers exhibiting MI, e.g., approximately 71% of gastric cancers[122] and 17% of endometrial carcinomas.[122] However approximately 82% of colorectal carcinomas with MI show this mutation,[118] suggesting that it may confer a specific as yet unidentified growth advantage to colonic cells.[123] However it should be noted that this particular cluster of cancers are already recognized as being linked in some way as Lynch syndrome II. Elucidation of the reason for such critical selection warrants further investigation.

Nevertheless, the demonstrations that primary human cancers generate such mutations at all confirms that acquisition of TGFβ resistance is an important fundamental event selected for during tumor progression.[75,105,106,118,122] Moreover, as reconstitution of TGFβ activity by re-expressinion of RII can reverse malignancy in colon cancers with MI a direct link between tumor progression and loss of RII expression has been confirmed.[75] This would indicate that the TGFβ receptor complex may function as a tumor suppressor gene in human malignancy.[99] This proposal represents the first example of a cell surface growth factor receptor acting as a tumor suppressor and is in contrast to the role of other putative tumor suppressors described in the literature such as *p53* and the retinoblastoma protein, which are thought to act primarily at the nuclear level.[99] Moreover, in a human colon carcinoma cell line GEO, shown to express low levels of RI and be relatively resistant to TGFβ, transfection of RI but not RII increased the inhibitory effect of TGFβ and delayed tumorigenicity in nude mice.[124] This indicates that functional activity of RI may also be a candidate for tumor suppressor function.[99]

b) TGFβ1 Signaling Using Smad Proteins

By natural extrapolation TGFβ and the entire downstream signaling pathway including the newly identified human mad (mothers against dpp) homologs termed Smads[125,126,127] are also potential tumor suppressor gene candidates.[99] Signal transduction of the TGFβ ligand following the activation of the RI/RII receptor complex is now thought to include the phosphorylation of specific pathway restricted Smads followed by oligomerization with the common mediator Smad4 and subsequent nuclear localization.[127] This is presumably followed by multiple targeted transcriptions of the appropriate growth regulatory genes to elicit the required cellular response.[127,128] Identification of these downstream components has provided for the first time a pivotal link between the membrane receptors and the target genes. At least 9 members of this family have now been identified.[128] Different members appear to have different roles in signaling: some are antagonistic (Smad6 and 7) and seemingly act as negative feedback controls.[129,130] Others have been shown to be targets for multiple growth factors (Smad1) suggesting that ultimately opposing regulatory inputs may ultimately determine Smad activity.[131] Smad 4, a mutual and essential partner of pathway restricted Smads, has been found to be altered in a significant number of pancreatic cancers and approximately 20% of colorectal cancers.[125,126,128,132] Loss of Smad4 expression has now been identified in various TGFβ resistant cancer cell lines and restoration of expression has been shown to rescue response to TGFβ as befits a true tumor suppressor gene.[133-135] Inactivating Smad2 mutations also affect TGFβ signal transduction and appear to be specifically associated with sporadic colorectal carcinoma, mutated in approximately 6% of cases.[136] Intriguingly, the Smad2 gene has been located on chromosome 18q, a site thought be important in colorectal carcinoma.[3,136,137] Elucidation of the precise functions of these and other as yet unidentified Smad proteins should prove a very fruitful task. Certainly the remarkable progress made in this area already in such a short time portends an explosion of information about the mechanism of TGFβ signaling in the colon and epithelial systems in general.

v) *TGFβ1* and the Regulation of Apoptosis in the Colon

a) *The Role of Apoptosis in the Colon*
The intestine is typified by high cell turnover rates and a well defined architecture of repetitive proliferative subunits. As a population capable of continuous renewal the regulation of cell number must be strictly controlled, hence a critical balance is maintained between cell gain through mitosis and cell loss by differentiation, cell migration and cell death. In the colonic crypt, cell proliferation is confined to the lower two thirds. There is a continuous migration up the crypt that is tightly linked to differentiation and subsequent loss of epithelial cells from the luminal surface of the colonic crypt. The exfoliation of these cells into the colonic lumen is thought to be a consequence of apoptosis, at a rate estimated to entirely offset new cell production within the crypt.[138-141]

Most colorectal carcinomas arise essentially from an abnormal focus of epithelial proliferation, where the immature proliferative cells are not limited to the base of the crypt and occupy the entire crypt length, appearing within the surface epithelium.[142] This suggests an uncoupling of the process of proliferation and differentiation and also raises the possibility that some of the genes involved in carcinogenesis reduce the rate at which cell loss occurs through apoptosis.[143] Indeed, transition of intermediary to late stage adenoma has now been shown to correlate with suppression of apoptosis.[144] Loss/inactivation of apoptotic signals would indeed produce an enlarged cell population, whilst the consequent extended cell survival could also increase the opportunity to acquire additional genetic defects that may contribute to malignancy.[145,146] Earlier studies on colonic proliferation observed that as colonic epithelial cells progressed towards malignancy, impaired differentiation also led to decreased cell shedding into the intestinal lumen as benign and malignant tumors arose.[147] This would suggest that the promotion of differentiation and apoptosis may be causally linked in some way in the normal regulation of the colon.

In the keratinocyte system, apoptosis has been demonstrated to occur as the final stage of terminal differentiation,[148] where the trigger to undergo differentiation is thought to be due to, at least in part, loss of contact with the basement membrane. Disruption of epithelial cell matrix interactions has also been shown to induce apoptosis.[149] In the colon apoptosis may also form part of a terminal differentiation pathway, again possibly initiated by the depletion of cell-cell contact. This could conceivably act as a fail-safe mechanism, to ensure that cells normally shed into the colonic lumen would be subsequently incapable of reattachment and growth.[75] In addition depletion/accumulation of extracellular matrix components or cytokines may also serve as trigger factors.[150] As increased expression of TGFβ1 in the nondividing differentiating cells creates a concentration gradient within the crypt similar to that seen with other apoptotic regulatory proteins, there may also be a role for TGFβ1 in influencing enterocyte differentiation and/or apoptosis.[62,66,163]

b) *TGFβ1 and Apoptosis in the Colon*
TGFβ1 has been demonstrated to induce a variety of differentiation-like responses in some human colon carcinoma cells including growth inhibition, morphological alteration and increased carcinoembryonic antigen expression.[38,61,151-153] Yet other studies have discovered no evidence to suggest that TGFβ1 induces a more differentiated phenotype in intestinal epithelial cells.[62,154] There are also conflicting reports as to whether TGFβ1 is involved in the maturation of fluid transporting enterocytes which comprise about 80% of

the colonic crypt[61,62,155] although it is thought to be involved in the regulation of intestinal epithelial barrier function by countering the effect of a T cell cytokine.[156]

Nevertheless, there is substantial evidence to indicate that TGFβ1 may participate in the enhancement and induction of apoptosis in a variety of epithelial cells in culture.[157-162] Now both adenoma and human carcinoma colorectal cell lines have also been shown to spontaneously undergo apoptosis in vitro in the form of cells shed into the culture medium.[163] Experimental evidence suggests that the process of apoptosis is in all likelihood initiated in the adherent cell population[164] although detachment occurs relatively early in the process.[165] The colonic floating cells were demonstrated to be morphologically apoptotic[163] and exhibit characteristic apoptotic DNA internucleosomal fragmentation.[166] The floating apoptotic cells retained high levels of colonic differentiation markers suggesting that differentiation took place prior to apoptosis.

Treatment with TGFβ1 did not induce apoptosis in two adenoma cell lines S/RG/C2 or PC/AA/C1 as calculated by the proportional increase of cells in the medium, although both cell lines were growth inhibited.[163] However subsequent studies have proceeded to show the induction of apoptosis by TGFβ1 in two specific adenoma cell lines: PC/BH/C1[154] and VACO-330.[75] Induction of apoptosis in PC/BH/C1 occurred *via* a differentiation independent pathway as compared to the differentiating agent sodium butyrate.[154] How can these discrepancies be resolved? If the role of TGFβ as an endogenous regulator of intestinal epithelial growth is acknowledged, it is then possible to understand that as such it would be unlikely to inhibit growth and then induce immediate apoptosis under normal circumstances. It may be that TGFβ has a "priming" role of the sort that it may maintain a stable nonproliferative state in order to allow the subsequent induction of a differentiated phenotype by additional growth and/or dietary factors.[154] Induction of delayed apoptosis by TGFβ1 may then be a normal physiological response after allowing cells in vivo to perform active functions as differentiated cells (Fig. 6.1). Alternatively TGFβ1 induced apoptosis may also occur in the presence of conflicting growth signals which in itself could partially explain the huge variation in response to this factor.[79,154] In support of this, inappropriately high levels of c-*myc* in the context of growth inhibitory signals have indeed been shown to trigger apoptosis.[143] Nonetheless it would appear that in colonic tumors development of resistance to TGFβ1 may involve two separate stages: resistance to growth inhibition and resistance to TGFβ1 induced apoptosis.[154]

c) Mechanisms of TGFβ1 Induced Apoptosis

Though, little is known regarding the mechanisms by which TGFβ induces apoptosis, TGFβ1 has recently been found to reduce the levels of expression of the apoptotic regulatory protein Bcl-2 in association with apoptosis induction in a colonic adenoma cell line (Hague et al manuscript in preparation). The Bcl-2 protein, a cell 'death protector', is primarily expressed in the base of the crypt and is restricted to the proliferative zone.[167,168] In contrast, the 'death promoting' homologs Bax and Bak are expressed at highest levels in the upper regions of the crypt.[169,170] Bcl-2 is expressed in many colorectal tumors[168] and now further investigations suggest that Bcl-2 expression may be less common in carcinomas than in adenomas.[170-172] As the ratio of Bcl-2 to Bax has been suggested to determine cell viability, a decrease in only Bcl-2 levels may be sufficient to induce apoptosis.[173] Elevated expression of Bcl-2 has previously been shown to block TGFβ induced apoptosis but not growth arrest in myeloid leukemia cells, neatly separating these two functions of TGFβ by linking apoptosis induction with Bcl-2.[174]

In addition, it is accepted that apoptosis depends upon the availability of certain key proteins such as calcium dependent endonucleases and transglutaminases. These proteins are not normally present in every cell in a tissue, and their synthesis may be regulated by specific controller genes. Studies with human gastric carcinoma cells[161] have suggested that exogenous TGFβ1 may induce endonuclease activity at a very early step in the process of apoptosis, possibly by regulating intracellular calcium homeostasis. Indeed, this would seem feasible with the cloning of a new ryanodine receptor calcium channel regulated by TGFβ.[175] Interestingly, TGFβ1 has been shown to alter the calcium influx in rat fibroblasts,[176] whilst directly inhibiting the efflux of calcium in the mouse keratinocyte BALB/MK cell line.[177] Coincidentally Bcl-2 has been also been shown to regulate calcium fluxes within various intracellular compartments including the nucleus, cytoplasm, endoplasmic reticulum and mitochondria.[178-180] With a link already established between Bcl-2 and TGFβ (Hague et al manuscript in preparation) it is noteworthy that recent studies indicate how Bcl-2 regulatory proteins may localize within mitochondria,[181] the site of significant amounts of TGFβ in other cells.[182] It is thus conceivable that a wide spectrum of intracellular physiology is mediated by TGFβ independently of the known cell surface receptors[183] (see Fig. 6.2).

d)p53 Mediated Apoptosis

In such a tightly controlled tissue as the colon, there are likely to be a number of independent pathways to apoptotic cell death to encompass not only routine tissue regulation as discussed above, but also response to abnormal stresses such as cell injury. In this context, the transfection of wild type *p53* into the human colon tumor-derived cell line EB has been reported to induce apoptosis.[138] A possible role for wild type *p53* in DNA synthesis inhibition and apoptosis was suggested by experiments showing that levels of the wild type protein increased after DNA damage.[184-186] Developing tumor cells pass through periods of DNA damage or stress brought on by anoxia and/or aneuploidy. Wild type *p53* protein may be involved in restricting growth by monitoring DNA damage and initiating apoptosis in cells too severely damaged to be repaired.[185-188] Studies with colorectal carcinomas have ascertained that alterations in *p53* detected by immunocytochemical stabilization preceded and facilitated the divergence of aneuploid subclones, confirming a role for *p53* in the regulation of abnormal replication.[189]

However, colorectal adenoma and carcinoma cell lines with mutant *p53* have been shown to have a relatively high frequency of spontaneous apoptosis and in some cases to allow modulation of apoptosis following treatment with TGFβ1 and/or the differentiating agent sodium butyrate.[154,163] A number of groups have now reported *p53* independent apoptotic pathways.[190,191] Certainly experiments in the colorectum indicate that *p53* is only one of the genes that determine the incidence of apoptosis in colon cancer[144,163,192] and imply that failure of *p53* mediated apoptosis is probably not the primary effect of *p53 loss* during colorectal tumor progression.[144]

vi) TGFβ and Metastatic Competence

Neoplasms tend to become increasingly and irreversibly aggressive in their behavior over the course of time, with the emergence of clonal subpopulations with the ability to spread to distant sites and form secondary tumors. These metastatically competent tumor cell variants have a pronounced growth advantage within the primary neoplasm, producing a similar phenomenon to that seen with the initial production of the tumor.[193] It is possible that a growth factor secreted by nonmetastatic carcinoma cells could preferentially stimulate these more aggressive and invasive variants to explain this second clonal expansion.[1] Equally the acquisition of metastatic competence may be promoted by a change from growth inhibition to growth stimulation by the same factor (Fig. 6.2).[72]

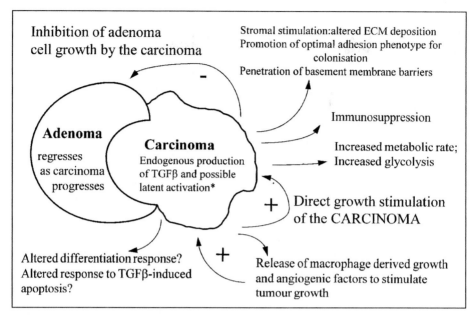

Fig. 6.2. Possible roles for TGFβ in tumor promotion. *Carcinoma cells produce TGFβ, which may be activated by the acidic micro-environment of the tumor. Regression of the residual adenoma tissue may, in part, be due to the inhibition of adenoma cell proliferation by TGFβ produced by the carcinoma, whereas carcinoma cells are often resistant to the growth inhibitory effects of TGFβ and may become growth stimulated by it.

a) TGFβ1 and the Stimulation of Epithelial Cell Growth

Studies in the colon have been instrumental in illustrating the latter hypothesis with respect to the effects of TGFβ1. It is feasible that the capacity of an epithelial cell within a tumor to positively respond to TGFβ1 could contribute to the invasive/aggressive capabilities of that tumor.[194] Accordingly, the colon carcinoma cell line PC/JW/FI has been observed to be weakly but consistently stimulated by TGFβ1.[195] Experiments by Fan et al[76] have demonstrated growth stimulation of 11 out of 13 colonic metastatic variants by TGFβ1, whilst Schroy et al[153,196] reported stimulation of 9 out of 20 resected colonic carcinomas including 3 out of 4 liver metastases. These results suggest that TGFβ1 can stimulate or maintain growth of colon carcinomas in vivo. In addition, positive growth regulation of the colon carcinoma cell line U9 (derived from the HT29 cell line) correlated with increased tumorigenicity in vivo and invasive behavior in vitro.[197] Such a switch from growth inhibition to growth stimulation in response to TGFβ1 has also been reported to occur in several other cell systems[1,198-201] indicating a potential role for TGFβ1 in the modulation of metastasis. TGFβ1 resistant nonmetastatic cells could release active TGFβ1 that stimulates the growth of a metastatically competent variant.[1] It is therefore of interest that concordant inactivation of several tumor suppressor genes implicated in the transduction of the TGFβ inhibitory signal have been associated with the acquisition of metastatic potential of colorectal carcinomas.[202]

b) Additional Roles for TGFβ

The loss of response to the inhibitory effect of TGFβ or gain in stimulatory response by epithelial cells represent aspects of TGFβ functions that may contribute to the malignant phenotype. Tissues as well as individual cells should be regarded as targets for cytokine action.[203,204] TGFβ is known to stimulate growth of stromal elements which constitute a major component of many solid tumors particularly colorectal carcinomas.[205] Experiments by Lieubeau et al[206] have demonstrated that TGFβ1 produced by colon cancer cell lines from progressive tumors in rat can stimulate myofibroblasts to deposit a specific peritumoral extracellular matrix, providing a permissive environment for tumor development and spread. TGFβ1 is well documented to affect the extracellular matrix and to induce the expression of cell adhesion molecules including fibronectin, laminin, carcinoembryonic antigen, collagen and integrins.[63,207-213] TGFβ may interact with the extracellular matrix in vivo to regulate carcinoma cell adhesion during the process of extravasation and attachment at secondary sites of metastasis.[213] Indeed TGFβ has been shown to stimulate mammary cell invasion and metastatic potential by facilitating penetration of basement membrane barriers.[214] The acquisition of an optimal adhesion phenotype may be important for the rapid and successful colonization of the immediate environment by the tumor cell, thereby enhancing survival chances in vivo.[215]

In addition, TGFβ1 produced by tumors may also promote escape from immune surveillance[216] whilst the observed recruitment and activation of monocytes by tumors via TGFβ1 may also serve to stimulate tumor growth by the release of macrophage derived growth and angiogenic factors.[217,218] Furthermore, since TGFβ is secreted from most cells in a latent form, mechanisms of activation provide another mode of regulation.[99] The possibility of latent TGFβ activation within the physiologically acidic environments characteristic of colonic tumors provides a further mechanism by which the full range of responses to TGFβ could be potentially exploited in the colon in particular (Fig. 6.2).[66,163]

Independent experiments using both human endometrial and colorectal carcinoma cells have demonstrated that loss of response to the inhibitory influence of exogenously added TGFβ correlates with increased expression of TGFβ mRNA.[77,219] Recent experiments by Pierce Jr et al[220] have suggested that although overexpression of TGFβ in vivo markedly suppressed mammary tumor development in the early stages of progression, increased expression of TGFβ in later stages may have paracrine effects on the host that favor tumor growth and spread and enhance the rate of malignant progression. Conversely, studies using *ras* transformed keratinocytes derived from mice with a targeted deletion of the β1 gene have shown accelerated multifocal progression to squamous cell carcinoma compared to wild type cells, although these tumor derived cells remained sensitive to exogenous TGFβ in vitro.[221,222] That many transformed cell types exhibit increased expression of TGFβ[223-225] that may be associated with disease progression[214,215,218,226,227] indicates that this growth factor does play a permissive role in tumor progression that may eventually eclipse any earlier role as a growth inhibitor (see Fig. 6.2).

vii) Future Applications, Research and Anticipated Developments

Despite being the one of the principle causes of death from malignant disease, marked variations in colorectal cancer incidence rates worldwide allude to dietary and environmental factors suggesting that many cases might be potentially avoidable. However there has been no significant reduction in mortality over the past 40 years emphasizing that research efforts into more effective treatment, earlier diagnosis and prevention should be intensified. Colorectal cancer is relatively refractory to chemotherapy and interest has recently focused on the role of endogenous growth regulation as a potential mechanism to control tumor growth. The analysis of soluble factors in the tumor microenvironment should provide an insight into cellular behavior in normal and diseased states whilst also being useful prognostically, as demonstrated for breast carcinoma.[228] Genetic changes collectively associated with tumor progression in colorectal neoplasia are now beginning to define abnormal pathology at the genetic level that may lead to new approaches to the treatment of cancer.

Though the multiplicity of genetic lesions discovered thus far may confound therapeutic strategies, not all genetic faults need to be corrected to achieve clinical benefit.[229] Studies by Goyette et al[92] suggest that despite numerous defects in tumor suppressor genes being ssociated with progression to malignancy in colorectal carcinogenesis, correction of only a single defect was capable of causing a reversion to a less tumorigenic phenotype. This supported previous observations by Baker et al[15] who reported similar results following transfection of wild type *p53* into colorectal carcinoma cells. Therefore whilst there are multiple molecular targets for the design of cancer therapies, only a sinular molecular strategy might need to be successful in order to suppress the malignant behavior of cancerous cells, providing fresh optimism for selective gene therapy.

Although the differential sensitivity of premalignant adenoma and tumorigenic carcinoma colorectal cell lines points to potential applications for use of TGFβ as a chemoprotective agent for cycle active drugs,[42,73,230] the expanding array of TGFβ functions and the ever increasing complexity of downstream signaling events suggest that this may be a simplistic view. Nevertheless, the possibility of reversing tumor cell resistance to inhibitory growth factors by manipulating the microenvironment is a realistic objective.[231] Newman showed that tumor cell lines only minimally inhibited by exposure to high concentrations of TGFβ1 in vitro could be severely suppressed by exposure to TGFβ1 in serum free medium in the presence of polyunsaturated fatty acids. Moreover as both normal and cancer tissue represent a composite of cell types and micro-environments, cooperative interactions between different cell types in response to TGFβ are liable to be of increasing importance in the critical regulation of tissue response to homeostasis or injury.[183]

The importance of disruption of TGFβ signaling pathways in promoting tumorigenesis is being increasingly recognized. The recent discovery of a mutation of the RII gene producing a detectable truncated receptor in a subset of colon cancers points to another possible target for gene therapy in restoring critical deleted functions together with potential use as a sensitive tool for screening.[99] Indeed, reconstitution of the TGFβ1 receptor system in cells lacking functional RII has already been demonstrated reversing malignant potential in systems where TGFβ signal transduction remained intact.[75,105] Furthermore, cell fusion experiments have shown that restoration of TGFβ mediated growth inhibition to carcinoma cell lines correlated with an increase in cross-linked RII.[43] These observations suggest that RII may be a valuable target for therapeutic intervention. Continued progress with unraveling of the TGFβ signaling pathway will yield increased understanding of involvement of TGFβ in disease states in the future and provide the ability to manipulate these pathways to favorably influence cell behavior.

The possibility of regulating apoptosis in certain circumstances is also important therapeutically and enables precise targeting of neoplastic tissue with tumor specific signals which can activate the expression of apoptotic genes in malignant cells.[232] This is particularly relevant in colon tissue which is exposed to a large number of dietary mutagens.[79] The ability of TGFβ to modulate apoptotic regulatory genes is a significant observation and further investigations in this area are warranted.

The colorectal cancer model is likely to prove relevant to other common human neoplasms for which processes of tumor development are less well defined, and will provide greater understanding of the cellular and molecular biology of cancer in general. Further isolation of colorectal adenoma and carcinoma cell lines is ongoing and will permit comparisons between newly generated cell lines and those which have been established in culture for many years and have been subject to phenotypic drift. This will include characterization of novel chromosomal abnormalities and signature combinations of genetic and phenotypic markers.[79] Studies with such cell lines will remain instrumental in linking basic molecular studies with clinical applications and permit further alucidation of mechanisms of colorectal carcinogenesis and involvement of TGFβ.

The role of TGFβ in colonic, as in other epithelial neoplasias is undoubtedly manifold. The challenge for the future is to harness properties of this unique factor for diagnostic and therapeutic gain.

Acknowledgments

Work from the Authors' laboratory is supported by the Cancer Research Campaign.

References

1. Theodorescu D, Caltabiano M, Greig R et al. Reduction of TGF-beta activity abrogates growth promoting tumor cell-cell interactions in vivo. J Cell Physiol 1991; 148:380-390.
2. Muto T, Bussey JR, Morson BC. The evolution of cancer of the colon and rectum. Cancer 1975; 36:2251-2270.
3. Vogelstein B, Fearon ER, Hamilton SR et al. Genetic alterations during colorectal tumor development. New Engl J Med 1988; 319:525-532.
4. Fearon ER, Vogelstein B. A genetic model for colorectal tumorigenesis. Cell 1990; 61:759-767.
5. Kinzler KW, Vogelstein B. Lessons from hereditary colorectal cancer. Cell 1996; 87:159-170.
6. Vogelstein B, Fearon ER, Kern SE et al. Allelotype of colorectal carcinoma. Science 1989;244:207-211.
7. Baker SJ, Fearon ER, Nigro JM et al. Chromosome 17 deletions and p53 gene mutations in colorectal carcinomas. Science 1989; 245:217-221.
8. Nigro JM, Baker SJ, Presinger AC et al. Mutations in the p53 gene occur in diverse human tumour types. Nature 1989; 342:705-707.
9. Fearon ER, Cho KR, Nigro JM et al. Identification of a chromosome 18q gene that is altered in colorectal cancers. Science 1990; 247:49-56.
10. Paraskeva C, Finerty S, Powell S. Immortalisation of a human colorectal adenoma cell line by continuous in vitro passage: Possible involvement of chromosome I in tumour progression. Int J Cancer 1988; 41:908-912.
11. Hague A, Hanlon KA, Paraskeva C. Clonal evolution and tumour progression in two human colorectal adenoma-derived cell lines in vitro: The involvement of chromosome 1 abnormalities. Int J Oncol 1992; 1:201208.
12. Sasaki M, Okamoto M, Sato C et al. Loss of constitutional heterozygosity in colorectal tumours from patients with familial polyposis coli and those with nonpolyposis colorectal carcinoma. Cancer Res 1989; 49:4402-4406.
13. Cunningham C, Dunlop MG, Wyllie AH et al. Deletion mapping in colorectal cancer of a putative tumour suppressor gene in 8p22-8p21.3. Oncogene 1993; 8:1391-1396.
14. Levine AJ, Momand J. Tumor suppressor genes: The p53 and retinoblastoma sensitivity genes and gene products. Biochim et Biophys Acta 1990; 1032:119-136.
15. Baker SJ, Markowitz S, Fearon ER et al. Suppression of human colorectal carcinoma cell growth by wild-type p53. Science 1990; 249:912-914.
16. Nishisho I, Nakamura Y, Miyoshi Y et al. Mutations of chromosome 5q21 genes in FAP and colorectal cancer patients. Science 1991; 253:665-669.
17. Smith KJ, Johnson KA, Bryan TM et al. The APC gene product in normal and tumour cells. Proc Natl Acad Sci USA 1993; 90:2846-2850.
18. Fearon ER. Genetic alterations underlying colorectal tumorigenesis. Cancer Surveys 1992; 12:119-136.

19. Cannon-Albright LA, Skolnick MH, Bishop T et al. Common inheritance of susceptibility to colonic adenomatous polyps and associated colorectal cancers. New Engl J Med 1988; 319:533-537.
20. Bodmer WF, Bailey CJ, Bodmer J et al. Localisation of the gene for familial adenomatous polyposis on chromosome 5. Nature 1987; 328:614-616.
21. Leppert M, Dobbs M, Scambler P et al. The gene for familial polyposis coli maps to the long arm of chromosome 5. Science 1987; 238:1411-1413.
22. Groden J, Thliveris A, Samowitz W et al. Identification and characterisation of the familial adenomatous polyposis coli gene. Cell 1991; 66:589-600.
23. Bishop DT, Thomas HJW. The genetics of colorectal cancer. Cancer Surveys 1990; 9:585-604.
24. Leach FS, Nicolaides NC, Papadopoulos N et al. Mutation of a muts homolog in hereditary nonpolyposis colorectal cancer. Cell 1993; 75:1215-1225.
25. Aaltonen LA, Peltomaki P, Leach FS et al. Clues to the pathogenesis of familial colorectal cancer. Science 1993; 260:812-816.
26. Aaltonen LA, Peltomaki P, Mecklin J-P et al. Replication errors in benign and malignant tumors from hereditary nonpolyposis colorectal cancer patients. Cancer Res 1994; 54:1645-1658.
27. Bronner CE, Baker SM, Morrison PT et al. Mutation in the DNA mismatch repair gene homologue hMLH1 is associated with hereditary nonpolyposis colon cancer. Nature 1994; 368:258-261.
28. Papadopoulos N, Nicolaides NC, Wei Y-F et al. Mutation of a mutL homolog in hereditary colon cancer. Science 1994; 263:1625-1629.
29. Ahiquist DA. Aggressive polyps in hereditary nonpolyposis solorectal cancer: Targets for screenig. Gastroenterology 1995; 108:1590-1592.
30. Buset M, Winawer S, Friedman E. Defining conditions to promote the attachment of adult human colonic epithelial cells. In Vitro Cell Dev Biol 1987; 23:403-412.
31. Berry RD, Powell SC, Paraskeva C. In vitro culture of fetal colonic epithelial cells and their transformation with origin minus SV40 DNA. Br J Cancer 1988; 57:287-289.
32. Siddiqui KM, Chopra DP. Primary and long-term epithelial cell cultures from human foetal normal colonic mucosa. In Vitro 1984; 20:859-868.
33. Paraskeva C, Buckle BG, Sheer D et al. The isolation and characterization of colorectal epithelial cell lines at different stages in malignant transformation from familial polyposis coli patients. Int J Cancer 1984; 34:49-59.
34. Paraskeva C, Harvey A, Finerty S et al. Possible involvement of chromosome 1 in in vitro immortalisation: Evidence from progression of a human adenoma derived cell line in vitro. Int J Cancer 1989; 43:743-746.
35. Willson JKV, Bittner GN, Oberley TD et al. Cell culture of human colon adenomas and carcinomas. Cancer Res 1987; 47:2704-2713.
36. Williams AC, Harper SJ, Marshall CJ et al. Specific cytogenetic abnormalities and Ki-ras mutations in two new human colorectal adenoma-derived cell lines. Int J Cancer 1992; 52:785-790.
37. Williams AC, Harper SJ, Paraskeva C. Neoplastic transformation of a human colonic epithelial cell line: In vitro evidence for the adenoma to carcinoma sequence. Cancer Res 1990; 50:4724-4730.
38. Hoosein NM, Brattain DE, McKnight MK et al. Characterisation of the inhibitory effects of transforming growth factor β on a human colon carcinoma cell line. Cancer Res 1987; 47:2950-2954.
39. Hoosein NM, McKnight MK, Levine AE et al. Differential sensitivity of subclasses of human colon carcinoma cell lines to the growth inhibitory effects of transforming growth factor β1. Exp Cell Res 1989; 181:442-453.
40. Moses HL, Yang EY, Pietenpol JA. TGFβ stimulation and inhibition of cell proliferation: New mechanistic insights. Cell 1990; 63:245-247.
41. Massague J. The transforming growth factor β family. Annu Rev Cell Biol 1990; 6:597-641.
42. Manning AM, Williams AC, Game S et al. Differential sensitivity of human colonic adenoma and carcinoma cells to transforming growth factor b:conversion of an adenoma cell

line to a tumourigenic phenotype is accompanied by a reduced response to the inhibitory effect of TGF-β. Oncogene 1992; 6:1471-1476.

43. Geiser AG, Burmester JK, Webbink R et al. Inhibition of growth by transforming growth factor β following fusion of two nonresponsive human carcinoma cell lines. J Biol Chem 1992; 267:2588-2593.

44. Wu S, Theodorescu D, Kerbel RS et al. TGF-β1 is an autocrine-negative growth regulator of human colon carcinoma FET cells in vivo as revealed by transfection of an antisense expression vector. J Cell Biol 1992; 116:187-196.

45. Filmus J, Kerbel R. Development of resistance mechanisms to the growth inhibitory effects of transforming growth factor-β during tumor progression. Curr Opin Oncol 1993; 90:770-774.

46. Markowitz SD, Myeroff L, Cooper MJ et al. A benign cultured colon adenoma bears three genetically altered colon cancer oncogenes but progresses to tumorigenicity and transforming growth factor-beta independence without activating the p53 tumor suppressor gene. J Clin Invest 1994; 93:1005-1013.

47. Levine AE, McRae LJ, Hamilton DA et al. Identification of endogenous inhibitory growth factors from a human colon carcinoma cell line. Cancer Res 1985; 45:2248-2254.

48. Murthy U, Anzano MA, Greig RG. Expression of TGF-alpha/EGF and TGF-b receptors in human colon carcinoma cell lines. Int J Cancer 1989; 44:110-115.

49. Sizeland AM, Burgess AW. The proliferative and morphologic responses of a colon carcinoma cell line (LIM1215) require the production of two autocrine growth factors. Mol Cell Biol 1991; 11:4005-4014.

50. Coffey Jr RJ, Shipley GD, Moses HL. Production of transforming growth factors by human colon cancer lines. Cancer Res 1986; 46:1164-1169.

51. Rodeck U, Herlyn M, Herlyn D et al. Tumor growth modulation by a monoclonal antibody to the epidermal growth factor receptor: Immunologically mediated and effector cell-independent effects. Cancer Res 1987; 47:3692-3696.

52. Pertovaara L, Sistonen L, Bos TJ et al. Enhanced jun gene expression is an early genomic response to transforming growth factor stimulation. Mol Cell Biol 1989; 9:1255-1262.

53. Game SM, Stone A, Scully C et al. Tumor progression in experimental oral carcinogenesis is associated with changes in EGF and TGF-β receptor expression and altered responses to these growth factors. Carcinogenesis 1990; 11:965-973.

54. Rollins BJ, O'Connell TM, Bennett G et al. Environment-dependent growth inhibition of human epidermal keratinocytes by recombinant human transforming growth factor beta. J Cell Physiol 1989; 139:455-462.

55. Hebert CD, Birnbaum. Lack of correlation between sensitivity to growth inhibition and receptor number for transforming growth factor β in human squamous carcinoma cell lines. Cancer Res 1989; 49:3196-3202.

56. Jetten AM, Shirley JE, Stoner G. Regulation of proliferation and differentiation of respiratory tract epithelial cells by TGF-β1. Exp Cell Res 1986; 167:539-549.

57. McMahon JB, Richards WL, Delcampo AA et al. Differential effects of transforming growth factor beta on proliferation of normal and malignant rat liver epithelial cells in culture. Cancer Res 1986; 46:4665-4671.

58. Berchuck A, Rodriguez G, Olt G et al. Regulation of growth of normal ovarian epithelial cells and ovarian cancer cell lines by transforming growth factor-β. Am J Obstet Gynecol 1992; 166:676-684.

59. Wyllie FS, Dawson T, Bond JA et al. Correlated abnormalities of transforming growth factor β1 response and p53 expression in thyroid epithelial cell transformation. Mol Cell Endocrinol 1991; 76:13-21.

60. Coffey Jr RJ, Kost LJ, Lyons RM et al. Hepatic processing of transforming growth factor β in the rat. Clin Invest 1987; 80:750-757.

61. Kurokowa M, Lynch K, Podolsky DK. Effects of growth factors on an intestinal epithelial cell line: Transforming growth factor β inhibits proliferation and stimulates differentiation.Biochem Biophys Res Commun 1987; 142:775-782.

62. Barnard JA, Beauchamp RD, Coffey RJ et al. Regulation of intestinal epithelial cell growth by transforming growth factor type beta. Proc Natl Acad Sci USA 1989; 86:1578-1582.
63. Roberts AB, Sporn M. Peptide growth factors and their receptors. In: Sporn M, Roberts A, eds. Handbook of Experimental Pharmacology. Heidelberg: Springer, 1990:419-472.
64. Park K, Kim S-J, Bang Y-J et al. Genetic changes in the transforming growth factor β type II receptor gene in human gastric cancer cells: Correlation with sensitivity to growth inhibition by TGF-β. Proc Natl Acad Sci USA 1994; 91:8872-8876.
65. Migdalska A, Molineux G, Demuynck H et al. Growth inhibitory effects of TGF-β1 in vivo. Growth Factors 1991; 4:239-245.
66. Avery A, Paraskeva C, Hall P et al. TGF-β expression in the colon: Differential immunostaining along crypt epithelium. Br J Cancer 1993; 68:137-139.
67. Glick AB, McCune BK, Abdulkarem N et al. Complex regulation of TGF-β expression by retinoic acid in the vitamin-A deficient rat. Dev 1991; 111:1081-1086.
68. Shipley GD, Pittelkow MR, Wille Jr JJ et al. Reversible inhibition of normal human prokeratinocyte proliferation by type β transforming growth factor growth inhibitor in serum-free medium. Cancer Res 1986; 46:2068-2071.
69. Knabbe C, Lippman ME, Wakefield LM et al. Evidence that transforming growth factor β is a hormonally regulated negative growth factor in human breast cancer cells. Cell 1987; 48:417-428.
70. Masui T, Wakefield LM, Lechner JF et al. Type β transforming growth factor is the primary differentiation-inducing serum factor for normal bronchial epithelial cells. Proc Natl Acad Sci USA 1986; 83:2438-2442.
71. Coffey Jr RJ, Sipes NJ, Bascom CC et al. Growth modulation of mouse keratinocytes by transforming growth factors. Cancer Res 1988; 48:1596-1602.
72. Moses HL, Tucker RF, Leof EB et al. Type β transforming growth factor is a growth stimulator and a growth inhibitor. Cancer Cells 1985; 3:65-71.
73. Goustin AS, Leof EB, Shipley GD et al. Growth factors and cancer. Cancer Res 1986; 46:1015-1029.
74. Roberts AB, Thompson NL, Heine U et al. Transforming growth factor β: Possible roles in carcinogenesis. Br J Cancer 1988; 57:594-600.
75. Roberts AR, Anzono MA, Wakefield LA et al. Type beta transfroming growth factor: A bifunctional regulator of cellular growth. Proc Natl Acad Sci USA 1984; 82:119-123.
76. Fan D, Chakrabarty S, Seid C et al. Clonal stimulation or inhibition of human colon carcinomas and human renal carcinomas mediated by transforming growth factor β1. Cancer Comm 1989; 1:117-125.
77. Suardet L, Gaide A-C, Calmes J-M et al. Responsiveness of three newly established human colorectal cancer cell ines to transforming growth factors β1 and β2. Cancer Res 1992; 52:3705-3712.
78. Wang J, Sun L, Myeroff L et al. Demonstration that mutation of the type II transforming growth factor β receptor inactivates its tumor suppressor activity in replication error-positive colon carcinoma cells. JBC 1995; 270:22044-22049.
79. Williams AC, Hague A, Elder DJE et al. In vitro models for studying colorectal carcinogenesis: Cellular and molecular events including APC and Rb cleavage in the control of proliferation, differentiation and apoptosis. BBA 1996; 1288:F9-F19.
80. Haddows S, Fowlis DJ, Parkinson K et al. Loss of growth control by TGF-β1 occurs at a late stage of mouse skin carcinogenesis and is independent of ras gene activation. Oncogene 1991; 6:1465-1470.
81. Hubbs AF, Hahn FF, Thomassen DG. Increased resistance to transforming growth factor beta accompanies neoplastic progression of rat tracheal epithelial cells. Carcinogenesis 1989; 10:1599-1605.
82. Terzaghi-Howe M. Changes in response to, and production of, transforming growth factor beta during neoplastic progression in cultured rat tracheal epithelial cells. Carcinogenesis 1989; 10:973-980.
83. Farr CJ, Marshall CJ, Easty DJ et al. A study of ras gene mutations in colonic adenomas from familial polyposis coli patients. Oncogene 1988; 3:673-678.

84. Bos JL, Fearon ER, Hamilton SR et al. Prevalence of ras gene mutations in human colorectal cancers. Nature 1987; 327:293-297.
85. Forrester K, Al,oguera C, Han Ket al. Detection of high incidence of Ki-ras oncogenes during human colon tumourigenesis. Nature 1987; 327:298-303.
86. Houck KA, Michalopoulos GK, Strom SC. Introduction of a Ha-ras oncogene into rat liver epithelial cells and parenchymal hepatocytes confers resistance to the growth inhibitory effects of TGF-β. Oncogene 1989; 4:19-25.
87. Longstreet M, Miller B, Howe PH. Loss of transforming growth factor β1 (TGF-β1) induced growth arrest and p34cdc2 regulation in ras-transfected epithelial cells. Oncogene 1992; 7:1549-1556.
88. Filmus J, Zhao J, Buick RN. Overexpression of Ha-ras oncogene induces resistance to the growth-inhibitory action of transforming growth factor beta 1 (TGF-β1) and alters the number and type of TGF-β1 receptors in rat intestinal epithelial cell clones. Oncogene 1992; 7:521-526.
89. Parkinson K, Balmain A. Chalones revisited-a possible role for transforming growth factor β in tumor promotion. Carcinogenesis 1990; 11:1950198.
90. Rodrigues NR, Rowan A, Smith MEF et al. P53 mutations in colorectal cancer. Proc Natl Acad Sci USA 1990; 87:7555-7559.
91. Baker SJ, Markowitz S, Fearon ER et al. Suppression of human colorectal carcinoma cell growth by wild-type p53. Science 1990; 249:912-915.
92. Goyette MC, Cho K, Fasching CL et al. Progression of colorectal cancer is associated with multiple tumor suppressor gene defects but inhibition of tumorigenicity is accomplished by correction of any single defect via chromosome transfer. Mol Cell Biol 1992; 12:1387-1395.
93. Gerwin BI, Spillare E, Forrester K et al. Mutant p53 can induce tumorigenic conversion of human bronchial epithelial cells and reduce their responsiveness to a negative growth factor, transforming growth factor beta 1. Proc Natl Acad Sci USA 1992; 89:2759-2763.
94. Reiss M, Vellucci VF, Zhou Z-L. Mutant p53 tumor suppressor gene causes resistance to transforming growth factor β1 in murine keratinocytes. Cancer Res 1993; 53:899-904.
95. Williams AC, Browne SJ, Manning AM et al. Transfection and expression of mutant p53 protein does not alter the in vivo or in vitro growth characteristics of the AA/C1 human adenoma derived cell line, including sensitivity to transforming growth factor-β1. Oncogene 1994; 9:1479-1485.
96. Williams AC, Miller JC, Collard TJ et al. Mutant p53 is not fully dominant over endogenous wild type p53 in a colorectal adenoma cell line as demonstrated by induction of MDM2 protein and retention of a p53 dependent G1 arrest after γ irradiation. Oncogene 1995; 11:141-149.
97. Forrester K, Lupold SE, Ott VL et al. Effects of p53 mutants in wild-type p53-mediated transactivation are cell type dependent. Oncogene 1995; 10:2103-2111.
98. Sporn MB, Roberts AB. Peptide growth factors are multifunctional. Nature 1988; 332:217-219.
99. Markowitz SD, Roberts AB. Tumor suppressor activity of the TGF-β pathway of human cancers. Cytokine and Growth Factor Reviews 1996; 7(1):93-102.
100. Alexandrow MG, Moses HL. Transforming growth factor β and cell cycle regulation. Cancer Res 1995; 55:1452-1457.
101. Wakefield LM, Smith DM, Masui T et al. Distribution and modulation of the cellular receptor for transforming growth factor beta. J Cell Biol 1987; 105:965-975.
102. Kimchi A, Wang X-F, Weinberg RA et al. Absence of TGF-β receptors and growth inhibitory responses in retinoblastoma cells. Science 1988; 240:196-199.
103. Damstrup L, Rygaard K, Spang-Thomsen M et al. Expression of transforming growth factor beta receptors and expression of TGF-beta 1, TGF beta 2, TGF-beta 3 in human small cell lung cancer cell lines. Br J Cancer 1993; 67:1015-1021.
104. Norgaard P, Damstrup L Rygaard K et al. Growth suppression by transforming growth factor beta 1 of human small-cell lung cancer cell lines is associated with expression of the type II receptor. Br J Cancer 1994; 69:802-808.

105. Sun L, Wu G, Willson JKV et al. Expression of transforming growth factor β type II receptor leads to reduced malignancy in human breast cancer MCF-7 cells. JBC 1994; 269:26449-26455.
106. Markowitz S, Wang J, Myeroff L et al. Inactivation of the type II TGF-β receptor in colon cancer cells with microsatellite instability. Science 1995; 268:1336-1338.
107. Wrana JL, Attisano L, Wieser R et al. Mechanism of activation of the TGF-β receptor. Nature 1994; 370:341-347.
108. Massague J, Weis-Garcia F. Serine/threonine kinase receptors: Mediators of transfoming growth factor beta family signals. Cancer Surveys 1996: 27:41-64.
109. Takenoshita S, Tani M, Nagashima M et al. Mutation analysis of coding sequences of the entire transforming growth factor beta type II receptor gene in sporadic human colon cancer using genomic DNA and intron primers. Oncogene 1997; 14:1255-1258.
110. Eshelman J, Markowitz S. Microsatellite instability in inherited and sporadic neoplasms. Curr Opin Oncol 1995; 7:83-89.
111. Han H-J, Yanagisawa A, Kato Y et al. Genetic instability in pancreatic cancer and poorly differentiated types of gastric cancer. Cancer Res 1993; 53:5087-5089.
112. Risinger JI, Berchuck A, Kohler MF et al. Genetic instability of microsatellites in endometrial carcinoma. Cancer Res 1993; 53:48-53.
113. Thibodeau SN, Bren G, Schaid D. Microsatellite instability in cancer of the proximal colon. Science 1993; 260:816-819.
114. Ionov Y, Peinado MA, Malkhosyan S et al. Ubiquitous somatic mutations in simple repeated sequences reveal a new mechanism for colonic carcinogenesis. Nature 1993; 363:558-561.
115. Kim H, Jen J, Vogelstein B et al. Clinical and pathological characteristics of sporadic colorectal carcinomas with DNA replication errors in microsatellite sequences. Am J Path 1994; 145:148-156.
116. Liu B, Nicolaides N Markowitz S et al. Mismatch repair gene defects in sporadic colorectal cancers with microsatellite instability. Nature Genet 1995; 9:48-53.
117. Samowitz WS, Slattery MS, Kerber RA. Microsatellite instability in human colonic cancer is not a useful indicator of familial colorectal cancer. Gastroenterology 1995; 109:1765-1771.
118. Parsons R, Myeroff LL, Liu B et al. Microsatellite instability and mutations of the transforming growth factor β type II receptor gene in colorectal cancer. Cancer Res 1995; 55:5548-5550.
119. Konishi M, Kikuchi-Yanoshita R, Tanaka K et al. Molecular nature of colon tumors in hereditary nonpolyposis colon cancer, familial polyposis, and sporadic colon cancer. Gastroenterology 1996; 111:307-317.
120. Akiyama Y, Iwanaga R, Ishikawa et al. Mutations of the transforming growth factor-β type II receptor gene are strongly related to sporadic proximal colon carcinomas with microsatellite instability. Cancer 1996; 78:2478-2484.
121. Akiyama Y, Iwanaga R, Saitoh K et al. Transforming growth factor β receptor gene mutations in adenomas from hereditary nonpolyposis colorectal cancer. Gastroenterology 1997; 112:33-39.
122. Myeroff LL, Parsons R, Kim S-J et al. A transforming growth factor β receptor type II gene mutation common in colon and gastric but rare in endometrial cancers with microsatellite instability. Cancer Res 1995; 55:5545-5547.
123. Samowitz WS, Slattery ML. Transforming growth factor-β receptor type 2 mutations and microsatellite instability in sporadic colorectal adenoma and carcinomas. Am J Path 1997; 151(1):33-35.
124. Wang J, Han WXW et al. Reduced expression of transforming growth factor-β type 1 receptor contributes to the malignancy of human colon carcinoma cells. J Biol Chem 1996; 271(29):17366-17371.
125. Hahn SA et al. DPC4, a candidate tumor suppressor gene at human chromosome 18q21.1 Science 1996; 271:350-353.
126. Riggins GJ, Kinzler KW, Vogelstein B et al. Frequency of Smad gene mutations in human cancers. Cancer Res 1997; 57:2578-2580.

127. Heldin C-H, Miyazono K, ten Dijke P. TGF-β signalling from cell membrane to nucleus through SMAD proteins. Nature 1997; 390:465-471.
128. Massague J, Hata A, Liu F. TGF-β signalling through the Smad pathway. Trends in Cell Biology 1997; 7:187-192.
129. Nakao A, Afrakhte M, Moren A et al. Identification of Smad7, a TGF-β inducible antagonist of TGF-β signalling. Nature 1997; 389:631-635.
130. Imamura T, Takase M, Nishihara A et al. Smad6 inhibits signalling by the TGF-β superfamily. Nature 1997; 389:622-626.
131. Kretzschmar M, Doody J, Massague J. Opposing BMP and EGF signalling pathways converge on the TGF-β family member Smad1. Nature 1997; 389:618-622.
132. Thiagalingam S, Lengauer C, Leach FS et al. Evaluation of chromosome 18q in colorectal cancers. Nat Genet 1996; 13:343-346.
133. Zhang Y, Feng X-H, Wu R-Y et al. Receptor-associated Mad homologues synergize as effectors of the TGF-β response. Nature 1996; 383:168-172.
134. Schutte M, Hruban RH, Hedrick L et al. DPC4 gene in various tumor types. Cancer Res 1996; 56:2527-2530.
135. DeCaestecker MP, Hemmati P, Larisch-Bloch S et al. Characterization of functional domains within Smad4/DPC4. JBC 1997; 272(21):13690-13696.
136. Eppert K, Scherer SW, Ozcellk H et al. MADR2 maps to 18q21 and encodes a TGFβ-regulated MAD-related protein that is functionally mutated in colorectal carcinoma. Cell 1996; 86:543-552.
137. Tanaka K, Oshimura M, Kikuchi R et al. Suppression of tumorigenicity in human colon carcinoma cells by introduction of normal chromosomes 5 or 18. Nature 1991; 349:340-342.
138. Shaw P, Bovey R, Tardy S et al. Induction of apoptosis by wild-type p53 in a human colon tumor-derived cell line. Proc Natl Acad Sci USA 1992; 89:4495-4499.
139. Gavrieli Y, Sherman Y, Ben-Sasson SA. Identification of programmed cell death in situ via specific labeling of nuclear DNA fragmentation. J Cell Biol 1992; 119:493-501.
140. Hall PA, Coates PJ, Ansari B et al. Regulation of cell number in the mammalian gastrointestinal tract: The importance of apoptosis. J Cell Sci 1994; 107:3569-3577.
141. Bedi A, Pasricha PJ, Akhtar AJ et al. Inhibition of apoptosis during development of colorectal cancer. Cancer Res 1995; 55: 1811-1816.
142. Jass JR. Diet, butyric acid and differentiation of gastrointestinal tract tumours. Medical Hypotheses 1985; 18:113-118.
143. Evan GI, Wyllie AH, Gilbert CS et al. Induction of apoptosis in fibroblasts by c-myc protein. Cell 1992; 69:119-128.
144. Fazeli A, Steen RG, Dickinson SL et al. Effects of p53 mutations on apoptosis in mouse intestinal and human colonic adenomas. Proc Natl Acad Sci USA 1997; 94:10199-10204.
145. Vaux DL, Corys S, Adams JM. Bcl-2 gene promotes haemopoietic cell survival and cooperates with c-myc to immortalise pre-B cells. Nature 1988; 335:440-442.
146. Korsmeyer SJ. Bcl-2: A repressor of lymphocyte death. Immunology Today 1992; 13:285-287.
147. Lipkin M, Higgins P. Biological markers of cell proliferation and differentiation in human gastrointestinal diseases. Adv Cancer Res 1988; 50:1-24.
148. McCall CA, Cohen JJ. Programmed cell death in terminally differentiating keratinocytes: Role of the endonuclease. J Invest Dermatol 1991; 97:111-114.
149. Frisch SM, Francis H. Disruption of epithelial cell-matrix interactions induces apoptosis. JCB 1994; 124:619-626.
150. Raff MC. Social controls on cell survival and cell death. Nature 1992; 356:397-400.
151. Chakrabarty S, Tobon A, Varani J et al. Induction of carcinoembryonic antigen secretion and modulation of protein secretion/expression and fibronectin/laminin expression in human colon carcinoma cells by transforming growth factor β1. Cancer Res 1988; 48:4059-4064.
152. Chakrabarty S, Jan Y, Brattain MG et al. Diverse cellular responses elicited from human colon carcinoma cells by transforming growth factor beta 1. Cancer Res 1989; 49:2112-2117.

153. Schroy P, Rifkin J, Cofffey RJ et al. Role of transforming growth factor beta in induction of colon carcinoma differentiation by hexamethylene bisacetamide. Cancer Res 1990; 50:261-265.
154. Butt AJ, Hague A, Paraskeva C. Induction of E-cadherin protein expression by sodium butyrate but not TGFβ in human colorectal adenoma and carcinoma-derived cell lines: Evidence for differentiation dependent and independent pathways to apoptosis. Cell Death and Diff 1997; 4:725-732.
155. Hafez MM, Infante D, Winwaer S et al. Transforming growth factor beta acts as an autocrine negative growth regulator in colon enterocytic differentiation but not in goblet cell maturation. Cell Growth Diff 1990; 1:617-626.
156. Planchon SM, Martins CAP, Guerrant RL et al. Regulation of intestinal epithelial barrier function by TGF-β1. J Immunol 1994; 153:5730-5739.
157. Kyprianou N, Isaacs JT. Expression of transforming growth factor in the rat ventral prostrate during castration-induced programmed cell death. Mol Endocrinol 1989; 3:1515-1522.
158. Rotello RJ, Lieberman RC, Purchio AF et al. Coordinated regulation of apoptosis and cell proliferation by transforming growth factor β1 in cultured uterine epithelial cells. Proc Natl Acad Sci USA 1991; 88:3412- 3415.
159. Oberhammer F, Bursch W, Parzefall W et al. Effect of transforming growth factor β on cell death of cultured rat hepatocytes. Cancer Res 1991; 51:2478-1485.
160. Lin J-K, Chou C-K. In vitro apoptosis in the human hepatoma cell line induced by transforming growth factor β1. Cancer Res 1992; 52:385-388.
161. Yanighara, Tsumuraya M. Transforming growth factor β1 induces apoptotic death in cultured human gastric carcinoma cells. Cancer Res 1992; 52:4042-4045.
162. Bursch W, Oberhammer F, Jirtle RL et al. Transforming growth factor β1 as a signal for induction of cell death by apoptosis. Br J Cancer 1993; 67:531-536.
163. Hague A, Manning AM, Hanlon KA et al. Sodium butyrate induces apoptosis in human colonic tumor cell lines in a p53-independent pathway-implications for the possible role of dietary fibre in the prevention of large bowel cancer. Int J Cancer 1993; 55:498-595.
164. Heerdt BG, Houston MA, Augenlicht LH. Potentiation by specific short-chain fatty acids of differentiation and apoptosis in human colonic adenoma cell lines. Cancer Res 1994; 54:3288-3294.
165. Arends MJ, Wyllie AH. Apoptosis: Mechanisms and roles in pathology. International Rev Exp Path 1991; 32:223-254.
166. Wyllie AH. Glucocorticoid-induced thymocyte apoptosis is associated with endogenous endonuclease activation. Nature 1980; 284:555-556.
167. Hockenberry D, Nunez G, Milliman C et al. Bcl-2 is an inner mitochondrial membrane protein that blocks programmed cell death. Nature 1990; 348:334-336.
168. Hague A, Moorghen M, Hicks DJ et al. Bcl-2 expression in human colorectal adenomas and carcinomas. Oncogene 1994; 9:3367-3370.
169. Krajewski S, Krajewska M, Shabaik A et al. Immunohistochemical determination of in vivo distribution of Bax, a dominant inhibitor of Bcl-2. Am J Pathol 1994; 145:1323-1336.
170. Krajewski S, Krajewska M, Reed JC. Immunohistochemical analysis of in vivo patterns of Bak expression, a proapoptotic member of the Bcl-2 protein family. Cancer Res 1996; 56:2849-2855.
171. Sinicrope FA, Ruan SB, Cleary KR et al. Bcl-2 and p53 oncoprotein expression during colorectal tumorigenesis. Cancer Res 1995; 55:237-241.
172. Watson AJM, Merritt AJ, Jones LS et al. Evidence for reciprocity of bcl-2 and p53 expression in human colorectal adenoma and carcinomas. Br J Cancer 1996; 73:889-895.
173. Oltvai ZN, Milliman CL, Korsmeyer SJ. Bcl-2 heterodimerizes in vivo with a conserved homolog, Bax, that accelerates programmed cell death. Cell 1993; 74:609-619.
174. Selvakumaran M, Lin H-K, Sijm RTT et al. The novel primary response gene MyDII8 and the protooncogenes myb, myc and bcl-2 modulate transforming growth factor β1-induced apoptosis of myeloid leukemia cells. Mol Cell Biol 1994; 14:2352-2360.
175. Giannini GE, Clementi R, Ceci G et al. Expression of a ryanodine receptor-Ca^{2+} channel that is regulated by TGF-beta. Science 1992; 257:91-94.

176. Muldoon LL, Rodland KD, Magun BE. Transforming growth factor β and epidermal growth factor alter calcium influx and phosphatidylinositol turnover in rat-1 fibroblasts. J Biol Chem 1988; 263:18834-18841.

177. Reiss M, Lipsey LR, Zhou Z-L. Extracellular calcium-dependent regulation of transmembrane calcium fluxes in murine keratinoytes. J Cell Physiol 1991; 147:281-291.

178. Marin MC et al. Apoptosis suppression by Bcl-2 is correlated with the regulation of nuclear and cytosolic Ca^{2+}. Oncogene 1996; 12:2259-2266.

179. Lam M, Dubyak G, Chen L et al. Evidence that Bcl-2 represses apoptosis by regulating endoplasmic reticulum-associated Ca^{2+} fluxes. Proc Natl Acad Sci USA 1994; 91:6659-6573.

180. Murphy AN, Bredesen DE, Cortopassi G et al. Bcl-2 potentiates the maximal calcium uptake capacity of neural cell mitochondria. Proc Natl Acad Sci USA 1996; 93:9893-9898.

181. Kroemer G. The protooncogene Bcl-2 and its role in regulating apoptosis. Nature Med 1997; 3(6):614-620.

182. Heine UI, Burmester J, Flanders KC et al. Localization of transforming growth factor-β1 in mitochondria of murine heart and liver. Cell Regulation 1991; 2:467-477.

183. Sporn MB, Roberts AB. Transforming growth factor-β: Recent progress and new challenges. JCB 1992; 119(5):1017-1021.

184. Kastan MB, Onyekwere O, Sidransky D et al. Participation of p53 protein in the cellular response to DNA damage. Cancer Res 1991; 51:6304-6311.

185. Kuerbitz SJ, Plunkett BS, Walsh WV et al. Wild-type p53 is a cell cycle checkpoint determinant following irradiation. Proc Natl Acad Sci USA 1992; 89:7491-7495.

186. Fritsche M, Haessler C, Brandner G. Induction of nuclear accumulation of the tumor suppressor protein p53 by DNA damaging agents. Oncogene 1993; 8:307-318.

187. Yonish-Rouach E, Resnitzky D, Lotem J et al. Wild-type p53 induces apoptosis of myeloid leukaemic cells that is inhibited by interleukin-6. Nature 1991; 352:345-347.

188. Lane DP. P53, guardian of the genome. Nature 1992; 358:15-16.

189. Carder P, Wyllie AH, Purdie CA et al. Stabilised p53 facilitates aneuploid clonal divergence in colorectal cancer. Oncogene 1993; 8:1397-1401.

190. Clarke AR, Purdie CA, Harrison DJ et al. Thymocyte apoptosis induced by p53 dependent and independent pathways. Nature 1993; 362:849-852.

191. Lowe SW, Schmitt EM, Smith SW et al. P53 is required for radiation-induced apoptosis in mouse thymocytes. Nature 1993; 362:847-849.

192. Bracey TS, Miller JC, Preece A et al. g-Radiation induced apoptosis in human colorectal adenoma and carcinoma cell lines can occur in the absence of wild type p53. Oncogene 1995; 10:2391-2396.

193. Kerbel RS, Waghome C, Korczak B et al. Clonal dominance of primary tumors by metastatic cells: Genetic analysis and biological implications. Cancer Surveys 1988; 7:597-629.

194. Yan Z, Hsu S, Winawer S et al. Transforming growth factor β1 (TGF-β1) inhibits retinoblastoma gene expression but not pRB phosphorylation in TGF-β1-growth stimulated colon carcinoma cells. Oncogene 1992; 7:801-805.

195. Hague A, Manning AM, van der Stappen JWJ et al. Escape from negative regulation of growth by transforming growth factor β and from the induction of apoptotsis by the dietary agent sodium butyrate may be important in colorectal carcinogenesis. Cancer Met Rev 1993; 12:227-237.

196. Schroy PC, Carnright K, Winawer SJ et al. Heterogenous responses of human colon carcinomas to hexamethylene bisacetamide. Cancer Res 1988; 48:5487-5494.

197. Hsu S, Huang F, Hafez M et al. Colon carcinoma cells switch their response to transforming growth factor β1 with tumor progression. Cell Growth and Diff 1994; 5:267-275.

198. Jetten AM, Shirley JE, Stoner G. Regulation of proliferation and differentiation of respiratory tract epithelial cells by TGF-β1. Exp Cell Res 1986; 167:539-549.

199. Schwartz LC, Gingras M-C, Goldberg G et al. Loss of growth factor dependence and conversion of transforming growth factor β1 inhibition to stimulation in metastatic Ha-ras transformed murine fibroblasts. Cancer Res 1988; 48:6999-7003.

200. Yan Z, Winawer S, Friedman E. Two different signal transduction pathways can be activated by transfoming growth factor β1 in epithelial cells. JBC 1994; 269(18):13231-13237.

201. Cui W et al. TGFβ1 inhibits the formation of benign skin tumors, but enhances progression to invasive spindle carcinoma in transgenic mice. Cell 1996; 86:531-542.
202. Ookawak K, Sakamoto M, Hirohashi S et al. Concordant p53 and DCC alterations and allelic losses on chromosomes 13q and 14q associated with liver metastases of colorectal carcinoma. Int J Cancer 1993; 53:382-387.
203. Nathan C, Sporn MB. Cytokines in context. J Cell Biol 1991; 113:981-986.
204. Theodorescu D, Sheenan C, Kerbel RS. TGF-β gene expression depends on tissue architecture In Vitro. Dev Biol 1993; 29A:105-108.
205. Peres R, Betsholtz C, Westermark B et al. Frequent expression of growth factors for mesenchymal cells in human mammary carcinoma cell lines. Cancer Res 1987; 47:3425-3429.
206. Lieubeau B, Garrigue L, Barbieux I et al. The role of transforming growth factor β1 in the fibroblastic reaction associated with rat colorectal tumor development. Cancer Res 1994; 54:6526-6532.
207. Ignotz RA, Massague J. Transforming growth factor β stimulates the expression of fibronectin and collagen and their incorporation into the extracellular matrix. J Biol Chem 1986; 261:4337-4345.
208. Pignatelli M, Bodmer WF. Integrin cell adhesion molecules and colorectal cancer. J Path 1990; 162:95-97.
209. Nugent MA, Newman MJ. Inhibition of normal rat kidney growth by transforming growth factor β is mediated by collagen. J Biol Chem 1989; 264:18060-18067.
210. Chakrabarty S, Fan D, Varani J. Modulation of differentiation and proliferation in human colon carcinoma cells by transforming growth factor beta 1 and 2. Int J Cancer 1990; 46:493-499.
211. Massague J. The transforming growth factor β family. Annu Rev Cell Biol 1990; 6:597-641.
212. Huang S, Chakrabarty S. Regulation of fibronectin and laminin receptor expression, fibronectin and laminin secretion in human colon cancer cells by transforming growth factor-β1. Int J Cancer 1994; 57:742-746.
213. Chakrabarty S. Role of protein kinase C in transforming growth factor β1 induction of carcinoembryonic antigen in human colon carcinoma cells. J Cell Physiol 1992; 152P494-499.
214. Welch DR, Fabra A, Nakajima M. Transforming growth factor β stimulates mammary adenocarcinoma cell invasion and metastatic potential. Proc Natl Acad Sci USA 1990; 87:7678-7682.
215. Arrick BA, Lopez AR, Elfman F et al. Altered metabolic and adhesive properties and increased tumorigenesis associated with increased expression of transforming growth factor β1. JCB 1992; 118:715-726.
216. Torre-Amoine G, Beauchamp RD, Koeppen H et al. A highly immunogenic tumour transfected with a murine transforming growth factor type β1 cDNA escapes immune surveillance. Proc Natl Acad Sci USA 1990; 87:1486-1490.
217. Wiseman DM, Polverini PJ, Kamp DW et al. Transforming growth factor beta (TGF-β) is chemotactic for human monocytes and induces their expression of angiogenic activity. Biochem Biophys Res Commun 1988; 157:793-800.
218. Arteaga CL, Carty-Dugger T, Moses H et al. Transforming growth factor-β(1) can induce estrogen-independent tumorigenicity of human breast cancer cells in athymic mice. Cell Growth Differ 1993; 4:193-201.
219. Boyd JA, Kaufman DG. Expression of transforming growth factor β1 by human endometrial carcinoma cell lines: Inverse correlation with effects on growth rate and morphology. Cancer Res 1990; 50:3394-3399.
220. Pierce Jr DF, Gorska AE, Chytil A et al. Mammary tumor suppression by transforming growth factor β1 transgene expression. Proc Natl Acad Sci USA 1995; 92:4254-4258.
221. Glick AB, Kulkarni AB, Tennenbaum T et al. Loss of expression of transforming growth factor β in skin and skin tumors is associated with hyperproliferation and a high risk for malignant conversion. Proc Natl Acad Sci USA 1993; 90:6076-6080.

222. Glick AB, Lee MM, Darwiche N et al. Targeted deletion of the TGF-β1 gene causes rapid progression to squamous cell carcinoma. Genes Devel 1994; 8:2429-2440.
223. Anzano MA, Roberts AB, De Larco JE et al. Increased secretion of type β transforming growth factor accompanies viral transformation of cells. Mol Cell Biol 1985; 5:242-247.
224. Derynck R, Goeddel DV, Allrich A et al. Synthesis of messenger RNAs for transforming growth factors alpha and beta and the epidermal growth factor receptor by human tumors. Cancer Res 1987; 47:707-712.
225. Sporn MB, Roberts AB, Wakefield LM et al. Some recent advances in the chemistry and biology of transforming growth factor beta. J Cell Biol 1987; 105:1039-1045.
226. Gorsch SM, Memoli VA, Stukei TA et al. Immunohistochemial staining for TGF-β1 associates with disease progression in human breast cancer. Camcer Res 1992; 52:6949-6952.
227. Kawamata H, Azuma M, Kameyama S et al. Effect of epidermal growth factor, transforming growth factor alpha, and transforming growth factor β1 on growth in vitro of rat urinary bladder carcinoma cells. Cell Growth and Differ 1992; 3:819-825.
228. Marrogi AJ, Munshi A, Merogi AJ et al. Study of tumor infiltrating lymphocytes and transforming growth factor-β as prognostic factors in breast carcinoma. Int J Cancer 1997; 74:492-501.
229. Bishop DT, Thomas HJW. The genetics of colorectal cancer. Cancer Surveys 1990; 9:585-604.
230. Goey H, Keller JR, Back T et al. Inhibiton of early murine haemopoeitic progenitor cell proliferation after in vivo locoregional administration of transforming growth factor beta 1. J Immunol 1989; 43:877-880.
231. Newman MJ. Inhibition of carcinoma and melanoma cell growth by type I transforming growth factor β is dependent on the presence of polyunsaturated fatty acids. Proc Natl Acad Sci USA 1990; 87:5543-5547.2.
232. Fesus L. Apoptosis. Immunology Today 1992; 13:A16-17.

CHAPTER 7

Role of TGFβ in Carcinogenesis and Mediation of Therapeutic Response in Breast Cancer

J.R. Benson

i) Introduction

Transforming growth factor β (TGFβ) has potent inhibitory effects upon both normal and transformed mammary epithelial cells, and malignant progression may be associated with breakdown of the autocrine and paracrine inhibitory loops in which TGFβ participates. In particular, transformed cells may at some critical stage loose their inhibitory growth response to TGFβ. Extensive in vitro studies with breast carcinoma cell lines indicate that most retain sensitivity to TGFβ growth inhibition. This may provide a window of opportunity whereby strategies based on boosting local endogenous levels of TGFβ could yield therapeutic benefit in the early stages of carcinogenesis. This chapter outlines evidence in support of TGFβ being a proximate effector in mediation of the anti-neoplastic effects of anti-estrogens and related therapeutic agents. The effects of anti-estrogens on stromal production of TGFβ is emphasized to illustrate how such agents may have clinical value irrespective of ER status of breast tumors, thereby broadening potential therapeutic targets.

A hallmark of TGFβ is its complex, pleiotropic functional profile; its growth inhibitory effects may dominate in the early stages of carcinogenesis, but as a tumor evolves, and possibly as epithelial responsiveness to autocrine inhibition wanes, TGFβ of both epithelial and stromal origin may indirectly promote tumor growth by collective enhancement of stroma formation, angiogenesis and immune suppression. The balance of these opposing influences will determine whether TGFβ declares itself as friend or foe.

ii) Anti-Estrogens

A) Clinical and Biological Actions

Anti-estrogens are primary agents of choice for the treatment of early and advanced breast cancer in both pre- and postmenopausal women, and their prophylactic application is under investigation. Clinical trials of tamoxifen as an adjuvant therapy were begun in the 1970's' and initial results indicated that tamoxifen was effective in prolonging both disease-free survival (DFS) and overall survival (OS) in postmenopausal, node-positive patients with ER rich tumors.[1-3] Such preliminary results were consistent with the benefits of tamoxifen in ER positive advanced disease. However, with the passage of time and recruitment

---

of increasing numbers of patients, these adjuvant studies revealed benefits of tamoxifen in other subgroups. Tamoxifen was found to significantly improve either overall[1,2] and/or disease-free survival[1-3] in node-negative patients, including premenopausal cases.[2,3] Of particular interest were the findings of the NATO and Scottish trials suggesting that the efficacy of tamoxifen was independent of ER status. In the analysis of the NATO trial after 8 years of follow up, division of patients according to ER status did not eliminate the favorable effects of tamoxifen treatment, and multi-variate regression analysis showed no significant difference between ER positive and ER negative tumors. The 1992 overview by the Early Breast Cancer trialists Collaborative Group involving 30,000 patients treated with adjuvant tamoxifen confirmed many earlier conclusions on the efficacy of adjuvant tamoxifen in various subgroups, including patients with ER 'poor' tumors.[4]

This overview demonstrated a highly significant reduction in annual rates of disease recurrence (25%) and of mortality (17%). The duration of tamoxifen therapy in most of these trials was approximately 2 years, and results suggest that longer term regimens of at least 2 years are preferable to shorter ones of 12 months. Subgroup analysis reveals that tamoxifen is effective irrespective of nodal, ER and menopausal status, and any differences are largely of a quantitative rather than qualitative nature. Thus absolute improvements in DFS and OS are greater for node positive than node negative patients as the former have greater risk of relapse. When tamoxifen is used alone in premenopausal women, the benefits in both DFS and OS are comparable to those for women over 50 years of age, although such studies lack the same statistical power.

One quarter of women in the overview analysis were ER poor (ER < 10 fmol/mg cytosol), but adjuvant tamoxifen still produces a highly significant reduction in disease recurrence (13%), though this is less than for ER rich patients (32%). Similarly, the reduction in mortality for ER poor tumors (11%) is approximately half that of ER rich tumors, but still represents a clinically significant effect. However, the overview process, by combining confounded studies (chemotherapy alone versus chemotherapy plus tamoxifen) with unconfounded studies (control versus tamoxifen) has made interpretation of these data difficult.

Therefore this meta-analysis did not identify any subgroup of patients who would fail to benefit from adjuvant tamoxifen therapy, and re-affirmed the unequivocal benefits of tamoxifen in ER negative patients, node negative patients and premenopausal patients. Moreover, the incidence of contralateral breast cancer was reduced by 39%, confirming an earlier report by Cuzik and Baum[5] and pointing to a potential prophylactic role of tamoxifen in well women. The most recent analysis of data from the EBCTCG overview (as yet unpublished) has once again demonstrated benefits of adjuvant tamoxifen in ER poor categories, though these are of more modest magnitude than suggested by previous analyses of less mature data.[6]

The original group of anti-estrogens were triphenylethylene derivatives of which tamoxifen is the dominant member and clinical prototype. Other agents within this group have relatively restricted clinical use at present and include toremifene, droloxifene and idoxifene. Like tamoxifen, these each have in common a triphenylbutene core and a basic/polar side chain (Fig. 7.1). This fundamental structure imparts a complex functional profile to this group of compounds which behave as 'impure' anti-estrogens with mixed agonist/antagonist properties at the level of interaction with the estrogen receptor (ER). Thus in addition to acting as a competitive inhibitor for the ligand binding site of the ER and thereby blocking expression of certain estrogen regulated genes, these impure anti-estrogens can invoke an attenuated transcriptional response. In the absence of ligand, ER is associated with a 90kDal heat shock protein (hsp90) which interacts with the HBD.[7] Upon ligand binding, a conformational change is induced in the HBD with release of the hsp90.[8] The ligand/ER complex can then undergo dimerization as a prelude to DNA binding.[9] These dimers bind to short palindromic sequences of DNA termed estrogen response elements (ERE) which constitute enhancers located close to oestrogen regulated genes which possess a variety of contiguous promotor sequences (Fig. 7.2).[10,11]

Following binding of the ligand/ER dimer to the ERE, efficiency of transcriptional activation is determined by the individual transactivation functions of regions A/B and E, or TAF1 and TAF2 respectively. TAF1 has constitutive transactivating function which is not dependent upon binding of ligand to HBD, in contrast to TAF2 which is only hormone inducible. This constitutive nature of TAF1 permits an attenuated and variable transcriptional response.[12,13] The palindromic structure of the ERE facilitates binding of homodimeric ER/ligand complexes.

Pure anti-estrogens which possess only antagonist activity, bind to the ER and prevent any dimerization and hence DNA binding.[14] Therefore no activation of any estrogen responsive genes occurs. By contrast, impure anti-estrogens with some agonist activity, permit dimerization and DNA binding,[14] and despite defective signaling from TAF2 (hormone inducible), can promote transcription through the constitutive function of TAF1. Hence impure anti-estrogens are unable to evoke a full transcriptional response, but can induce expression of some genes normally stimulated by estrogens.[15] At present, few such genes have been identified, but impure anti-estrogens can both simultaneously inhibit and promote expression of estrogen regulated genes within the same cell. These intrinsic agonist properties may ultimately compromise the anti-tumor efficacy of these agents, and the newer 'pure' anti-estrogens which act exclusively as antagonists may offer clinical advantages.[16] Though much experimental and clinical data testifies to anti-estrogens mediating their effects principally via the ER, not all of the anti-tumor effects of tamoxifen can be accounted for by its competitive antagonism for the ligand binding site of the ER (Fig. 7.3). The clinical efficacy of tamoxifen in ER negative tumors, both in an adjuvant and to a lesser extent the advanced setting, implies the existence of ER independent pathways. In addition, tamoxifen is effective in premenopausal women despite high plasma levels of estradiol which might be expected to competitively overcome any conventional antagonist activity.[17]

Compelling evidence has now accrued for ER-independent mechanisms of action, for which enzyme inhibitory effects and paracrine growth factor modulation appear of paramount importance. Furthermore, pathways involving the conventional ER may interact with those for which ER/ligand activation is not an obligate step.

These effects may be relatively more important for 'impure' compared with 'pure' anti-estrogens, but they are not confined to compounds with a triphenylbutene core. Like tamoxifen and other triphenylethylene analogs, these pure anti-estrogens possess a side chain with basic/polar groups which have recently been shown to be essential for estrogen antagonist properties upon ER binding.[18] Nevertheless, this basic triphenylbutene structure may be partly responsible for the functional pleiotropy of impure anti-estrogens since its unique chemical structure may permit interaction with multiple and varied effector systems, not just those dependent upon ER interaction.

Evidence for a possible non-ER mediated effect of anti-estrogens first emerged from the work of Sutherland and colleagues who found a biphasic inhibition of MCF-7 cell growth, with an estrogen reversible effect at lower concentrations (up to 1μM) but an oestrogen-irreversible inhibition at higher concentrations of tamoxifen (2.5–10 μM).[17,19] They also identified anti-estrogen binding sites (AEBS) which appeared to be specific for anti-estrogens.[20] However, saturation levels did not correlate with physiological response, questioning their significance.

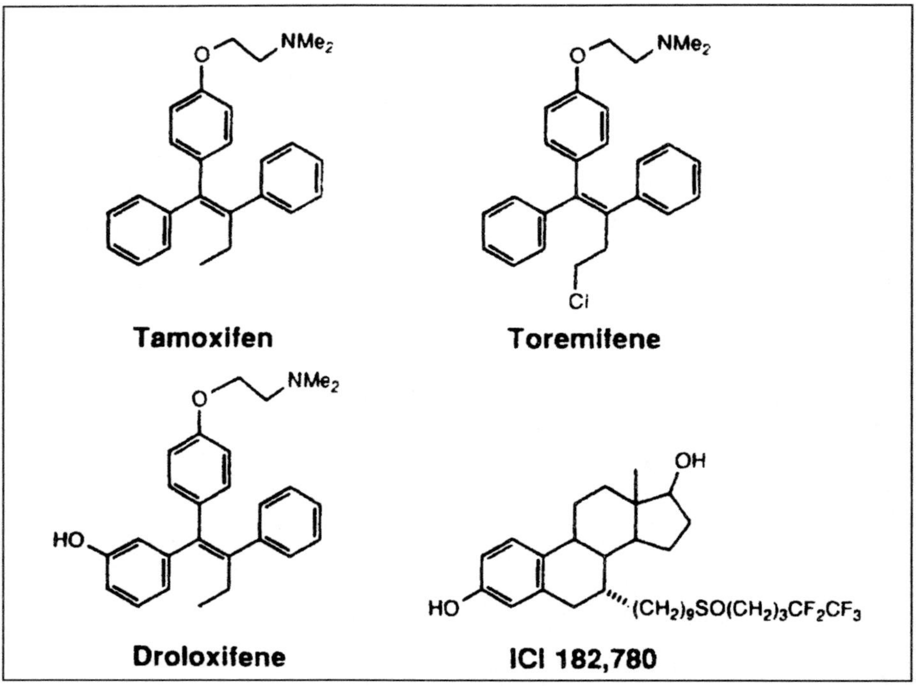

Fig. 7.1. Chemical structure of the triphenylethylene anti-estrogens. All compounds share the common feature of a triphenylbutene core together with a basic/polar side chain and possess both estrogenic antagonist and agonist properties at the level of the ER. Modifications of this fundamental structure yield agents with differing relative actions and hence anti-tumor, ureterotrophic and bone/cardiovascular effects. Addition The pure anti-estrogen ICI 164 384 is an estradiol derivative and is devoid of any partial agonist activity. Reprinted with permission from: Jordan VC. Breast Cancer Res Treat 1995; 31, No. 1:42. © Kluwer Academic Publishers.

The local induction of TGFβ constitutes one of these alternate modes of action of tamoxifen. Other mechanisms have been proposed and include: (a) enzyme inhibition (b) suppression of insulin-like growth factors and c) inhibition of angiogenesis.

1) Enzyme Inhibition

i) Inhibition of Protein Kinase C

Tamoxifen inhibits the enzyme protein kinase C (PKC) at micro-molar concentrations in a sub-cellular enzyme system.[21] This enzyme is a calcium and phospholipid dependent protein kinase which is normally activated by diacylglycerol, a product of hydrolysis of inositol triphosphate (IP3).[22] Evidence suggests that tamoxifen may interact with phospholipid in a competitive manner, thereby indirectly preventing activation of the enzyme. It may also interact with the regulatory domain of this enzyme, but not directly with its active site, as tamoxifen does not inhibit the Ca^{2+} and phospholipid independent function of PKC.[21,23] Growth inhibition of MCF-7 breast cancer cells by various triphenylethylene derivatives correlates with their ability to inhibit binding of radiolabeled phospholipid precursors in murine C3H/10T 1/2 cells.[23]

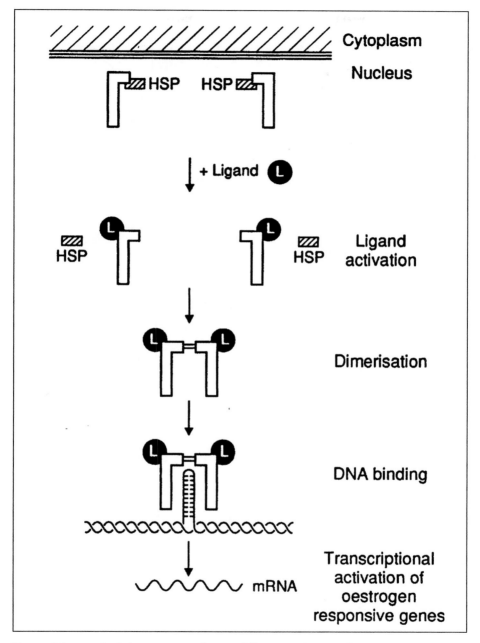

Fig. 7.2. Diagram depicting sequence of events following activation of ER by ligand, with concomitant release of heat shock protein (hsp 90). Note that receptor homodimers bind to a 13bp palindromic sequence or estrogen response element (ERE). Reprinted with permission from: Benson JR, Baum M, Colletta AA. In: deVita, Hellman, Rosenberg, eds. Biologic Therapy of Cancer, 2nd Edition. 1995:817-828. © Lippincott-Raven Publishers.

Fig. 7.3. In ER-positive cells, anti-estrogens act as competitive antagonists for the ligand binding site of the ER. "Pure" anti-estrogens completely block transcription of estrogen regulated genes, but "impure" anti-estrogens permit a partial transcriptional response driven by a constitutively active TAF-1. In ER negative cells, ER independent mechanisms for controlling estrogen responsive genes may be operative. Reprinted with permission from: Benson JR, Baum M, Colletta AA. Journal of Mammary Gland Biology and Neoplasia 1996; 1:381-389. © Plenum Publishing Corporation.

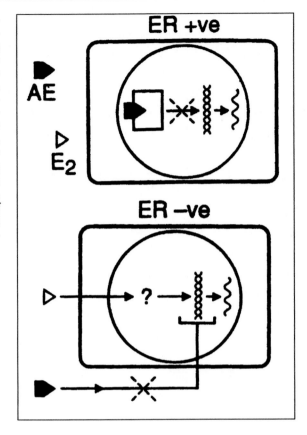

PKC participates in various pathways involved in cell proliferation and differentiation, and activation of this enzyme is likely to be a step in transduction of various cellular stimuli. Protein phosphorylation is a preeminent mechanism for regulation of extracellular stimuli. Phorbol esters, which are tumor promoters, usually stimulate PKC activity, hence interest in the apparent inhibition of this enzyme by tamoxifen. However, inhibition of PKC activity is not invariably associated with reduced proliferative activity, and enhanced PKC activity correlates with growth inhibition in MCF-7 cells.[24] Thus the precise role of PKC as a signal transducer in breast cancer cells, and the significance of any inhibition of PKC by tamoxifen remains unclear.

ii) Inhibition of Calmodulin Dependent cAMP Phosphodiesterase

Another enzyme inhibited by tamoxifen is calmodulin dependent cAMP phosphodiesterase (CPD) (Lam 1984).[25] Again, tamoxifen appears to interfere with the action of calmodulin, rather than directly inhibiting the enzyme. There is evidence that the ER and calmodulin may be involved in coupled signaling pathways controlling hormone dependent cellular proliferation.[26] The estrogen-irreversible effects of tamoxifen correlates with calmodulin inhibition in ER positive cells (Gulino et al 1986)[27] and the calmodulin antagonist, calmidazolium, blocks the MCF-7 cell cycle at the same point as tamoxifen.[28]

Therefore inhibition of CPD may only be of significance in ER positive cells, as binding of tamoxifen to the ER appears necessary for optimal inhibitory effects upon calmodulin.

2) Suppression of Insulin-Like Growth Factors

Agents such as tamoxifen may not only stimulate production and secretion of negative growth factors, but may also suppress production of positive ones such as insulin-like growth factors I and II. As discussed in the preceding chapter, there is evidence for modulation of both systemic and local levels of insulin-like growth factors by tamoxifen. [29-31] Breast tumor epithelium may participate in a positive paracrine pathway, whereby fibroblasts are stimulated by epithelial cells to secrete IGF-I and IGF-II which in turn act upon neighboring epithelial cells in a positive paracrine manner. [32] This could be a target for pharmacological suppression by tamoxifen in both ER positive and ER negative tumors as significant levels of type I IGF receptors are present in ER negative cells. [33]

3) Inhibition of Angiogenesis

Development of a tumor beyond the size of approximately 1 million cells is dependent upon an intact micro-vasculature. [34] Blood vessels not only support further tumor growth by encouraging adequate supplies of oxygen and nutrients to cells deep within a tumor bolus, but also provide opportunity for metastasis, especially as newly formed vessels tend to be fragile and leaky. Inhibition of angiogenesis is therefore a potentially important anti-tumor strategy. Tumor vessel count/grade has been correlated with lymph node status and survival, with higher vessel counts being associated with poorer clinical outcome. [35,36] Tamoxifen has been shown to inhibit angiogenesis in a chick chorio-allantoic membrane model. [37] This effect was not reversible with estrogen, suggesting an ER independent mechanism. TGFβ is a potent anti-angiogenic agent and inhibits endothelial cell mitosis, [38] and can reduce endothelial cell proliferation in the early stages of vascular regeneration following trauma. [39] In the study of Gagliardi and Collins, no measurements of TGFβ1 immunoreactivity were carried out and the role of TGFβ in mediation of this anti-angiogenic effect is purely speculative. However, tamoxifen decreases the rate of proliferation of vascular smooth muscle cells in vitro which is associated with a 50-fold increase in secretion of TGFβ into the conditioned medium. Rates of proliferation remained unchanged in the presence of anti-TGFβ antibodies, suggesting that this effect was mediated via induction of TGFβ. [40] Therefore induction of TGFβ by tamoxifen may involve not only a direct anti-proliferative effect upon epithelial cells, but also an indirect effect on tumor growth secondary to inhibition of angiogenesis. Notwithstanding these potential anti-angiogenic effects of TGFβ, in vivo developmental studies demonstrate a positive correlation between TGFβ immunoreactivity and sites of active neo-vascularization. [41] These pro-angiogenic effects of TGFβ are discussed in chapter 3 and may include indirect effects of TGFβ upon other cytokines such as fibroblast growth factor (FGF) which are liberated from fibroblasts and components of the reticulo-endothelial system such as monocytes. [42,43] Of interest, work with bovine endothelial cells in vitro have provided insight into the potential dichotomous function of TGFβ in angiogenesis. Thus TGFβ exerts growth inhibitory effects in cultures of endothelial cells which remain sub-confluent, but upon and beyond confluency, TGFβ appeared to stimulate proliferation with attempts by cells to form a quasi-network of duct-like structures. These growth promotory effects may have been encouraged by the operation of a positive autocrine loop involving TGFβ as this growth factor was secreted in active form by bovine epithelial cells. [44]

B) *Local Induction of TGFβ by Anti-Estrogens*

There is evidence from both in vivo and in vitro studies for induction of TGFβ in response to a variety of agents including anti-estrogens. When assessing the significance of any altered TGFβ expression in breast cancer it is important to distinguish between the roles of TGFβ in carcinogenesis per se, and that of mediating a response to therapeutic agents. [45]

Changes in TGFβ expression may precede or accompany neoplastic progression, or be a consequence of drug exposure. In analyzing the expression of TGFβ in breast tissue, especially in response to tamoxifen therapy, particular controversy relates to the origin of both non- and pharmacologically induced TGFβ. The following section discusses the evidence for induction of TGFβ in epithelial versus stromal tissue components.

1) Epithelial Induction of TGFβ

Both ER positive and ER negative breast cancer cell lines produce and secrete TGFβ isoforms in vitro,[46] and these cells are growth inhibited by exogenous TGFβ. This together with the ubiquity of TGFβ receptors suggests that TGFβ may participate in an autocrine inhibitory loop involving epithelial cells. Knabbe and co-workers reported that secretion of TGFβ into the conditioned media of ER positive MCF-7 cells was increased by tamoxifen, and conversely that estrogen treatment of these cells resulted in decreased levels of secretion.[47] These responses were confined to ER positive cells and the effect of tamoxifen was estrogen reversible and so presumably occurred via a classical ER mediated mechanism. ER negative cells could be growth inhibited by tamoxifen if cocultured with ER positive cells in a system permitting interchange of conditioned media. Anti-TGFβ antibodies largely abolished this effect, providing evidence that tamoxifen induced TGFβ1 from ER positive cells served as a negative paracrine factor for ER negative cells. Despite these and other in vitro studies confirming the induction of TGFβ protein in ER positive cell lines, an in vivo study by Butta and co-workers revealed no significant increase in epithelial expression of TGFβ1 in response to primary tamoxifen therapy, despite dramatic stromal induction of TGFβ1 (see section iii (b)).[48] Moreover, most immunohistochemical studies of TGFβ expression in both malignant and normal mammary tissue reveal predominantly epithelial immunoreactivity relative to expression of TGFβ1, TGFβ2 and TGFβ3 in stromal elements. However, these 'static' immunohistochemical studies may betray complex secretory dynamics in vivo, and confirm neither source nor site of action of TGFβ.[49,50]

Other discrepant data exist in relation to the role of epithelial sources of TGFβ in breast cancer. For example, ER negative cell lines, which are more tumorigenic than ER positive ones, constitutively secrete higher levels of TGFβ1. Arteaga and co-workers reported that 4 strains of ER negative breast cancer cell lines were growth inhibited by exogenous TGFβ, but 3 strains of ER positive cells with an apparent absence of TGFβ receptors showed no inhibitory response to picomolar concentrations of TGFβ.[51] Despite higher constitutive levels of secretion of TGFβ by ER negative cell lines, proliferation of these cells was enhanced in vitro with an anti-TGFβ antibody, implying the existence of a functional autocrine inhibitory loop. Similarly, in a related study, proliferation of the ER negative cell lines MDA-MB-231 and HS578T was stimulated by sera containing neutralizing anti-TGFβ1 and anti-TGFβ2 antibodies. There was concomitant upregulation of TGFβ binding sites on cells and reduced steady-state expression of TGFβ1mRNA levels.[51] MCF-7 cells transfected with the v-Ha ras oncogene exhibit enhanced growth despite a resultant increase in constitutive levels of TGFβ1,[52] and human breast cancer cells stably transfected with the TGFβ1 gene have an unaltered response to estrogen and anti-estrogens despite greatly enhanced expression of TGFβ1. Furthermore, these cells have increased tumorogenicity and display estrogen independence when grown in athymic mice.[53] A relatively high level of TGFβ1 production by these cell lines would not be expected if this growth factor is acting as a primary epithelial inhibitor. Immunohistochemical studies of breast tumors show no correlation between epithelial expression of TGFβ and ER status. Gorsch and co-workers have suggested that increased epithelial expression of TGFβ1 in vivo correlates with disease progression.[54] In their immunohistochemical study, sections of breast biopsy specimens were stained with isoform specific antibodies to TGFβ1, TGFβ2 and TGFβ3. Staining was predominantly epithelial for

TGFβ1 but stromal for TGFβ2. Univariate analysis showed a correlation between intensity of staining for TGFβ1 and disease progression (assessed as recurrence, progression or cancer related deaths). No such correlations were found for TGFβ2 or TGFβ3. Because the antibodies used in this study only recognized the intracellular form of TGFβ1, it is possible that release of epithelial TGFβ1 is defective in progressive disease and therefore higher intracellular levels would correlate with a worse prognosis. Several workers have examined TGFβ mRNA expression in both cell lines and breast tumors rather than the levels of TGFβ product. Increased TGFβ production and secretion in response to tamoxifen in MCF-7 cells and fetal fibroblasts was not associated with any concomitant increase in levels of mRNA.[47,55] This implies a post transcriptional control mechanism which may be operative in the physiological regulation of TGFβ production. Thus measurement of TGFβ mRNA levels may not be a valid reflection of TGFβ activity. Caution is therefore needed in interpretation of studies where only TGFβ mRNA levels are measured and correlated with various prognostic indices.

Thompson and co-workers found high levels of TGFβ1 gene expression in 45 out of 56 primary breast cancers, and levels were particularly high in a subgroup of patients who were resistant to tamoxifen administered in a preoperative schedule.[56] RNA was extracted from whole tumor specimens which thus contained both epithelial and stromal components. Were TGFβ mRNA to originate from the epithelial cells, then these results could suggest breakdown of a negative autocrine loop, due for example to failure of activation of TGFβ or loss of receptors. However, most cell lines demonstrate preservation of TGFβ receptors, and there is no evidence supporting widespread loss of receptors at any stage of carcinogenesis in breast cancer.

In many of these studies in which levels of TGFβ transcript have been analyzed, it is unclear whether the source of any identified TGFβ mRNA is epithelial or stromal, rendering interpretation difficult. If TGFβ were stromal in origin, then higher levels might be expected in patients receiving primary tamoxifen therapy as observed in vivo by Butta and co-workers (see section iii (b)). However, Thompson et al did not find higher tissue levels of TGFβ mRNA in patients who responded to tamoxifen therapy. Travers and co-workers examined TGFβ mRNA expression in benign and malignant breast tumors and found significantly higher levels of transcript in whole tissue samples from malignant tumors.[57] McCallum and co-workers examined expression of TGFβ1, TGFβ2 and TGFβ3 mRNA in 50 breast cancer specimens.[58] Patterns of expression between different tumors were variable, but all tumors contained at least one isoform of TGFβ. The β3 isoform was most widely expressed (94% of tumors) and TGFβ2 relatively least. Ninety percent of specimens expressed TGFβ1, and this study concluded that breast tumors expressing mRNA for all 3 isoforms of TGFβ were significantly more likely to be associated with lymph node involvement, suggesting an adverse influence of TGFβ expression in more advanced breast tumors.[59] This echoes the findings of an immunohistochemical study of 86 invasive breast carcinomas in which high levels of TGFβ1 immunoreactivity were associated with lymph node metastases and other parameters of invasive potential such as enhanced expression of tenascin and fibronectin.[60]

Expression of TGFβ isoforms following tamoxifen therapy is associated with variable and inconsistent changes, with some patients showing an increase in levels of TGFβ transcript and others a decrease.[59] In contrast to these results, Murray and co-workers measured TGFβ1 mRNA expression in breast tumor tissue from which total RNA extraction was performed.[61] Levels of TGFβ1 mRNA expression were inversely correlated with nodal status, but not with ER status, T-stage or menstrual status. Relapse-free survival was higher in patients deemed to have high TGFβ1 levels (arbitrary cut-off), but this was not an independent factor and accounted for by the correlation with nodal status. Mizukami also noted an association between higher levels of TGFβ expression and a more favorable prognosis, with a higher 2 year relapse-free survival in patients with TGFβ 'positive' tumors.[62] Like other studies with extraction of total RNA from tumor samples, these data on TGFβ mRNA expression in breast tumor tissue fail to permit any distinction between epithelial and stromal sources of TGFβ mRNA. The over-expression of TGFβ in an autocrine capacity by breast epithelial cells is difficult to reconcile with its inhibitory effects upon epithelium, and epithelial sources of TGFβ may serve primarily to promote stromal expansion (including angiogenesis) and hence tumor growth in the more advanced stages of carcinogenesis.

2) Stromal Induction of TGFβ

The counter-intuitive results of trials of adjuvant tamoxifen indicating the clinical efficacy of this anti-estrogen in ER poor tumors suggested that an ER independent mechanism of action might exist. The hypothesis was put forward that tamoxifen directly stimulates stromal fibroblasts to produce and secrete negative growth modulators which act upon neighboring epithelial cells in a negative paracrine manner (Fig. 7.4). Certain other observations contributed to formulation of this hypothesis; firstly, the timing of androgen receptor expression in the mesenchyme of the developing rodent prostate—androgen receptors are expressed on the mesenchyme of hormonally sensitive tissues prior to their expression on epithelial cells,[63] indicating that hormonal effects upon epithelial cells may be mediated indirectly via mesenchyme which possesses corresponding receptors and which alone is androgen responsive at this stage. Secondly, skin fibroblasts from patients with a family history of breast cancer display fetal-like characteristics, thus alluding to some systemic abnormality of fibroblasts[64,65] which may influence neoplastic development and/or progression or partly determine response to therapies aimed at manipulation of stromal behavior. Finally desmoids, which are pure mesenchymal tumors, undergo dramatic clinical response to tamoxifen and related triphenylethylenes, implying a direct effect of these agents upon fibroblasts.[66] Some of these observations are further elaborated in chapter 4.

Support for the hypothesis in mammary tissue is provided by experimental evidence demonstrating mesenchymal induction of the negative growth modulator TGFβ both in vitro[52] and in vivo[48] in response to tamoxifen.

Using human fetal fibroblasts as a model for breast tumor fibroblasts, secretion of the TGFβ1 isoform was shown to be increased between 3- and 30-fold by these cells in vitro in response to tamoxifen.[52] Two strains of human fetal fibroblasts (Flow 2000-lung and Flow 9000-pituitary) were exposed to sub-toxic concentrations of tamoxifen (500 nM), its chlorinated analog toremifene (500 nM) or the pure anti-estrogen ICI 164 384, an estradiol derivative. Analysis of conditioned media with an anti-TGFβ1 specific polyclonal antibody revealed significant, though variable induction of TGFβ by both these triphenylethylene derivatives. The pure anti-estrogen ICI 164 384 was less effective, whilst the presumed active metabolite of tamoxifen (the 4-OH derivative) was no more potent than the parent compound (Fig. 7.5 and Table 7.1). The TGFβ secreted by these fetal fibroblasts was growth inhibitory to CCL64 indicator cells, an effect which was reversed by specific anti-TGFβ1, but not anti-TGFβ2 antibodies. Immunoprecipitation of metabolically labeled conditioned media confirmed that fibroblasts synthesized TGFβ1 de novo, with no evidence for induction of the TGFβ2 isoform. Moreover, studies with fetal fibroblasts involving ligand binding assays, immunocytochemistry and ER mRNA analysis, did not demonstrate ER, suggesting that tamoxifen is interacting with some other protein in these fibroblasts.[52]

The induction of TGFβ1 has also been demonstrated in vivo in both ER positive and ER negative breast cancer patients following 3 months of primary tamoxifen therapy. In this immunohistochemical study, a series of 5 ER positive and 5 ER negative breast tumor sections were stained with antibodies recognizing either the extracellular (LC) or intracellular (CC) forms of TGFβ1. These polyclonal antibodies were produced in rabbits chal-

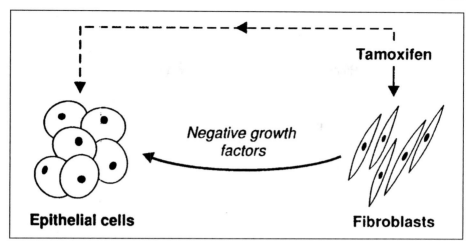

Fig. 7.4. Negative paracrine hypothesis. Tamoxifen may directly stimulate fibroblasts to produce and secrete negative growth factors which act in an inhibitory paracrine manner upon neighboring epithelial cells. Reprinted with permission from: Benson JR, Baum M, Colletta AA. In: deVita, Hellman, Rosenberg, eds. Biologic Therapy of Cancer, 2nd Edition. 1995:817-828. © Lippincott-Raven Publishers.

lenged with synthetic peptides as immunogens, and have been raised to peptides corresponding to the first 30 amino-acids of mature TGFβ1. One of these, anti-CC (1-30) reacts with the extracellular form of TGFβ1, whilst the other anti-LC (1-30) with the intracellular form. Differences in processing of these peptides is thought to have resulted in unique patterns of folding for each peptide, thus yielding different epitope characteristics which determine the observed differences in antibody reactivity.[67] These differential staining characteristics have been well documented and appear to be mutually exclusive.

Matched tumor samples taken before and after tamoxifen treatment were stained simultaneously, and conditions selected which maximized differences in staining intensity. In the posttreatment samples, marked upregulation of the extracellular form of TGFβ1 was observed between and around stromal cells, with little increase in the vicinity of epithelial cells. Moreover, staining for the intracellular form of the TGFβ1 antibody was predominantly confined to stromal cells, suggesting these to be the source of TGFβ1. No significant staining was observed for the TGFβ2 and TGFβ3 isoforms. These in vitro and in vivo findings are consistent with the proposed paracrine model, whereby tamoxifen stimulates production and secretion of a paracrine growth inhibitor from stromal cells which in turn acts upon neighboring epithelial cells, whether these be ER positive or ER negative. Despite small numbers, there appeared to be qualitatively greater induction of TGFβ1 in ER positive tumors in vivo,[48] which if corroborated may indicate the operation of a reciprocal paracrine effect whereby an activated ER/ligand complex can generate an intracellular signal which leads to secretion of a soluble factor which augments TGFβ1 production by fibroblasts. Though upregulation of TGFβ1 was seen in both ER positive and ER negative tumors in vivo, clinical response of ER positive tumors was 3- to 4-fold greater than for ER negative tumors. Patients in this study were a heterogeneous group, with some having more advanced disease for which the clinical response is known to be more closely related to ER status, compared with early breast cancer where tamoxifen is acting as an adjuvant. Induction of TGFβ1 may be quantitatively more important in early stage disease where tumor

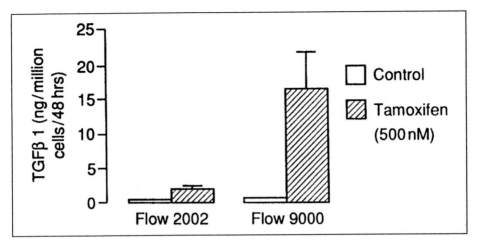

Fig. 7.5. Tamoxifen increases the rates of secretion of transforming growth factor β into the conditioned medium of 2 strains of human fetal fibroblasts derived from either lung (Flow 2002) or pituitary (Flow 9000) tissue. Reprinted with permission from: Benson JR, Baum M, Colletta AA. In: deVita, Hellman, Rosenberg, eds. Biologic Therapy of Cancer, 2nd Edition. 1995:817-828. © Lippincott-Raven Publishers.

Table 7.1. Rate of secretion of TGFß (ng/10 million cells/48 hrs)

	Flow 2002 cells	[Fold Induction]	*Flow 9000 cells*	[Fold Induction]
Control	0.4 ± 0.1	1.0	0.6 ± 0.0	1.0
10nM Estradiol	0.3 ± 0.1	0.8	1.2 ± 0.2	1.9
500nM Tamoxifen	2.0 ± 0.5	5.0	16.7 ± 5.3	27.4
500nM Toremifene	1.1 ± 0.2	2.7	6.8 ± 3.6	11.2

Rates of secretion of TGFß by two strains of fetal fibroblasts (Flow 2002 and Flow 9000). Rates of secretion expressed as ng per million cells per 48 hours in monolayer culture and are the mean values ± the standard deviations of triplicate estimates from duplicate experiments.

burden is small and epithelial cells can respond to subtle changes in levels of negative growth factors in their micro-environment. As a tumor evolves, cancer cells may become unresponsive to factors such as TGFβ1, thus precluding any anti-proliferative effect due to this paracrine mechanism. The role of TGFβ may change from that of an inhibitor of epithelial proliferation in early lesions, to a net promoter of growth in more advanced tumors. These results suggest that stromal fibroblasts can be pharmacologically manipulated to indirectly regulate epithelial proliferation via a negative paracrine effect.

Further evidence in support of such a mechanism comes from immunohistochemical studies of primary cultures of breast tumor fibroblasts using antibodies to the intracellular form of TGFβ1 and a secondary biotinylated antibody linked to a peroxidase labeled avidin-biotin system.[68] Following exposure of cells in vitro to tamoxifen at a concentration of 1μM for a period of 48 hrs, a marked increase in intracellular immunoreactivity for the β1 isoform was observed in treated cells compared to controls. Despite augmented intracellular levels of TGFβ1, analysis of levels of TGFβ secretion into the conditioned media using a sandwich ELISA technique did not reveal a concomitant increase in levels of the secreted protein product. This contrasted with previous studies with fetal fibroblasts (*vide supra*), and may indicate how complex reciprocal paracrine interactions with neighboring epithelial cells and/or extracellular matrix determine secretion dynamics and are mandatory for an optimal secretory response in vivo.

Intriguingly, using an anti-TGFβ1 antibody conjugated to an immunofluorescent detection system, this intracellular staining was found to be located predominantly in the nuclear region. These findings suggest that discrete nuclear and secreted forms of TGFβ1 may exist, with the former shorter peptide lacking the signaling sequence essential for secretion. Nuclear staining for growth factors which are considered to act classically by interaction with cell surface membrane receptors is not without precedent, and challenges this as an exclusive mechanism for mediating the action of certain growth factors.[68,69] Cells may produce growth factors and related proteins which are not only destined for secretion, but which may also be diverted to the nucleus where they can directly influence nuclear events independently of any cognate receptor. These two forms of TGFβ1 could be differentially induced by tamoxifen; relative amounts of the secretory form may be increased by tamoxifen in vivo[48] but isolated fibroblasts in vitro may respond aberrantly to tamoxifen with increased amounts of the nuclear form.

If indeed two discrete forms of intracellular TGFβ1 exist, then control of the relative amounts of secretory and nuclear forms may occur at the level of translation of the TGFβ mRNA molecule. The androgen regulated prostatic protein, probasin, exists as nuclear and secretory forms which are demonstrable immunohistochemically in the nuclei and secretory ducts respectively of prostatic epithelium in vivo.[70] These two distinct forms of probasin are encoded by a single, bifunctional mRNA molecule which contains two "in phase" AUG initiation codons within its coding region. Adjacent epithelial cells in histological sections showed preferential expression of either secreted or nuclear protein, but in situ hybridization revealed no difference in mRNA levels. As only a single probasin mRNA could be detected, there appeared to be translational regulation of a bifunctional mRNA. Using synthetic probasin mRNA's, these authors showed how two distinct proteins could be translated in vitro by initiation at two different AUG codon start sites. The protein destined for secretion was initiated from the upstream codon and contained a signal peptide sequence essential for secretion. Following processing of the secreted form, the final product would be identical to the nuclear form. By analogy with probasin, both nuclear and secretory forms of TGFβ1 could be encoded by a single mRNA molecule. Derynck and co-workers have shown that the TGFβ1 mRNA molecule has a long 5′ untranslated region (UTR), and in addition to the usual start codon located 82 nucleotides from the 5′ end, there is a second "in phase" initiation codon located downstream at position 954, which has a better sequence context for translational initiation.[71] The upstream AUG codon codes for the 391 amino-acid precursor molecule, but this second initiation codon would yield a smaller TGFβ1 precursor peptide of 354 amino-acids in length. Therefore initiation from this downstream AUG would eliminate the signal peptide and might allow trafficking to intracellular locations such as the nucleus. This smaller precursor would contain amino-acids 268—278 against which the precursor antibody was raised, and hence be detectable within the nucleus with the antibody employed in these experiments. Processing of this smaller precursor would occur after its arrival in the nucleus, and depend upon the presence of nuclear peptidases. These are known to be associated with the plasma membrane, but might also occur within the nuclear membranes. That the additional NH2-terminal sequences possessed by the 391 amino-acid precursor do in fact contain a signal peptide is supported by data on sequence analysis in this region. A sequence of 16 hydrophobic residues (8–23) exist within this NH2-terminus which may constitute the hydrophobic core of a signal peptide.[72] Thus the TGFβ1 precursor initiated at the downstream AUG codon would be shorter by only 37 amino-acids which corresponds with the average length of a signal peptide (20–30 amino-acids). Omission of a signal peptide may be insufficient per se to permit trafficking to the nucleus. Specific nuclear translocation sequences have been identified for several polypeptides which normally function within the nucleus (c-*erb*-A, c-*myc*, N-*myc*, p53).[73] Imamura and co-workers have elegantly demonstrated that acidic FGF not only lacks a signal peptide for secretion but also contains a sequence which is similar to the specific nuclear translocation sequences of these nucleoproteins.[74] Mutant forms of FGF with this sequence deleted were unable to elicit a mitogenic response. Furthermore, creation of a chimeric protein by addition of a yeast nuclear translocation sequence restored this response, suggesting that nuclear translocation is important for a complete biological action of FGF. These nuclear transloca-tion sequences have also been found in the polypeptide chains of PDGF, which as noted above have been detected within the nucleus of SSV transformed cells.[75] It would be inter-esting to examine whether a similar sequence is also present in the TGFβ1 product. Of interest, fibroblast growth factor (FGF), platelet-derived growth factor (PDGF) and TGFβ are all potent mitogens for mesenchymal cells and have been localized within the nuclei of such cells.[76] An intracrine mechanism with nuclear translocation of these polypeptide prod-ucts may represent a more efficient method for "auto-stimulation" with rapid and direct interaction between growth factors and nuclear structures.

As for probasin, only one species of TGFβ1 mRNA has been identified, and the long 5′ UTR may confer upon the molecule an innate bi-functional character. Increased synthesis of TGFβ1 in these breast tumor fibroblasts is not associated with any concomitant elevation of TGFβ1 mRNA levels, implying that induction of TGFβ1 involves enhanced synthesis at a posttranscriptional level. It is conceivable that tamoxifen may interact with the stem-loop structures in the 5′UTR of the TGFβ1 mRNA to overcome any inhibitory effects upon trans-lation (see section ii(c)). Arrick's group have recently described a 5′ truncated transcript of TGFβ3 mRNA in human breast carcinoma cell lines (T47-D, ZR-75, BT-474). As for other isoforms, TGFβ3 has hitherto been considered to express only a single transcript of 3.5-kb in length. This novel TGFβ3 transcript is 870 nucleotides shorter within the 5′ noncoding region, and was shown to have approximately 7-fold greater translational efficiency than the full-length transcript.[77] The 2 stem-loop structures within the 5′UTR of TGFβ1 mRNA were located between bases +1 to +840.[78] Therefore this sequence omission of 870 nucle-otides in length may contain similar stem-loop structures which inhibit translation. The shorter transcript, lacking these structures, would display enhanced translational efficiency and ribosomal binding.

Immunohistochemical staining revealed that this intracellular induction of TGFβ1 by tamoxifen was not confined to fibroblasts derived from malignant breast tumors, but also those from benign fibroadenomas. However, this response was not observed in 'normal' skin fibroblasts suggesting that breast tumor fibroblasts may display peculiar phenotypic features which are not shared by other somatic fibroblasts. The development of abnormal fibroblasts secondary to epigenetic phenomena arising from primary oncogenic events in transformed epithelial elements is discussed in chapter 4 which focuses on stromal-epithe-lial interactions. These aberrant stromal phenotypes may be associated with two important sequelae. Firstly they may lead to deranged stromal-epithelial interactions and thereby pro-mote neoplastic progression. Secondly, they may fortuitously permit the pharmacological induction of TGFβ1 by agents such as tamoxifen.

In these studies with primary cultures of breast tumor fibroblasts, no functional dis-tinction has been made between possible subsets of fibroblasts. The normal breast contains both interlobular and intralobular fibroblasts. The latter are located within the functional unit of the breast and have a more intimate association with epithelial cells. Moreover, together with the epithelium of a terminal duct lobular unit, these intralobular fibroblasts alone undergo response to cyclical hormonal changes, implying a differential response to steroid hormones between these two subsets of fibroblasts.[79] Furthermore, only interlobular fibroblasts express the cell surface enzyme dipeptidyl peptidase IV.[80] Using a method of differential digestion and centrifugation Schor and co-workers have broadly isolated these 2 fibroblast types and shown functional heterogeneity with respect to both migratory phenotype and production of motility factors in both normal and cancerous breast tissue.[81] This fibroblast heterogeneity could result in different interactions with epithelial cells, and Caniggia and co-workers have reported that intralobular fibroblasts induced predominantly epithelial differentiation, whilst interlobular ones induced proliferation.[82] A pertinent question is whether pharmacological induction of TGFβ1 is confined to intralobular fibroblasts which are in closer proximity to epithelial cells and hence better placed for paracrine interactions. If there exists a different TGFβ functional profile between intra- and interlobular fibroblasts, then the observed wide variation in absolute rates of TGFβ secretion between strains could partially reflect differing proportions of each fibroblast subpopulation in primary cultures.

These aberrant fibroblasts may be amenable to pharmacological manipulation irrespective of whether their altered phenotype is inherited and systemic or acquired and induced epigenetically by local events. Of interest, intralobular fibroblasts derived from histologically normal tissue adjacent to sporadic breast carcinomas have been found to display a fetal-like phenotype which is manifest, and persists in vitro in the absence of the primary tumor.[81] Whether these are inductive effects from the latter ("extended field effect")[83] or a response to other stimuli which precede tumor development is unknown.

C) PostTranscriptional Mechanisms of Control

Whether induction of TGFβ by tamoxifen occurs in MCF-7 cells via the conventional ER or in fibroblasts via some other binding protein, this appears to occur via a posttranscriptional mechanism, as there is no observed concomitant increase in TGFβ mRNA.[47,52,68] Furthermore, nonpharmacological (physiological) modulation of TGFβ1 may also involve a posttranscriptional mechanism. Levels of TGFβ1 mRNA are similar in unstimulated monocytes compared to those activated to become macrophages with accompanying secretion of TGFβ1 protein.[84] Conversely, in keratinocytes treated with retinoic there is an increase in TGFβ message but not levels of protein product, further illustrating how a disparate correlation may exist between level of transcript and protein product.[85]

In an attempt to elucidate a possible posttranscriptional mechanism of control, attention has focused on the unusually long 5′ untranslated region (5′UTR) of the TGFβ mRNA molecule.[86] Computer analysis of sequences of this region which are rich in GC content reveals 2 potential highly stable stem-loop structures (Fig. 7.6.).[87] Selective deletion of portions of this 5′ UTR and incorporation of deletion mutants into a heterologous human growth hormone reporter system have shown these structures to be potent inhibitors of translation.[87] This inhibition is not observed in all cell types, and specificity may be conferred by binding of cell-type specific cytoplasmic proteins to these stem-loop structures. Where tamoxifen induces TGFβ by an ER-independent mechanism, it may be directly interacting with these stem-loop structures to overcome their inhibitory effects on translation. The receptor for tamoxifen could be a cytoplasmic protein which normally binds to these stem-loop structures, and augments translational inhibition. Tamoxifen could enhance translation by combining with and displacing this protein. Of interest, the 5′UTR of ferritin mRNA contains a stem-loop structure[88] which inhibits translation in vitro.[89] A protein which binds to this 'iron-responsive element' has been characterized.[90] The 5′UTR of TGFβ mRNA contains the palindromic motif AGAAGA just upstream of the second translational start site. This motif appears to be involved in the ER-independent translational control of the basic myelin protein by estradiol.[91]

Perry and co-workers have reported that tamoxifen at concentrations of 10 μM can modulate expression of TGFβ1 in breast cancer cell lines in vitro. Incubation for periods exceeding 12 hours was associated with increased levels of both TGFβ1 protein and transcript.[92] It has been pointed out in recent correspondence[93] that concentrations in these experiments were much higher than in previous studies demonstrating pharmacological induction of TGFβ1 where concentrations of tamoxifen were typically ≤ 1μM (Knabbe et al, 1987[47]; Colletta et al 1990[52]; Colletta et al 1991[98]). Nonetheless, these observations raise the intriguing possibility that tamoxifen may act by a posttranscriptional mechanism at lower concentrations and a transcriptional one at higher concentrations.

iii) Progestins

Progesterones together with estrogens dominate the endocrine environment of human breast tissue. Though there is cogent evidence implicating estrogens in the growth of established breast cancers, there is conflicting evidence regarding progesterone whose precise roles in both mammary neoplasia and normal breast function remain unresolved. Despite the elusive function of progestins in human breast cancer, it is apparent that high dose progestins can induce remission in some advanced breast cancers, thus implying an antiproliferative or 'good' effect upon malignant breast epithelium. However, it is not valid to extrapolate from the clinical use of these high doses of synthetic progesterone analogs to the physiological setting, where endogenous progesterones may have a different functional profile. In animal tumor models, natural progesterone and synthetic progestins can either inhibit or stimulate DMBA-induced tumors in rats depending on whether they are administered before or after the initiating dose of DMBA.[94] In vitro studies with breast cancer cell lines are slightly confusing; thus progestins can inhibit proliferation of cells in vitro when these are grown in the presence of phenol red,[95] but in the absence of this estrogenic indicator, progestins can stimulate growth. Growth inhibitory effects of progestins may be due to an anti-estrogenic action, but ER negative/PR positive cells are also growth inhibited.[96] If progestins are only stimulatory in an estrogen free environment, then growth inhibitory effects may dominate in vivo where some estrogen is invariably present. From a therapeutic viewpoint, it is crucial to be certain of the action of progestins in vivo, as this will dictate whether a progestin or anti-progestin strategy is employed clinically. Progestins may have differential effects depending on age. If they are protective in premenopausal women, then a chemopreventive strategy based on a progestin contraceptive would be logical. Interestingly, the use of progestins in women with benign breast disease has been associated with a reduced breast cancer risk.[97]

Gestodene is a synthetic ∂15 progestin which is inhibitory to a range of ER positive and ER negative cells in a dose-dependent manner. It is thought to mediate its effect via a specific gestodene binding protein (GBP) which is expressed in breast cancer cells irrespective of their ER status.[98] Moreover, at growth inhibitory concentrations, gestodene induces up to a 90-fold increase in levels of TGFβ detected by radioreceptor assay and sandwich enzyme-linked immunoassay (SELISA) in conditioned media of both ER positive (T47-D; MCF-7) and ER negative (MDA-MB-231; BT-20) breast cancer cell lines. Furthermore, levels of induction of TGFβ1 are proportional to levels of GBP and are unrelated to expression of progesterone receptor. These findings suggest that gestodene can mediate its growth inhibitory effects by induction of TGFβ which is part of a negative autocrine loop. This is analogous to the effects of tamoxifen on MCF-7 cells.[47] Support for such a mechanism comes

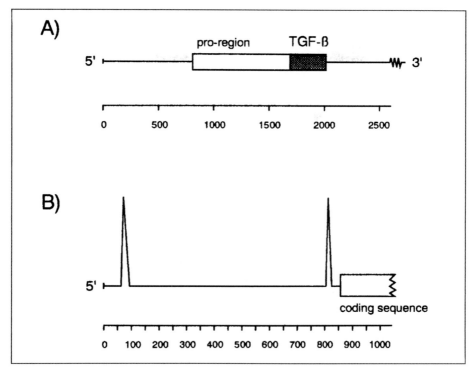

Fig. 7.6. (A) Schematic diagram showing nucleotide sequence of the TGFβ mRNA molecule. The boxed area represents the coding sequence for the precursor molecule with hatching indicating the sequences coding specifically for the 112 a-a peptide monomer of the mature moeity. Note the relatively long 5′ untranslated region (5′ UTR). (B) Location of 2 highly stable stem-loop structures within the 5′ UTR identified by computer analysis (sequences between +49 and +77 and between +750 and +786). These stem-loops may hinder the association of the mRNA molecule with ribosomal subunits and restrict translational efficiency.

from recent data showing abrogation of a response to gestodene in T47-D cells which have been transfected with a TGFβ1 dominant negative mutant and no longer produce significant amounts of this inhibitory growth factor (K. Wells—personal communication). Similarly, in the experiments of Colletta and colleagues, gestodene induced inhibition of T47D cells was partially blocked by anti-TGFβ neutralizing antibodies.[98]

Thus it may be feasible to harness these inductive effects of progestins on TGFβ1 to produce a bifunctional agent which has combined contraceptive and chemopreventive actions. This would be particularly relevant to women with a strong family history of breast cancer development at a young age. Of interest, in the above experiments, the majority of the TGFβ secreted by T47-D cells in response to gestodene appeared to be in the biologically active form with neither transient acidification nor heating significantly increasing the amount of receptor reactive TGFβ in unprocessed conditioned media.[98] However, contradictory results from current trials of progestin only oral contraceptive preparations must be resolved before such pharmacological idealism is translated into clinical reality. A large survey by the WHO Collaborative Study published in 1990[99] found no overall increased risk of breast cancer in users of the contraceptive medroxyprogesterone acetate as a depot preparation, and similar conclusions apply to combined estrogen and progestin oral contraceptives.[100] However, closer analysis of these studies reveals that younger women taking either a combined or progestin only preparation for prolonged periods are at increased risk.[101,102] It is possible that this increase reflects the action of these agents on breast tissue with a relatively higher average mitotic activity.[103]

iv) Retinoids

Retinoids are naturally occurring derivatives of vitamin-A which exert a key role in maintenance of epithelial homeostasis through regulation of cellular proliferation and differentiation. In the first quarter of this century Wolbach and Howe reported that vitamin-A deficient animals exhibited increased rates of proliferation and mitotic activity within retinoid deficient epithelia.[104] The effects of vitamin A deficiency were not confined to proliferative activity *per se*, but were also manifest as alterations in normal patterns of differentiation. Thus the usual pathway of differentiation of stem cells into mature epithelial cells was interrupted and cells frequently expressed an over-abundance of keratin. Certain similarities between the tissues of vitamin-A deficient states and those of neoplasia were apparent; these authors observed that the metaplastic epithelium associated with vitamin-A deficiency shared common features with malignant lesions. Furthermore, it was noted that squamous metaplasia in hamster tracheal epithelium had similar histological appearances whether it be induced by vitamin-A deficiency or the known carcinogen, benzo[a]—pyrene-ferric oxide.[105] Thus vitamin-A deficiency can lead to changes which are morphologically similar to carcinogen-induced changes in epithelium.

These results suggest that oncogenic events may disrupt normal control of epithelium by retinoids, the latter being endogenous morphogens which are essential for control of normal cellular proliferation and differentiation. Epithelia which are dependent upon retinoids for this "epithelial homeostasis" often have minimal proliferative activity under resting conditions, with low levels of thymidine uptake by basal cells. However, despite low proliferative activity in basal states, these epithelia can respond to an insult promptly with rapid increases in cell turnover. Moreover, both carcinogens and vitamin-A deficiency can evoke a proliferative response, suggesting that the normal function of retinoids is to suppress DNA synthesis and replication in these epithelia. Mutations resulting in malignant progression may interfere with regulation of epithelial cells by retinoids.

Therefore if retinoids act as a physiological restraint, can they counteract specific adverse influences upon epithelia which may promote oncogenic change? As a corollary, this could provide the rationale for the therapeutic development of retinoids for treatment and prevention of cancer. In particular, such interventions with retinoids are likely to be most important in the preneoplastic and early stages of carcinogenesis where subtle disturbances of cellular regulatory mechanisms and stromal-epithelial interactions could be rectified. Thus epithelial homeostasis could be restored and the transition from preneoplastic to in situ and possibly in situ to invasive states aborted.

Early studies by Fell and Melanby in the 1950s provided the first evidence that exogenous retinoids (retinol and retinyl acetate) could determine the phenotypic expression of epithelia.[106] In organ cultures of chick epidermis, exposure to retinoids resulted in replacement of normal keratinized epithelium of the skin by one containing mucus-producing ciliated cells. Though these experiments indicated that retinoids could directly produce phenotypic changes in epithelium, they did not involve any reversal of a neoplastic process. Subsequent work with mouse prostatic tissue showed not only that epithelial atypia induced by the carcinogen methylcholanthracene resembled vitamin-A deficient epithelium, but that retinoids could partially reverse a premalignant phenotype. Thus organ cultures of prostatic tissue which had undergone prior exposure to methylcholanthracene were composed of epithelium showing atypical features. A normal epithelium could be restored by subsequent treatment of these organ cultures with retinoids.[107] Similarly, the retinoid 4-hydroxyphenylretinamide (4-HPR) can partially reverse the oncogenic effects of 7,12 dimethylbenzanthracene on mammary epithelium in organ culture.[108] The capacity of retinoids to suppress malignant transformation in vitro has also been demonstrated in isolated cell lines. Initial studies focused on cells of mesenchymal origin,[109,110] but suppressive effects of retinoids on various epithelial cell lines in vitro have since been confirmed. Though retinoids have consistent inhibitory effects upon the mesenchymally derived cell lines 10T 1/2 fibroblasts and human myeloid leukemia cells (HL60), the effects upon DNA synthesis are variable. Decreases in rates of proliferation of human breast cancer cell lines may be associated with either a decrease[111] or increase[112] in thymidine uptake. Retinoic acid has properties of a cytostatic rather than a cytotoxic agent which is consistent with its role as a growth regulator in maintenance of epithelial homeostasis. It appears to act in a 'holding capacity' and may exert its effect in the G1 phase of the cell cycle.[113] Of interest, in experiments where retinoids have suppressed development of a malignant phenotype in cells previously exposed to a carcinogen, this effect is only maintained whilst retinoids are present within the culture medium.[110]

The molecular basis for the action of retinoids remain to be elucidated, but initial events involve interaction with discrete intracellular receptors which are members of the steroid hormone receptor superfamily. The transduction pathway between activated retinoid receptor and changes in gene expression are unknown. However, one type of retinoid receptor termed RXR appears to interact directly with nuclear elements and indeed possesses discrete DNA and hormone binding domains. Furthermore, it can form complexes with retinoic acid receptor (RAR) and interact with other nuclear receptors within this superfamily.[114] It may therefore function as a ligand activated transcription factor in a manner analogous to the estrogen receptor (section ii). Whatever the proximal steps in retinoid signaling, there is evidence that modulation of TGFβ expression may be an important component in mediating the actions of retinoids in normal tissues in vivo. As discussed in chapter 3, TGFβ has potent inhibitory effects upon a wide range of epithelial types,[115-117] and has an important role in developmental processes with specific patterns of spatial and temporal expression and inhibitory effects upon developing end buds in mammary glands.[118-120] TGFβ may therefore constitute a key element in fundamental regulatory pathways linking retinoids with cellular proliferation and differentiation.

There is now evidence for induction of TGFβ both in vitro and in vivo in response to retinoid treatment. Glick has shown that all-*trans*-retinoic acid induces secretion of the TGFβ2 isoform in primary cell cultures of mouse keratinocytes.[123] Maximal induction occurred at concentrations similar to the median effective dose resulting in inhibition of DNA synthesis. This retinoid-induced TGFβ was in the biologically active form and levels of both TGFβ product and transcript were modulated. Moreover, expression of the β2 isoform was also increased in vivo within the epidermis of retinoid treated animals, suggesting that TGFβ might mediate some of the effects of retinoic acid on this tissue, including hyperproliferation of the epidermis. In vitro studies employing anti-TGFβ2 antibodies indicated that almost one-third of the inhibitory effects of retinoic acid on DNA synthesis was attributed to the activity of TGFβ2. Induction of TGFβ2 has also been observed in A549 cells and normal rat NRK fibroblasts, though these effects being of lesser magnitude than in keratinocytes.[121] Studies in vivo have been extended to examine the effects of retinoids on expression of TGFβ isoforms in various tissues of the vitamin-A deficient rat model.[122] In this immunohistochemical study, polyclonal antibodies raised against peptides corresponding to the three isoforms of TGFβ were used to stain different tissues in rats exposed to systemic all-*trans*-retinoic acid administered orally at a dose of 100μg. All three isoforms of TGFβ were induced in epidermis within 24 to 48 hours of an oral dose of retinoic acid. Interestingly, the hyperproliferative response observed in mice following local application of retinoic acid was not seen in rodent epidermis,[123] indicating that such a response is not an obligatory sequela of TGFβ induction. Marked induction of TGFβ2 and TGFβ3 were observed at 2 and 4 days posttreatment respectively in both the bronchial and tracheal epithelium. Immunoreactivity was most intense in the basal regions of regenerating squamous epithelium and the cell bodies of newly formed ciliated epithelium. Induction of these 2 isoforms was also seen in the alveolar cells where once again minimal changes in expression of TGFβ1 were evident. In all respiratory tissues levels of expression had fallen to those of vitamin-A deficient tissues at 8 days post treatment. Inductive effects of all-*trans*-retinoic acid on intestinal mucosa was almost exclusively confined to the β2 isoform. Increased TGFβ2 staining was seen in the lamina propria of both small intestine and colon within 24 hours of systemic administration of retinoid. After 4 days, staining was most intense in cells along the villi, perhaps indicative of progressive differentiation. Staining for the β3 isoform was seen in the colonic mucosa and lamina propria. In contrast to the above tissues, expression of all 3 isoforms was intense in vitamin-A deficient vaginal epithelium, and this was suppressed by retinoid treatment. This down-regulation of TGFβ expression was associated with partial restoration of a normal stratified epithelium. The expression of TGFβ isoforms within these various tissues was highly dependent upon intrinsic retinoid levels, with levels of the TGFβ2 isoform being most sensitive to changes in retinoid status.

These studies suggest that changes in TGFβ expression involving all 3 isoforms occurs *parri-passu* with excess or deficiency of retinoic acid. There is a positive correlation between tissue retinoid levels and TGFβ isoform expression in the epidermis together with respiratory and intestinal epithelia. The putative roles of TGFβ within these latter tissues are discussed in detail in chapter 8. In brief, TGFβ can cause almost complete growth arrest in lung epithelial cells[124,125] and inhibit proliferation of colonic adenoma cell lines.[126] Similarly, TGFβ can also induce differentiation in these respiratory and intestinal cell lines.[127] Although these immunohistochemical studies do not prove that retinoic acid directly induces expression of TGFβ, they indicate that retinoic acid can regulate expression of TGFβ in a wide range of tissues, with induction being observed in both epithelial and mesenchymal elements. In turn, TGFβ is known to have potent effects upon cellular proliferation and differentiation. However, alteration in expression of TGFβ isoforms could be secondary to any proliferative response. Though induction of TGFβ may accompany retinoic acid treatment, exogenous TGFβ may be insufficient to mimic the net results of such treatment.[128] Furthermore, with some physiological processes, TGFβ and retinoic acid appear to have antagonistic effects. For example, TGFβ generally stimulates synthesis and inhibits degradation of extracellular matrix proteins whereas retinoic acid can have the opposite effects.[129] The capacity of retinoic acid to induce TGFβ in several different tissues may prove to be a clinical handicap when systemic therapy is employed. The retinoid X receptor has several structurally distinct isoforms which have been found in mammalian tissues and these appear to exhibit a degree of tissue specificity in their pattern of expression. It may be possible to develop retinoid derivatives whose action is restricted to RXR responsive pathways, the predominant effects of which are confined to a limited spectrum of tissue types.

In addition to the possible mechanistic interactions between retinoids and the TGFβ system during development,[118-120,128] there is likely continued interaction in the mature tissues of the adult organism. It may be feasible to exploit this functional relationship between retinoids and polypeptide growth factors such as TGFβ for therapeutic purposes. Many of the more common epithelial tumors arise from epithelia which are dependent upon retinoids for maintenance of 'epithelial homeostasis', suggesting that disordered cellular growth may be averted/abhorted by manipulation of the local retinoid environment.

v) Chemoprevention

Chemoprevention is by definition, the use of natural substances, analogs thereof or other synthetic agents to interfere with development of the neoplastic process, up to the stage of in situ carcinoma. Early neoplastic events may involve intrinsic changes in levels of TGFβ and substances such as retinoids within the local micro-environment of tissues. Strategies which directly booster local endogenous TGFβ production constitute a realistic objective for both chemoprevention and treatment of early stage cancer. Moreover, the source of induced TGFβ, be it stromal or epithelial, would not matter as target cells could respond to TGFβ from both autocrine and paracrine sources within the local micro-environment of tissues. Optimal strategies might involve a dual local induction of TGFβ from both stromal and epithelial cells, with the latter being exposed to both paracrine and autocrine inhibitory effects. In the case of breast cancer, this could be achieved by a combination of tamoxifen with a retinoid which would induce TGFβ from stromal and epithelial cells respectively. Retinoids have potent effects on cells of mesenchymal origin[130] and a dual inductive action on TGFβ by a combination of triphenylethylenes and retinoids may not be mutually exclusive. The former may modulate autonomic inhibitory loops in epithelial cells, whilst the latter could enhance stromal expression of TGFβ and in turn act in a negative paracrine manner upon epithelial cells.

This mutually complementary approach would maximize endogenous TGFβ production in response to pharmacological intervention. This "combination chemoprevention" approach is supported by data from studies on animal tumor models in which retinoids can act synergistically with estrogen ablation to suppress development of mammary carcinoma. McCormick and co-workers reported that ovariectomized rats receiving oral retinyl acetate had a lower incidence of second cancers than controls.[131] Moreover, rats undergoing ovariectomy alone or receiving retinoid alone had an incidence of tumor formation intermediate between controls and combination therapy. Further animal experiments have confirmed that a combination of the retinoid 4-hydroxyphenylretinamide (4-HPR) and nonsurgical estrogen ablation using the anti-estrogen tamoxifen is likewise synergistic for suppression of NMU-induced mammary tumors in rodents.[132] Combined therapy with these agents was much more effective than either modality alone in preventing the appearance of further mammary tumors following excision of primary mammary tumors. Furthermore, this effect was evident upon both early and late onset lesions, and the apparent efficacy of a combination of 4-HPR and tamoxifen on later tumor development may be a consequence of the estrogen agonist component of the latter coupled with its pharmacokinetics.[133] By contrast, ovariectomy results in immediate estrogen ablation and its physiological consequences therefore evident much earlier. This combination chemoprevention strategy is being explored clinically; like tamoxifen, 4-HPR is well tolerated clinically with minimal side-effects.[134] Trials are currently in progress to evaluate a combination of these two agents in prevention of breast cancer.[135]

vi) TGFβ and Carcinogenesis

Much evidence has accrued indicating that TGFβ is a potent and preeminent inhibitor of both normal mammary epithelial cells and their malignant, transformed counterparts. Experimental and clinical data cited in this chapter provides circumstantial evidence for the participation of TGFβ in both autocrine and paracrine growth inhibitory loops with resultant net suppression of epithelial proliferation. TGFβ is a component of the complex language of intercellular communication and may serve as a cellular 'switch'. It is proposed that these inhibitory growth factor loops are operative in vivo in normal tissues of the developing and adult organism. Moreover, at some point along the neoplastic continuum functional disruption occurs and epithelial cells no longer exhibit sensitivity to the growth inhibitory effects of TGFβ, or at best demonstrate an attenuated response. It seems likely that this reduced sensitivity involves multiple mechanisms. including loss of functional TGFβ receptors.

More direct evidence for an important growth inhibitory effect of TGFβ in vivo comes from studies in the developing organism. Silberstein and Daniel demonstrated that exogenous TGFβ administered as slow-release implants induced dramatic regression of the proliferating stem cell layer of end-buds with concomitant involution and resultant inhibition of ductal growth in the developing mouse mammary gland.[119] Moreover, these inhibitory effects upon duct elongation only occurred when TGFβ implants were placed in the vicinity of advancing end buds. During normal development, TGFβ is not located at these sites, but is present within the epithelium of growth quiescent ducts.[136] Over-expression of TGFβ in the mammary glands and skin of transgenic mice confers increased resistance to chemically induced carcinogenesis. Conversely, *ras*-transformed keratinocytes from TGFβ " knock out" mice in which expression of the TGFβ gene has been functionally deleted are tumorigenic in nude mice with formation of malignant lesions, whilst similarly transformed keratinocytes from normal mice form benign tumors. This accelerated tumor formation in null mice suggests that TGFβ1 suppresses the process of carcinogenesis via autocrine inhibitory loops, and that reduced expression of TGFβ favors development of malignant tumors.[138] Interestingly, immunohistochemical studies of skin tumors in mice have revealed that TGFβ1 immunoreactivity is an inverse prognostic factor for malignant transformation.[139] TGFβ can therefore determine the ultimate phenotype of cells subjected to oncogenic manipulation, once again illustrating the importance of the net balance of opposing influences impinging upon cells.

Elegant experiments employing transgenic mice which over-express TGFβ1 provide further support for potent growth inhibitory effects of TGFβ upon normal mammary epithelium being operative in vivo.[140] These animals were generated by introducing a constitutively active mutant TGFβ1 gene directly into one-cell mouse embryos. This construct was created by linking a mutant 1.4kb simian TGFβ1 gene to the 1.5kb mouse mammary tumor virus (MMTV) promoter/enhancer. Of note, the simian TGFβ1 gene contained mutations at codons 223 and 225 resulting in production and secretion of active TGFβ1.[141] Tissue specific expression of the transgene was confirmed by immunohistochemistry using TGFβ1 antibodies;[142] transgenic mice at 13 weeks showed strong immunoreactivity in mammary ductal epithelial cells with less intense staining of stromal elements. By contrast, age-matched controls revealed very weak staining in both epithelial and stromal compartments. Over-expression of TGFβ1 resulted in pronounced ductal hypoplasia with poor ductal arborization and lateral branching. Bromodeoxyuridine staining revealed marked suppression of labeling index, suggesting that stunted ductal development resulted from inhibition of cell proliferation in transgenic animals. Direct augmentation of an autocrine inhibitory loop involving mammary epithelial cells would be consistent with these results, which are also in accordance with the aforementioned studies employing exogenous TGFβ.[120,136] The paradigm that epithelial proliferation is controlled by the net balance of positive and negative growth factors within the local micro-environment of cells is supported by a related group of experiments involving cross-breeding of transgenic mice. By analogous methodology, transgenic mice can be generated which over-express the mitogenic growth factor TGF alpha.[143,144] By contrast with TGFβ1 transgenics, mice over-expressing TGF alpha (MMTV—TGF alpha transgene) demonstrate mammary ductal hyperplasia and implantation of exogenous TGF alpha into regressed mammary glands reverses the changes of involution.[145]

Furthermore, MMTV-TGF alpha transgenic mice display a marked increase in the rate of spontaneous tumor formation which is accelerated by administration of the carcinogen 7,12-dimethylbenzanthracene (DMBA).[146] MMTV-TGFβ1 transgenic mice have not been reported to exhibit spontaneous tumor formation and indeed appear resistant to DMBA induced carcinogenesis. This observation suggests that TGFβ1 can suppress events initiating tumor formation and are consistent with an important role in the early phases of tumor development when subtle changes in levels of growth factors within the local micro-environment may portend and promote neoplastic progression. Interestingly, cross-breeding experiments between MMTV-TGFβ1 and MMTV TGF alpha transgenic mice allude to the potential interplay between positive and negative growth factors in determining overall proliferative proclivities of cells. Thus animals possessing both transgenes fail to develop tumors, implying that over-expression of a potent inhibitory growth factor can overcome the growth stimulatory and transforming capacity of oncogenic events. The potential importance of such a "malignancy-resistant phenotype" in chemoprevention of breast cancer is discussed in the concluding section of this chapter. In the context of the present discussion, these experiments lend further support to the existence of functional TGFβ growth inhibitory loops in vivo, disruption of which provides one mechanism for malignant progression.

The action of various agents in hormone-dependent systems both in vitro and in vivo provides circumstantial evidence for the operation of growth factor loops. Despite relatively high constitutive production of TGFβ by more tumorigenic, hormone-independent ER negative breast cancer cell lines,[53] stimulation of growth by neutralizing anti-TGFβ antibodies implies the operation of autocrine inhibitory loops within these cells. An inactivating mutation has been found in the type II TGFβ receptor of colonic carcinoma cells.[147] Though most breast cancer cell lines remain sensitive to the growth inhibitory effects of TGFβ, malignant transformation of colonic adenoma cells is associated with loss of TGFβ responsiveness.[126] Moreover, restoration of an inhibitory response in both colonic[147] and breast cancer cell lines[149,150] which are devoid of functional wild-type receptor can be accomplished by transfection of the TGFβ type II receptor subunit into these cells. The transfectants display a nontumorigenic phenotype, and this observation coupled with the association of this type II receptor mutation with a DNA repair defect (micro-satellite instability) implies an important role in carcinogenesis, perhaps by permitting cells to escape from negative regulatory influences. Similar findings have been documented for the breast cancer cell line MCF-7. Sun and co-workers reported that transfectants possessing a re-expressed type II TGFβ receptor less readily formed tumors in athymic mice.[150] The crucial issues relating to these TGFβ receptor defects as a mechanistic step in carcinogenesis are 2-fold. Firstly, what is the relative frequency of these mutations amongst various tumors, and secondly, at what stage in carcinogenesis do they occur ? As previously emphasized, in vitro studies suggest that loss and/or defective function of TGFβ receptors does not appear to be a widespread phenomenon in breast cancer compared with colonic or gastric malignancies (see chapters 6 and 8).[53,117,148] However, in an immunohistochemical study involving staining of breast tumor specimens with antibodies against the type II TGFβ receptor, 93% of invasive breast carcinomas revealed none or only minimal staining of cells (< 10%), with only 3% of sections showing staining of more than 50% of cells.[151]

There is an apparent contradiction in the multi-functional character of TGFβ and its potential role in carcinogenesis. Though interrelated, it is important to distinguish between changes in expression of TGFβ which are a consequence of therapeutic intervention, and those which occur *pari-passu* with malignant progression. The latter may in turn be incidental or causative. It is proposed that in normal tissues and the early period immediately following malignant transformation, mammary epithelial cells retain a growth inhibitory response to TGFβ. Epithelial and stromal cells may produce and secrete this inhibitory growth factor which can thus act in either an autocrine or paracrine manner respectively. As cells progress along the neoplastic continuum, these regulatory mechanisms may become compromised either due to a loss of negative cell signaling or a fundamental change in the TGFβ "switch" whose function is so highly context dependent. The net result of these changed physiological circumstances is loss of growth inhibition and a concomitant stimulation of stromal development by TGFβ. Epithelial sources of TGFβ would effectively stimulate fibroblasts, and possibly reticulo-endothelial cells in a positive paracrine manner to elaborate extracellular matrix proteins and release angiogenic factors respectively (Fig. 7.7). Moreover, the role of TGFβ in carcinogenesis is further complicated by the possible existence of a functional dichotomy *apropos* the effects of this growth factor upon epithelial proliferation. In a skin-grafting model system using oncogenically activated (v-Ha-*ras*) keratinocytes and fibroblasts from TGFβ1 'knockout' mice, Glick and co-workers, have studied the relative contributions of autocrine and paracrine sources of TGFβ to epithelial growth and differentiation in the context of neoplastic progression.[152] In the absence of functional deletion of the TGFβ1 gene, benign papillomas develop in mouse epidermis, but these rarely undergo malignant transformation to squamous cell carcinomas. Xenografts of null keratinocytes rapidly progressed to squamous cell carcinomas with a multi-focal distribution within highly dysplastic papillomas. This enhanced tumorogenicity was attributable to loss of TGFβ1 expression within keratinocytes and not to mutations involving v-Ha-ras or p53. Furthermore, there was no evidence for diminished sensitivity due to loss of TGFβ receptors. Coimplantation experiments with dermal fibroblasts revealed interesting results; Combinations of null keratinocytes with wild type fibroblasts yielded tumors with relatively a high cell labeling index. By contrast, labeling indices were lower for all tumors constituted of null fibroblasts, i.e., those in which both epithelial and stromal cells had deletion of the TGFβ1 gene. It was concluded from these experiments that autocrine TGFβ1 suppressed both rate and frequency of malignant progression, whilst paracrine sources of TGFβ1 increased rates of proliferation within tumors but not malignant conversion. This apparent compartmental dependence of TGFβ function is likely to add a further dimension to the relation of function to stage of carcinogenesis. In early stage lesions, both autocrine and paracrine sources of TGFβ may be inhibitory to epithelial growth, but as malignancy progresses, paracrine sources of TGFβ may switch from being inhibitory to stimulatory in accordance with other documented growth promotory effects of TGFβ in more advanced tumors. Thus evidence has already been cited from immunohistochemical and molecular biological studies suggesting a positive association between increased TGFβ expression and adverse prognosis.[56,59,60,153-155] Furthermore, in vitro studies indicate that TGFβ can promote invasion by stimulating degradation of the basement membrane and lung metastases. A possible direct role for TGFβ in tumor invasion is suggested by an immunohistochemical study which revealed staining for extracellular TGFβ1 to be most intense at the periphery of primary tumors than the central portions. This localization of TGFβ1 to the advancing edge of tumors may reflect is role in tumor invasion. Moreover, in the same study, patients with axillary nodal metastases invariably showed greater immunoreactivity for both intra- and extracellular TGFβ in nodal tissue compared with the primary tumor.[153]

TGFβ has well documented suppressive effects on the immune system, including regulation of T cell activation[157] and suppression of both proliferation and differentiation of B lymphocytes.[158] In addition TGFβ appears to control processes of deactivation of cell of the monocyte system such as macrophages.[159] These effects may collectively add to the overall tumor growth promotory characteristics of TGFβ in the more advanced stages of malignancy. This duality of TGFβ function also presents a dilemma regarding appropriate therapeutic strategies. This issue of whether to boost or suppress local levels of TGFβ is discussed further in the next section.

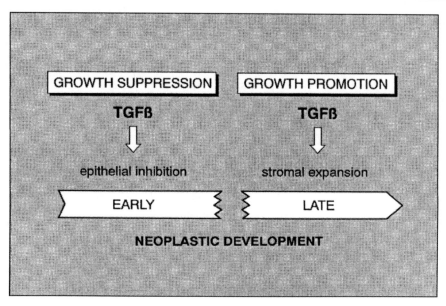

Fig. 7.7. The role of TGFβ may change as a tumor evolves. In the early stages of carcinogenesis the epithelial inhibitory effects of TGFβ dominate, whilst in the more advanced stages this growth factor may serve to promote tumor growth by stimulating angiogenesis and elaboration of extracellular matrix proteins resulting in stromal expansion and support for malignant elements of a carcinoma.

vii) Prospects for Therapy

There is circumstantial evidence for the preservation of functional TGFβ inhibitory loops in the earlier stages of malignant transformation, with production of TGFβ by normal and some transformed mammary epithelial cells. These growth inhibitory effects of TGFβ could therefore be harnessed and exploited therapeutically at a stage in the neoplastic continuum where subtle changes in the balance of growth factors within the local microenvironment of cells is an important determinant of cell behavior, especially proliferative potential. The pharmacological manipulation of growth factor loops represents a realistic strategy for modulating local endogenous levels of growth factors. There is much experimental data in support of the pharmacological induction of TGFβ in hormone dependent systems. However, this response is not confined to hormone sensitive tissues and indeed may be mediated by mechanisms which are partially independent of conventional receptors.[47,48,52,98,123]

Though evidence has been presented in support of TGFβ participating in epithelial autocrine inhibitory loops in vivo, evidence for direct of enhancement of such autocrine inhibitory effects by administration of anti-estrogens is at present inconclusive. Not only are any breast cancer cell lines reported to be unresponsive to TGFβ, but increased intracellular expression of TGFβ within epithelial cells following some pharmacological intervention provides no indication of where the ligand will be targeted, i.e., an autocrine or paracrine action. Therefore it remains unclear whether ER dependent growth inhibition by anti-estrogens involves direct augmentation of a TGFβ inhibitory loop in malignant breast epithelial cells. In fact, studies with the ER positive breast cancer cell line CAMA-1 suggest that modulation of TGFβ is not an obligatory step in tamoxifen mediated growth inhibition; these cells express neither TGFβ receptors nor the corresponding transcript yet are strongly growth inhibited by tamoxifen at a concentration of 1μM.[160] Furthermore, studies examining the potential role of TGFβ1 as a proximate effector in mediation of growth inhibition of T47D cells by progestins cast doubt on the relevance of this growth factor *apropos* induction of growth arrest. Inhibition of these ER positive cells is not associated with increased expression of TGFβ1 and the response is not abrogated by anti-TGFβ1 neutralizing antibodies. As in CAMA-1 cells, mRNA for TGFβ type II receptor is lacking in these cells, thus precluding any autocrine, or indeed paracrine, epithelial inhibitory response.[161] Similarly, cell cycle events associated with growth inhibition in tamoxifen sensitive MCF-7 and T47-D cells are not blocked by anti-TGFβ antibodies.[162]

Despite uncertainty over direct modulation of autocrine inhibitory loops both in vitro and in vivo, evidence has been presented supporting stromal induction of TGFβ in response to pharmacological intervention (Fig. 7.8). This enhancement of paracrine inhibitory loops is dependent upon maintenance of epithelial responsiveness to TGFβ which remains a contentious issue.[53] Furthermore, current data does not permit any assessment of the relative quantitative contribution of TGFβ1 induction to the overall anti-tumor effects of agents such as anti-estrogens. In the study of Butta and colleagues, though upregulation of TGFβ1 was seen in both ER positive and ER negative tumors in vivo, clinical response of ER positive tumors was 3- to 4-fold greater than for ER negative tumors. Induction of TGFβ1 may be quantitatively more important in early stage disease where tumor burden is small and epithelial cells are more responsive to subtle changes in levels of negative growth factors in their micro-environment. It is crucial that the magnitude of TGFβ induction is correlated with parameters of clinical response. Such assessments will also permit comparisons between different therapeutic agents. In situ hybridization studies will aid clarification of the source of TGFβ and indicate whether strategies for boosting endogenous levels of TGFβ should focus on stromal versus epithelial cells as the more appropriate target for induction.

Local induction within individual tissues is the optimal approach for increased exposure of target cells to TGFβ. This growth factor has a relatively short plasma half-life which precludes it from acting at a site distant from its origin, and animal studies indicate that systemically administered forms of TGFβ are generally toxic and the pharmacokinetics of distribution of any dose complex.[163] The latent form of TGFβ has a longer plasma half-life than the active form, and could travel in the circulation to act at a site distant from its origin. Little is known of local tissue levels of TGFβ and their correlation with plasma levels. Moreover, plasma forms of TGFβ may be preferentially sequestered by tissues other than the target organ and local bioavailability restricted even further by binding of TGFβ to extracellular matrix components of target tissues. Plasma levels of TGFβ1 have been found to be greatly elevated in some patients with advanced breast cancer, but the physiological significance of this is unclear.[164]

In most of the systems investigating pharmacological induction of TGFβ, the assayed product was in the biologically active form. This is a coincidental advantage and would obviate the need for specific prior activation which might be a rate-limiting step. Functionally active forms of TGFβ may therefore be available to a wider spectrum of potential target cells.[47,52,123]

There is scope for refinement and development of current approaches for boosting local endogenous production of TGFβ; specificity could be increased by enhancing sensitivity of target tissues to any locally induced TGFβ, permitting levels of TGFβ induction which maximize therapeutic ratios and minimize adverse effects of TGFβ upon healthy tissues.[165] Retinoids have been shown to render a previously resistant MCF-7 cell line responsive to exogenous TGFβ, perhaps involving modulation of receptor density.[166] The latent TGFβ

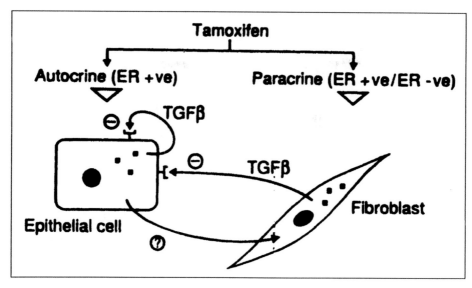

Fig. 7.8. TGFβ can be locally induced in tissues by agents such as tamoxifen. Both epithelial and stromal elements are potential sources of pharmacologically induced TGFβ, which may be secreted in the biologically active form where it can inhibit epithelial cell growth without the requirement for prior activation. Reprinted with permission from: Benson JR, Colletta AA. Clinical Immunotherapeutics 1995; 4:249-258. © ADIS International Publications Limited.

complex is bound to the ECM via the LAP and LTBP, suggesting that the local bioavailability of TGFβ could be augmented by manipulating levels of these specific binding proteins.

Studies with transgenic mice indicate that gene therapy may be a feasible method for enhancing local TGFβ production where there is an identifiable target lesion. This could involve introduction of multiple copies of the TGFβ gene, or manipulation of its promoter region. Transcriptional efficiency could be increased by modifying the transactivating potential of transcription factors such as the early growth response 1 (EGR-1) gene. This binds to GC rich regulatory elements in the promoter region of the TGFβ1 gene and stimulates secretion of the protein product in the fibrosarcoma cell line HT 1080 whose growth is suppressed by TGFβ1.[167] This stimulation of transcription is counteracted by repressor factors which bind to specific regions of the EGR-1 gene. Mutant forms of EGR-1 which lack these repressor domains exhibit enhanced rates of transcription. Thus gene therapy could be employed to increase transactivation by EGR-1 directly using EGR-1 expression vectors or indirectly by abrogating repressor activity. The stem-loop structures in the 5′ UTR of the TGFβ1 mRNA molecule could be modified genetically such that any inhibitory effects upon rates of translation are attenuated.[87] Both epithelial and stromal cells would constitute targets for gene therapy, though genetic manipulation of epithelial cells *per se* might in some circumstances promote malignant change. Moreover, as stromal cells are amenable to pharmacological induction of TGFβ, they may represent the optimal target for gene therapy which can complement and augment induction by more conventional therapeutic agents Dr. Benson wants to change this, but I can't read his writing. As discussed in the previous section, TGFβ1 transgenic mice which express augmented levels of TGFβ1 within mammary duct epithelium fail to produce spontaneous tumors and are resistant to chemically induced carcinogenesis. Therefore enhancement of local TGFβ levels may constitute an important strategy for generation of a "malignancy-resistant phenotype". Furthermore, altered expression of TGFβ within tissues could be a useful surrogate biomarker for assessing response to potential chemopreventive agents and thus avoiding reliance on extensive and prolonged animal/clinical studies to determine efficacy.

Invasive breast carcinomas have been reported to express low levels of the type II TGFβ receptor on immunohistochemical assays.[151] Were a TGFβ receptor defect to develop in the relatively early stages of carcinogenesis and to occur in a high percentage of cells within a particular tumor (e.g., colorectal carcinoma), it may be feasible to apply gene therapy to correct this defect and restore an inhibitory response to TGFβ. Such therapy could be combined with the above strategies for enhancing local endogenous levels of TGFβ. This combination of local induction of TGFβ and augmentation of cellular sensitivity might maximally exploit the specific growth inhibitory effects of TGFβ upon epithelial cells.

This strategy of pharmacological manipulation of growth factor loops accords with the concept of 'cancer control' rather than 'cancer kill' whereby the therapeutic goal shifts from cell kill to re-regulation.[168] Improvements in disease-free and overall survival may ensue from effectively rendering the behavior of a tumor more benign. Furthermore, this pharmacological manipulation of so-called "biological response modifiers" in the early stages of neoplastic development might abort the transition from premalignant to in situ change, or possibly in situ to invasive disease. This echoes the philosophy espoused by Wellings and colleagues 20 years ago:[169]

> " *More emphasis might be shifted now to elucidation of the remote and early conditions that precede human breast cancer. This is perhaps the best approach to prevention, early diagnosis and cure.*"

It has been stated that TGFβ can potentially function either as friend or foe; despite it's potent growth inhibitory effects, other aspects of TGFβ action are associated with growth stimulation. This complex pathophysiological profile casts uncertainty over the optimal therapeutic approaches for manipulating components of the TGFβ system. It seems clear that in the preneoplastic and early stages of tumor development, boosting of local endogenous levels of TGFβ seems appropriate and targeting of neoplastic tissues should help minimize the adverse effects of TGFβ on normal tissues, such as pulmonary fibrosis. Several studies have implied a direct association between increased tissue expression or plasma levels of TGFβ, and tumor progression. These tumor promoting properties of TGFβ are likely to pertain in more advanced tumors and to result collectively from effects on extracellular matrix, angiogenesis and immune suppression coupled with loss of epithelial growth inhibitory effects. There is some evidence that TGFβ may also confer resistance to some conventional forms of chemotherapy. Huang and co-workers have hypothesized that aberrant expression of TGFβ may contribute to tumor progression by decreasing genetic stability of cells.[170] Murine fibroblast cell lines (10 1/2) were transfected with a TGFβ1 construct and transectants over-expressing active forms of TGFβ1 were resistant to the cytotoxic effects of N-(phosphonoacetyl)-L-aspartate (PALA) in colony-forming assays.[171] Fluctuation analysis performed on cell lines expressing the metallothionein promoter confirmed that resistance to PALA was proportional to TGFβ1 expression. Moreover, this resistance to cytotoxicity was associated with amplification of the gene coding for the target protein of PALA, termed CAD, a complex polypeptide with multiple enzymatic functions.

Thus TGFβ may indirectly promote tumor growth through gene amplification, thereby conferring resistance to cytotoxic agents. Of related interest, it has recently been shown that TGFβ can almost completely block efflux of drugs from glial cells within an in vitro system.[172] Such a mechanism would tend to counter innate drug resistance mechanisms and once again illustrates the complex functional profile of TGFβ. Though anti-TGFβ strategies have found useful application in noncancer treatments such as wound healing,[173-175] it is difficult to advocate such an approach at present in cancer therapy. Anti-sense technology employing oligo-deoxyribonucleotides which are complementary to TGFβ have proved effective in reducing the proliferative and metastatic potential of H-*ras*-transformed (10 1/2) fibrosarcomas for which TGFβ acts in a positive autocrine manner promoting tumor growth.[176] (See chapter 3 section viii.)

Within the framework of current understanding and perceived paradigms of TGFβ pathophysiology, those therapeutic endeavors which focus on the growth inhibitory properties of TGFβ, which appear operative in normal, preneoplastic states and early stage malignancy, are likely to be most rewarding as a 'translational' strategy. With this in mind, the challenge for the future is the development of agents which have more potent and specific effects upon synthesis, secretion and bioavailability of TGFβ from both epithelial and mesenchymal cells. Development of three-dimensional coculture systems in which fibroblasts and epithelial cells are embedded within an artificial extracellular matrix may permit expression and design of optimal functional responses, such as induction and secretion of cytokines. These models could be employed to test new agents including "designer" drugs with correspondingly greater inductive properties and clinical efficacy. Success with these therapeutic strategies will be dependent upon some assessment of the relative quantitative

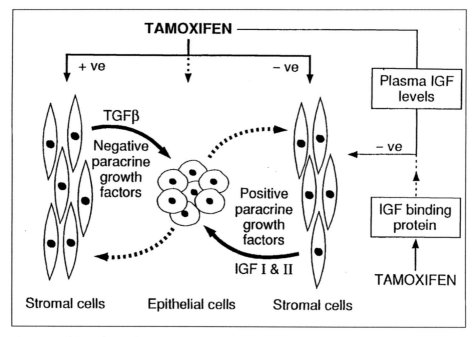

Fig. 7.9. Unifying schema showing the potential dual action of agents such as tamoxifen on growth factor levels. Thus tamoxifen may directly stimulate either stromal or epithelial cells to enhance secretion of the negative growth factor TGFβ. Conversely it may act upon these same cells to suppress production of stimulatory growth factors such as IGF I and IGF II. Furthermore, epithelial proliferation may be indirectly modulated by changes in systemic levels of growth factors and the local bioavailability of growth factors as dictated by levels of cognate binding proteins. Reprinted with permission from: Benson JR, Baum M, Colletta AA. In: deVita, Hellman, Rosenberg, eds. Biologic Therapy of Cancer, 2nd Edition. 1995:817-828. © Lippincott-Raven Publishers.

contributions of these various mechanisms to the overall anti-neoplastic action of these agents.

Complementary approaches include the use of related compounds which can also induce TGFβ in epithelial cells, and suppress production of positive growth factors such as IGF I and II from both stromal and epithelial tissue components (Fig. 7.9). Such agents must be of a specificity and potency to be clinically efficacious with minimal toxicity. This strategy may be especially pertinent in a chemopreventive setting and in the early stages of malignancy where epithelial load is modest, inductive effects have not been exhausted and malignant cells still possess corresponding receptors. Elucidation of the mechanisms by which TGFβ and other negative growth modulators deliver a growth inhibitory signal to epithelial cells may provide further potential targets for therapy.

References

1. Nolvadex Adjuvant Trial Organisation. Controlled trial of tamoxifen as a single adjuvant agent in the management of early breast cancer. Br J Cancer 1988; 57:608-611.
2. Medical Research Council Scottish Trials Office. Adjuvant tamoxifen in the management of operable breast cancer. Lancet 1987; 11:171-175.
3. Fisher B, Constantino J, Redmond C et al. A randomised clinical trial evaluating tamoxifen in the treatment of patients with node negative breast cancer who have estrogen receptor negative tumours. NEJM 1989; 320:479-484.
4. Early Breast Cancer Trialists Collaborative Group. Systemic treatment of early breast cancer by hormonal, cytotoxic or immune therapy. 133 randomised trials involving 31,000 recurrences and 24,000 deaths among 75,000 women. Lancet 1992; 339:1-15, 71-78.
5. Cuzik J, Baum M. Tamoxifen and contralateral breast cancer. Lancet 1985; (ii):282-282.
6a. Early Breast Cancer Trialists Collaborative Group. Tamoxifen for early breast cancer: an overview of randomised trials. Lancet 1998; 351:1451-67.
6b. Benson JR. Tamoxifen in early breast cancer. Lancet 1998; 352:404-405.
7. Denis M, Poellinger L, Wikstrom A-C et al. Requirement of hormone for thermal conversion of the glucocorticoid receptor to a DNA-binding state. Nature 1988; 333:686-688.
8. Parker MG. In: Cancer Surveys Vol 14. Growth regulation by nuclear hormone receptors. London: ICRF Press. 1992:1-4.
9. Miller MA, Mullik A, Green GL and Katzenellenbogen BS. Characterisation of the subunit nature of the nuclear oestrogen receptors by the chemical cross-linking and dense amino-acid labelling. Endocrinology 1985; 117:515-522.
10. Klein-Hitpass L, Schorpp M, Wagner U and Ryfell GU. An estrogen responsive element derived from the 5' flanking region of the xenopus vitellogen A2 gene functions in transfected human cells. Cell 1986; 46:1053-1061.
11. Klein-Hitpass L, Ryfell GU Heitlinger E, Cato ACB. A 13 bp palindrome is a functional estrogen responsive element and interacts specifically with estrogen receptor. Nucleic Acids Res 1988; 16:647-663.
12. Kumar V, Green S, Stack G et al. Functional domains of the human oestrogen receptor. Cell 1987; 51:941-951.
13. Tora L, White J, Brou C et al. The human estrogen receptor has two independent non-acidic transcriptional activation functions. Cell 1989; 59:477-487.
14. Fawell SE, Whiter, Hoare S et al. Inhibition of estrogen receptor-DNA binding by the pure anti-oestrogen ICI 164,384 appears to be mediated by impaired receptor dimerisation. Proc Natl Aca Sci (USA) 1990; 87:6883-6887.
15. Berry M, Metzger M and Chambon P. Role of two transactivating domains in the cell-type and promoter-context dependent agonist activity of the anti-estrogen 4-hydroxytamoxifen. EMBO J 1990; 9:2811-2818.
16. Wakeling AM, Dukes M, Bowler J. A potent specific pure anti-estrogen with clinical potential. Cancer Res. 1992; 52:3867-3873.

17. Sutherland RL, Hall RE, Taylor IW. Cell proliferation kinetics of MCF-7 human mammary carcinoma cells in culture and effect of tamoxifen on exponentially growing and plateau phase cells. Cancer Res 1983; 43:3998-4006.
18. Katzenellenbogen BS, Fang H, Avery Ance B et al. Estrogen receptors: ligand discrimination and anti-estrogen action. Br Cancer Res Treat 1993; 27:17-26.
19. Sutherland RL, Watts CKW, Reunitz PC. Definition of two distinct mechanisms of action of anti-estrogens on human breast cancer cell proliferation using hydroxytriphenylethylenes with high affinity for the estrogen receptor. Biochem Biophys Res Comm 1986; 140:523-529.
20. Sutherland RL, Murphy LC, Ming San Foo et al. High affinity anti-estrogen binding site distinct from the estrogen receptor. Nature 1980; 288:273-275.
21. O'Brian CA, Liskamp RM, Solomon DH, Weinstein IB. Inhibition of protein kinase C by tamoxifen. Cancer Res 1985; 45:2462-2465.
22. Berridge MJ, Irving RF. Inositol triphosphate, a novel second messenger in cellular signal transduction. Nature 1984; 312:315-321.
23. O'Brian CA, Liskamp RM, Solomon DH, Weinstein IB. Triphenylethylenes: A new class of Protein Kinase C inhibitors. J Natl Cancer Inst 1986; 76:1243-1246.
24. Guerrin M, Guilaud M, Valette A. Regulation par la proteine kinase C de l'expression due TGFβ1 dans les cellules d'adenocarcinoma mammaire en culture. Bull Canc 1992; 79:357-363.
25. Lam H-YP. Tamoxifen is a calmodulin antagonist in the activation of a cAMP phosphodiesterase. Biochem Biophys Res Comm 1984; 118:27-32.
26. Rowland MG, Parr IB, MacCague R et al. Variation of the inhibition of calmodulin dependent cyclic AMP phospho-diesterase among analogs of tamoxifen: Correlation with cytotoxicity. Biochem Pharmacol 1990; 40:283-289.
27. Gulino A, Barrera G, Vacca A et al. Calmodulin antagonism and growth inhibitory activity of triphenylethylene anti-estrogens in MCF -7 human breast cancer cells. Cancer Res 1986; 46:6274-6278.
28. Musgrove EA, Wakeling AE, Sutherland RL. Points of action of estrogen antagonists and a calmodulin antagonist within MCF-7 human breast cancer cell cycle. Cancer Res 1989; 49:2398-2404.
29. Pollak M, Huynh HT, Pratt Lefebre S. Tamoxifen reduces serum insulin-like growth factor I (IGF I). Br Cancer Res Treat 1992; 22:91-100.
30. Huynh HT, Tetenes E, Wallace L, Pollak M. In vivo inhibition of insulin-like growth factor I gene expression by tamoxifen. Cancer Res 1993; 53:1727-1730.
31. Pollak M. The Challenge of Breast Cancer. Brugge: Lancet Conference, 1994.
32. Cullen KJ, Smith HS, Hill S et al. Growth factor messenger RNA expression by human breast fibroblasts from benign and malignant lesions. Cancer Res 1991; 51:4978-4985.
33. Peyrat JP, Bonneterre J, Beuscart R et al. Insulin-like growth factor I receptors in human breast cancer and their relation to estradiol and progesterone receptors. Cancer Res 1988; 48:6429-6433.
34. Folkman J. What is the evidence that tumours are angiogenesis dependent? J Natl Cancer Inst 1990; 82:4-6.
35. Weidner N, Semple JP, Welch WR, Folkman J. Tumour angiogenesis and metastasis-correlation in invasive breast carcinoma. NEJM 1991; 324:1-8.
36. Horak E, Harris AL. Angiogenesis, assessed by platelet/endothelial cell adhesion molecule antibodies, as indicator of node matastses and survival in breast cancer. Lancet 1992; 340:1120-1124.
37. Gagliardi A, Collins DC. Inhibition of angiogenesis by anti-estrogens. Cancer Res 1993; 53:533-535.
38. Shultz GS, Grant MB. Neovascular growth factors. Eye (London) 1991; 5:178-180.
39. Heimark RL, Twardzik DR, Schwartz SM. Inhibition of endothelial regeneration by type-β transforming growth factor from platelets. Science 1986; 233:1078-1080.
40. Grainger DA, Weissberg PL, Metcalfe JC. Tamoxifen decreases the rate of proliferation of rat vascular smooth-muscle cells in culture by inducing production of transforming growth factor β. Biochem J 1993; 294:109-112.

41. Heine UI, Munoz EF, Flanders KC et al. Role of transforming growth factor β in the development of the mouse embryo. J Cell Biol 1987; 105:2861-2876.

42. Wiseman DM, Polverini PJ, Kamp DW et al. Transforming growth factor β is chemotactic for human monocytes and induces their expression of angiogenic activity. Biochem Biophysic Res Comm. 1988; 157:793-800.

43. Ueki N, Nakazato T, Ohkawa T et al. Excessive production of transforming growth factor β1 can play an important role in the development of tumorigenesis by its action for angiogenesis: Validity of neutralising antibodies to block tumor growth. Biochim Biophys Acta Mol Cell Res 1992; 1137:189-196.

44. Iruela-Arispe ML, Sage EH. Endothelial cells exhibiting angiogenesis in vitro proliferate in response to TGFβ1. J Cell Biochem 1993; 52:414-430.

45. Benson JR, Baum M. Transforming growth factor beta isoforms in breast cancer. Br J Cancer 1994; 70:1278-1278.

46. Dickson RB, Bates S, McManaway M et al. Characterisation of oestrogen responsive transforming activity in human breast cancer cell lines. Cancer Res 1986 (a); 46:1707-1713.

47. Knabbe C, Lippman ME, Wakefield LM et al. Evidence that transforming growth factor-beta is a hormonally regulated negative growth factor in human breast cancer. Cell 1987; 48:417-428.

48. Butta A, Maclennan K, Flanders KC et al. Induction of transforming growth factor beta 1 in human breast cancer in vivo following tamoxifen treatment. Cancer Res 1992; 52:4261-4264.

49. McCune BK, Mullin BR, Flanders KC et al. Localisation of transforming growth factor β isotypes in lesions of the human breast. Human Path 1992; 23:13-20.

50. Dublin EA, Barnes DM, Wang DY et al. TGF alpha and TGFβ expression in mammary carcinoma. J Path 1993; 170:15-22.

51. Arteaga CL, Coffey RJ, Dugger TC et al. Growth stimulation of human breast cancer cells with anti-transforming growth β antibodies: Evidence for negative autocrine growth regulation by transforming growth factor β. Cell Growth Diff 1990; 1:367-374.

52. Dickson RB, Kasid A, Huff KK et al. Activation of growth factor secretion in tumorigenic states of breast cancer induced by 17β estradiol or v-Ha-ras oncogene. Proc Natl Acad Sci (USA) 1987; 84:837-841.

53. Arteaga CL, Carty-Dugger T, Moses HL et al. Transforming growth factor beta 1 can induce estrogen -independent tumorogenicity of human breast cancer cells in athymic mice. Cell Growth and Diff 1993; 4:193-201.

54. Gorsch SM, Memoli V, Stukel TA et al. Immunohistochemical staining for transforming growth factor β1 associates with disease progression in human breast cancer. Cancer Res 1992; 52:6949-6952.

55. Colletta AA, Wakefield LM, Howell FV et al. Anti-oestrogens induce the secretion of active transforming growth factor beta from human foetal fibroblasts. Br J Cancer 1990; 62:405-409.

56. Thompson AM, Kerr DJ, Steel CM. Transforming growth factor β1 is implicated in the failure of tamoxifen therapy in human breast cancer. Br J Cancer 1991; 63:609-614.

57. Travers MT, Barrett-Lee PJ, Berger U et al. Growth factor expression in normal, benign and malignant breast tissue. BMJ 1988; 296:1621-1624.

58. MacCallum J, Bartlett JMS, Thompson AM et al. Expression of transforming growth factor β mRNA isoforms in human breast cancer. Br J Cancer 1994; 69:1006-1009.

59. MacCallum J, Bartlett JMS, Thompson AM et al. Change in TGFβ mRNA expression in breast cancer patients treated with tamoxifen (abstract). The Breast 1995; 4:No.3 255.

60. Walker RJ, Dearing SJ, Gallacher B. Relationship of transforming growth factor β1 to extracellular matrix and stromal infiltrates in invasive breast cancer. Br J Cancer 1994; 69:1160-1165.

61. Murray PA, Barrett-Lee P, Travers M et al. The prognostic significance of transforming growth factors in human breast cancer. Br J Cancer 1993; 67:1408-1412.

62. Mizukami Y, Nonomura A, Yamada T et al. Immunohistochemical demonstration of growth factors, TGF alpha, TGFβ, IGF-I and neu oncogene product in benign and malignant breast tissues. Anticancer Res 1990; 10:1115-1126.

63. Cunha GR, Donjacour A. Stromal-epithelial interactions in normal and abnormal prostatic development. Prog Clin Biol Res 1987; 239: 251-272.

64. Haggie JA, Sellwood RA, Howel A et al. Fibroblasts from relatives of patients with hereditary breast cancer show fetal-like behaviour in vitro. Lancet 1987; (i):1455-1457.

65. Schor SL, Haggie JA, Durning P et al. Occurrence of a fetal fibroblast phenotype in familial breast cancer. Int J Cancer 1986; 37:831-836.

66. Brooks MD, Ebbs SR, Colletta AA, Baum M. Desmoid tumours treated with triphenylethylenes. Eur J Cancer 1992; 28:1014-1018.

67. Flanders KC, Thompson NL, Cissel DS et al. Transforming growth factor β-histochemical localisation with antibodies to different epitopes. J Cell Biol 1989; 108:653-660.

68. Benson JR, LM Wakefield, MB Sporn et al. Synthesis and secretion of TGFβ isoforms by primary cultures of human breast tumour fibroblasts in vitro and their modulation by tamoxifen. Br J Cancer 1996; 74:352-358.

69. Cross M and Dexter TM. Growth factors in development, transformation and tumorigenesis. Cell 1991; 64:271-280.

70. Spence AM, Sheppard PC, Davie JR et al. Regulation of a bifunctional mRNA results in synthesis of secreted and nuclear probasin. PNAS(USA) 1989 86:7843-7847.

71. Derynck R, Jarrett JA, Ellson YC et al. Human transforming growth factor beta complementary DNA sequence and expression in normal and transformed cells. Nature 1985; 316:701-705.

72. Perlhman D, Halvorson HO. A putative signal peptidase recognition site and sequence in eukaryotic and prokaryotic signal peptides. J Mol Biol 1983; 107:391-409.

73. Dang CV, Lee WMF. Nuclear and nucleolar targeting sequences of c-erb-A, c-myb, N-myc, p53, HSP70 and HIV tat proteins. J Biol Chem 1989; 264:18019-18023.

74. Imamura T, Engleka K, Zhan X et al. Recovery of mitogenic activity of a growth factor mutant with a nuclear translocation sequence. Science 1990; 249:1567-1570.

75. Yeh H-J, Pierce GF, Deuel TF. Ultrastructural localisation of platelet-derived growth factor/v-sis related protein(s) in cytoplasm and nucleus of simian sarcoma virus-transformed cells. Proc Natl Aca Sci (USA) 1987; 84:2317-2321.

76. Sano H, Forough R, Maier JAM et al. Detection of high levels of heparin binding growth factor-1 in inflammatory arthritic joints. J Cell Biol 1986; 110:1417-1426.

77. Arrik BA, Grendell RL, Griffin LA. Enhanced translational efficiency of a novel transforming growth factor beta 3 mRNA in human breast cancer cells. Mol Cell Biol 1994; 14:619-628.

78. Kim S-Y, Park K, Koeller D et al. Posttranscriptional regulation of the human transforming growth factor β1 gene. J Biol Chem 1992; 267:13702-13707.

79. Ferguson JE, Schor AM, Howell A, Ferguson MWJ. Changes in the extracellular matrix of the normal human breast during the menstrual cycle. Cell Tissue Res 1992; 268:167-177.

80. Atherton AJ, Monaghan P, Warbuton MJ et al. Dipeptidyl peptidase IV expression identifies a functional sub-population of breast fibroblasts. Int J Cancer 1992; 50:15-19.

81. Schor AM, Rushton G, Ferguson JE et al. Phenotypic heterogeneity in breast fibroblasts: functional anomaly in fibroblasts from histologically normal tissue adjacent to carcinoma. Int J Cancer 1994; 59:25-32.

82. Caniggia I, Tseu I, Han RN et al. Spatial and temporal differences in fibroblast behaviour in fetal rat lung. Am J Physiol 1991; 261:424-443.

83. Nohammer G, Bajardi F, Benedetto C et al. Histophotometric quantification of the field effect and the extended field effect of tumors. Free Rad Res Comm 1989; 7:129-137.

84. Assosian RK, Fleurdelys BE, Stevenson HC et al. Expression and secretion of type β transforming growth factor by activated human macrophages. PNAS (USA) 1987; 84:6020-6024.

85. Glick AB, Flanders KC, Danielpour D et al. Retinoic acid induces transforming growth factor β2 in cultured keratinocytes and mouse epidermis Cell Reg 1989 (b); 1:87-97.

86. Derynck R, Jarrett JA, Ellson Y C et al. Human transforming growth factor beta complementary DNA sequence and expression in normal and transformed cells. Nature 1985; 316:701-705.
87. Kim S-Y, Park K, Koeller D et al. Posttranscriptional regulation of the human transforming growth factor β1 gene. J Biol Chem 1992; 267: 13702-13707.
88. Hentze MW, Rouault TA, Caughman SW et al. A cis-acting element is necessary and sufficient for translational regulation of human ferritin expression in response to iron. Proc Natl Aca Sci (USA) 1987; 84:6730-6734.
89. Caughman SW, Hentze MW, Rouault TA et al. The iron-responsive element is the single element responsible for iron dependent translational regulation of ferritin biosynthesis. J Biol Chem 1988; 263:19048-19052.
90. Rouault TA, Hentze MW, Haile DJ et al. The iron -responsive element binding protein: A method for the affinity purification of a regulatory RNA-binding protein. Proc Natl Aca Sci (USA) 1989; 86:5768-5772.
91. Verdi JM, Campagnoni AT. Translational regulation by steroids. J Biol Chem 1990; 265:20314-20320.
92. Perry RR, Kang Y, Greaves BR. Relationship between tamoxifen-induced transforming growth factor β1 expression, cytostasis and apoptosis in human breast cancer cells. Br J Cancer 1995; 72:1441-1446.
93. Benson JR, Colletta AA. Changes in expression of transforming growth factor beta mRNA isoforms in patients undergoing tamoxifen therapy (letter). Br J Cancer 1997; 75:776-778.
94. Russo J, Tay LJ, Russo IH. Differentiation of the mammary gland and susceptibility to carcinogenesis. Breast Cancer Res Treat 1981; 2:5-73.
95. Clarke CL, Sutherland RL. Progestin regulation of cellular proliferation. Endo Rev 1990; 11:266-301.
96. Horwitz KB, Wei LL, Sedlacek SM, D'Arville CN. Progestin action and progesterone receptor structure in human breast cancer: A review. Recent Progress in Hormonal Research 1985; 41:249-317.
97. Plu-Bureau G, Le MG, Sitruk-Ware R et al. Progestogen use and decreased risk of breast cancer on a cohort study of premenopausal women with benign breast disease. Br J Cancer 1994; 70:270-277.
98. Colletta AA, Wakefield LM, Howell FV et al. The growth inhibition of human breast cancer cells by a novel synthetic progestin involves the induction if TGFβ. J Clin Invest 1991; 87:277-283.
99. The WHO Collaborative Study of Neoplasia and Steroid contraceptives. Breast cancer and combined oral contraceptives: results from a multinational study. Br J Cancer 1990; 61:110-119.
100. Vessey MP, Doll R, Jones K et al. An epidemiological study of oral contraceptives and breast cancer BMJ 1979; I:1757-1760.
101. Pike MC, Henderson BE, Krako MD. Breast cancer in young women and use of oral contraceptives: possible modifying effect of formulation and age at use. Lancet 1983; 2:926-930.
102. Paul C, Skegg DCG, Spears GFS. Depot MPA and risk of breast cancer. BMJ 1989; 299:759-762.
103. Henderson BE, Ross R, Bernstein L. Estrogens as a cause of human cancer. Cancer Res 1988; 48:246-253.
104. Wolbach SB, Howe PR. Tissue changes following deprivation of fat soluble Vitamin A. J Exp Med 1925; 43:753-777.
105. Harris AL, Nicholson S. EGF receptors in human breast cancer. In: Lippman ME, Dickson RB, eds. Breast Cancer-Cellular and Molecular Biology. Boston: Kluwer Academic Publishers, 1988:343-362.
106. Fell HB, Mellanby E. Metaplasia produced in cultures of chick ectoderm produced by high Vit A. J Physiol 1953; 119:470-488.
107. Lasnitski I. Reversal of methylcholanthrene-induced changes in mouse prostates in vitro by retinoic acid and its analogs. Br J Cancer 1976; 34:239-248.

108. Chatterjee M, Banerjee MR. Influence of hormones on N-[4-hydroxyphenyl]-retinamide inhibition of 7,12-dimethylbenzanthracene transformation of mammary cells in organ culture Cancer Lett 1978; 16:239-245.
109. Todaro GJ, de Larco JE, Sporn MB. Retinoids block phenotypic cell transformation produced by sarcoma growth factor. Nature 1978; 276:272-274.
110. Merriman RL, Bertram JS. Reversible inhibition by retinoids of 3-methylcholanthrene-induced neoplstic transformation in C3H/10T 1/2 clone 8 cells. Cancer Res 1979; 39:1661-1666.
111. Ueda H, Takenawa T, Millan JC et al. The effects of retinoids on the proliferative capacities and macro-molecular synthesis in human breast cancer MCF-7 cells. Cancer 1980; 46:2203-2209.
112. Marth C, Mayer I, Daxenbichler G et al. Effect of retinoic acid and 4-hydroxytamoxifen on human breast cancer cell lines. Biochem Pharmacol 1984; 33: 2217-2221.
113. Dion LD, Blalock JE, Gifford GE. Retinoic acid and the restoration of anchorage -dependent growth to transformed mammalian cells. Exp Cell Res 1977; 117:15-22.
114. Kliewer SA, Umesono K, Mangelsdorf DJ, Evans RM. Retinoid X receptor interacts with nuclear receptors in retinoic acid, thyroid hormone and vitamin D3 signalling. Nature 1992; 355:446-449.
115. Roberts AB, Sporn MB. The transforming Growth Factor betas. In: Sporn MB, Roberts AB, eds. Peptide growth factors and their receptors. Handbook of Experimental Pharmacology, Vol. 95. Heidelberg: Springer Verlag, 1990:419-472.
116. Tucker RF, Shipley GD, Moses HL. Holley RW. Growth inhibitor from BSC-1 cells is closely related to the platelet type β transforming growth factor Science 1984; 226:705-707.
117. Arteaga CL, Tandon AK, von Hoff DD, Osborne CK. Transforming growth factor β: potential autocrine growth inhibition of estrogen receptor negative human breast cancer cells. Cancer Res 1988 (b); 48:3898-3904.
118. Heine UI, Munoz EF, Flanders KC et al. Role of transforming growth factor β in the development of the mouse embryo. J Cell Biol 1987; 105:2861-2876.
119. Silberstein GB, Daniel CW. Reversible inhibition of mammary gland growth by transforming growth factor β. Science 1987; 237:291-293.
120. Heine UI, Munoz EF, Flanders KC et al. Colocalisation of TGFβ1 and collagen I and III, fibronectin and GAG during lung branching morphogenesis. Dev 1990; 109:29-36.
121. Danielpour D, Kim K-Y, Winkur TS, Sporn MB. Differential regulation of the expression of TGFβs 1 and 2 by retinoic acid, epidermal growth factor and dexamethasone in NRK-49F and A549 cells. J Cell Physiol 1991; 148:235-244.
122. Glick AB, McCune BK, Abdulkarem N et al. Complex regulation of TGFβ1 expression by retinoic acid in the Vitamin A deficient rat. Dev 1991 (a); 111:1081-1086.
123. Glick AB, Danielpour D, Morgan DL et al. Induction and autocrine receptor binding of TGFβ2 during terminal differentiation of primary mouse keratinocytes. Mol Endo 1990; 4:46-52.
124. Shipley GD, Childs CB, Volkenant ME, Moses HL. Differential effects of epidermal growth factor, transforming growth factor and insulin on DNA and protein synthesis and morphology in serum-free cultures of AKR-2B cells. Cancer Res 1984; 44:710-716.
125. Tucker RF, Shipley GD, Moses HL, Holley RW. Growth inhibitor from BSC-1 cells is closely related to the platelet type β transforming growth factor. Science 1984; 226:705-707.
126. Manning AM, Williams AC, Game SM, Paraskeva C. Differential sensitivity of human colonic adenoma and carcinoma cells to transforming growth factor beta: conversion of an adenoma cell line to a tumorigenic phenotype is accompanied by a reduced response to the inhibitory effects of TGFβ. Oncogene 1993; 6:1471-1477.
127. Masui T, Wakefield LM, Lechner JF et al. Type β transforming growth factor is the primary differentiation inducing serum factor for normal human bronchial epithelial cells. Proc Natl Aca Sci (USA) 1986; 83:2438-2442.
128. Mummery CL, Slager H, Kruijer W. Expression of transforming growth factor β2 during the differentiation of murine embryonal carcinoma and embryonal stem cells. Develop Biol 1990; 137:161-170.

129. Moralis TI, Roberts AB. The interaction between retinoic acid and the transforming growth factors-β in calf articular cartilage organ cultures. Arch Biochem Biophys 1992; 293:79-84.

130. Danielpour D, Kim KY, Winokur TS et al. Differential expression of Transforming growth factors β1 and β2 by retinoic acid, epidermal growth factor and dexamethasone in NRK-49 and A549 cells J Cell Physiol 1991; 148:235-244.

131. McCormick DL, Sowell ZL, Thompson CA, Moon RC. Inhibition by retinoid and ovariectomy of additional malignancies in rats following surgical removal of the first mammary cancer. Cancer 1988; 51:594-599.

132. Ratko TA, Detrisac CJ, Dinger MN et al. Chemopreventive efficacy of combined retinoid and tamoxifen treatment following surgical excision of a primary mammary cancer in female rats. Cancer Res 1989; 49:4472-4476.

133. Jordan VC, Allen KE, Dix CJ. Pharmacology of tamoxifen in laboratory animals. Cancer Treat Rep 1980; 64:745-759.

134. Rotmensz N, DePalo G, Formelli F et al. Long term tolerability of fenretinide (4-HPR) in breast cancer patients. Eur J Cancer 1991; 27:1127-1131.

135. Costa A. Breast Cancer Chemoprevention. Eur J Cancer 1993; 29A:589-592.

136. Robinson SD, Silberstein GB, Roberts AB et al. Regulated expression and and growth inhibitory effects of transforming growth factor β isoforms in mouse mammary gland development. Dev 1991; 113:867-878.

137. Wu S, Theodorescu D, Kerbel RS et al. TGFβ1 is an autocrine-negative growth regulator of human colon carcinoma FET cells in vivo as revealed by transfection of an anti-sense expression vector. J Cell Biol 1992; 116:187-196.

138. Glick AB, Lee MM, Darwiche N et al. Targetted deletion of the TGFβ1 gene causes rapid progression to squamous cell carcinoma. Genes Dev 1994; 8:2429-2440.

139. Cui W, Kemp CJ, Duffie E et al. Lack of TGFβ1 expression in benign skin tumors of p53 null mice is prognostic for a high risk of conversion. Cancer Res 1994; 54:5831-5836.

140. Pierce DF, Johnson MD, Matsui Y et al. Inhibition of mammary duct development but not alveolar outgrowth during pregnancy in transgenic mice expressing active TGFβ1. Genes Dev 1993; 7:2308-2317.

141. Brunner N, Zugmaier G, Bano M et al. Endocrine therapy of human breast cancer cells: the role of secreted polypeptide growth factors. Cancer cells 1989; 1:81-86.

142. Pelton RW, Saxena B, Jones M et al. Immunohistochemical localisation of TGFβ1, TGFβ2 and TGFβ3 in the mouse embryo: expression patterns suggest multiple roles during embryonic development. J Cell Biol 1991; 115:1091-1095.

143. Matsui Y, Halter SA, Holt JT et al. Development of mammary hyperplasia and neoplasia in MMTV-TGF alpha transgenic mice. Cell 1990; 61:1147-1156.

144. Halter SA, Dempsey P, Matsui Y et al. Distinctive patterns of hyperplasia in transgenic mice with mammary tumor virus transforming growth factor alpha. Characterisation of mammary gland and skin proliferation. Am J Path 1992; 140:1131-1146.

145. Snedeker SM, Brown CF, Diaugustine RP. Expression and functional properties of TGF alpha and EGF during mouse mammary gland ductal morphogenesis. Proc Natl Aca Sci (USA) 1991; 88:276-280.

146. Coffey RJ, Meise K S, Matsui Y et al. Acceleration of mammary neoplasia in transforming growth factor alpha transgenic mice by 7,12 dimethylbenzanthracene. Cancer Res 1994; 54:1678-1683.

147. Markowitz S, Wang J, Myeroff L et al. Inactivation of the type II TGFβ receptor in colon cancer cells with microsatellite instability. Science 1995; 268:1336-1338.

148. Wakefield LM, Colletta AA, McCune BK, Sporn MB. Roles for transforming growth factors β in the genesis, prevention and treatment of breast cancer. In: Dickson RB, Lippman ME, eds. Genes, Oncogenes and Hormones: Advances in Cellular and Molecular Biology Breast Cancer. Boston: Kluwer Academic Publishers, 1991:97-136.

149. Geiser AG, Burmester JK, Webbink R et al. Inhibition of growth by TGFβ following fusion of two nonresponsive human carcinoma cell lines. Implication of the type II receptor in growth inhibitory responses. J Biol Chem 1992; 267:2588-2593.

150. Sun L, Wu G, Willson JKV et al. Expression of transforming growth factor β type II receptor leads to reduced malignancy and in human breast cancer MCF-7 cells. J Biol Chem 1994; 269:26449-26455.

151. Younes M, Fernandez L, Laucirica R. Transforming growth factor β type II receptor is infrequently expressed in human breast cancer. Breast J 1996; 2:150-153.

152. Glick AB, Lee MM, Darwiche N et al. Targeted deletion of the TGFβ1 gene causes rapid progression to squamous cell carcinoma. Genes Dev 1994; 2429-2439.

153. Dalal DI, Keown PA, Greenberg AH. Immunocytochemical localisation of secreted transforming growth factor β1 to the advancing edges of primary tumors and to lymph node metastases of human mammary carcinoma. Am J Path 1993; 43:381-389.

154. Walker RA, Dearing SJ. Transforming growth factor β1 in ductal carcinoma in situ and invasive carcinomas of the breast. Eur J Cancer 1992; 28:641-644.

155. Daly RJ, King RJB, Darbre PD. Interaction of growth factors during progression towards steroid independence in T47-D human breast cancer cells. J Cell Biochem 1990; 43:199-211.

156. Oda K, Hori S, Itoh H et al. Immunohistochemical study of transforming growth factor β, fibronectin and fibronectin receptor in invasive mammary carcinomas. Acta Path Jap 1992; 42:645-650.

157. Kehrl JH, Wakefield LM, Roberts AB et al. Production of transforming growth factor β by human T lymphocytes and its potential role in the regulation of T cell growth. J Exp Med 1986; 163:1037-1050.

158. Kehrl JH, Taylor AS, Delsing GA et al. Further studies of the role of transforming growth factor β in human B cell function. J Immunol 1989; 143:1868-1874.

159. Tsunawaki S, Sporn M, Ding A et al. Deactivation of macrophages by transforming growth factor β. Nature 1988; 334:260-262.

160. Ji H, Stout LE, Zhang Q et al. Absence of transforming growth factor β responsiveness in the tamoxifen growth-inhibited human breast cancer cell line CAMA-1. J Cell Biochem 1994; 54:332-342.

161. Kalkhoven E, Kwakkenbos-Isbrucker L, Mummery CL et al. The role of TGFβ production in growth inhibition of breast-tumour cell by progestins. In J Cancer 1995; 61:80-86.

162. Dugger TC, Meggouth F, CL Arteaga. Blockade of TGFβ1, -β2 and β3 does not abrogate tamoxifen induced growth inhibition of human breast carcinoma cells. Proc Amer Assoc Cancer Res 1994; 35:265.

163. Coffey R, Kost L, Lyons R. et al. Hepatic processing of transforming growth factor β in the rat liver. J Clin Invest 1987; 80:750-757.

164. Wakefield LM, Letterio JJ, Chen T et al. Transforming growth factor β1 circulates in normal human plasma and is unchanged in advanced metastatic breast cancer. Clinical Cancer Res 1995; 1:129-136.

165. Anscher MS, Murase T, Prescott DM et al. Changes in plasma TGFβ levels during pulmonary radiotherapy as a predictor of the risk of developing radiation pneumonitis. Int J Radiat Oncol Biol Physic 1994; 30:671-676.

166. Valette A, Botanche C. Transforming growth factor beta potentiates the inhibitory effect of retinoic acid on human breast carcinoma (MCF-7)cell proliferation. Growth Factors 1990; 2:283-287.

167. Lui C, Adamson E, Mercola D. Transcription factor EGR-1 suppresses the growth and transformation of human HT-1080 fibrosarcoma cells by induction of transforming growth factor β. Proc Natl Aca Sci 1996; 93:11831-11836.

168. Schipper H. Shifting the Cancer Paradigm: Must we Kill to Cure? (Editorial) J Clin Oncol 1995; 13 No.4: 801-807.

169. Wellings SR, Jensen HM, Marcum RG. An atlas of subgross pathology of the human breast with special reference to precancerous lesions. J Natl Cancer Inst 1975; 55:231-273.

170. Huang A, Jin H, Wright JA. Drug resistance and gene amplication potential regulated by transforming growth factor β1 expression. Cancer Res 1995; 55:1758-1762.

171. Schwarz LC, Gingras M-C, Goldberg G et al. Loss of growth factor dependence and conversion of transforming growth factor β inhibition to stimulation in metastatic H-*ras*- transformed murine fibroblasts. Cancer Res 1988; 48:6999-7003.

172. Schluesener HJ, Meyermann R. Spontaneous multidrug transport in human glioma cells is regulated by transforming growth factors type β. Acta Neuropathol 1991; 81:641-648.

173. Rowe PM. Clinical potential for TGFβ. The Lancet 1994; 344:72-73.

174. Roberts AB, Sporn MB. Physiological actions and clinical applications of transforming growth factor-β. Growth Factors 1993; 8:1-9.

175. Shah M, Foreman DM, Ferguson MWJ. Control of scarring in adult wounds by neutralising antibody to TGFβ. Lancet 1992; 339:213-214.

176. Spearman M, Taylor WR, Greenberg AH et al. Anti-sense deoxyribonucleotide inhibition of TGFβ1 gene expression and alterations in the growth and malignant properties of mouse fibrosarcoma cells. Gene 1994; 149:25-29.

CHAPTER 8

TGFβ and Cancer in Other Organs

J.R. Benson, H.S. Poulsen , S. Hougaard, P. Norgaard

i) Introduction

In addition to colonic and breast carcinoma which are discussed in chapters 6 and 7 respectively, there are other epithelial tumors for which TGFβ appears implicated in disordered processes of cell proliferation and differentiation. These include cancers of the stomach, lung and prostate, which like breast and colon constitute relatively common tumors. The role of TGFβ in malignancies of the gastrointestinal tract has been extensively investigated, and there may be differences in TGFβ action between hormone dependent tumors such as the breast and prostate, and those derived from nonendocrine responsive tissues. However, there are common themes which apply to the role of TGFβ within different organ systems permitting some parallels and analogies to be legitimately drawn. For example, the apparent dichotomous behavior of TGFβ in breast tissue may appertain in gastric tumors. Thus evidence has accrued from both in vivo and in vitro studies of gastric cancer suggesting that on the one hand this growth factor can act as a potent inhibitor of epithelial proliferation, whilst on the other it can promote stromal expansion and thereby support tumor growth. Once again, the precise role of TGFβ may be dependent upon the stage of tumor development, with epithelial inhibitory effects dominating in early stage tumors where subsequent loss of growth inhibition may contribute to malignant progression and acquisition of a transformed phenotype. Gastric carcinoma cells produce other (mitogenic) growth factors which can act in an autocrine/paracrine manner with the balance of these determining net proliferative activity.[1] Moreover, carcinogenesis in gastric tissue is a multi-step process,[2] but loss of responsiveness to the inhibitory effects of TGFβ appears to be a common step in the initial stages of malignant transformation. Point mutations of the *ras* oncogene and the tumor suppressor gene p53 have been identified in gastric cancers, together with amplification of genes such as c-*met*, k-*sam*, *cerbB2/neu* and loss of heterozygosity at sites corresponding to the *bcl-2*, APC and DCC genes.[3]

Of particular interest is data indicating that loss of responsiveness to the negative growth regulator, TGFβ may be secondary to a mutation involving it's receptor complex[4] or a defect in postreceptor signalling.[5] Furthermore, TGFβ can induce apoptosis (programmed cell death) in some gastric carcinoma cells implying that not all growth inhibitory effects are reversible and hinting at a potentially important therapeutic strategy.[6-8]

ii) Gastric Cancer

Several gastric carcinoma cell lines have been established in culture, with some such as HSC-39[9] and HSC-43[10] being derived from scirrhous type carcinomas (associated with excessive collagen deposition), whilst others are from nonscirrhous type tumors (MKN-1, adenosqamous cell carcinoma; MKN-7, MKN-28 and MKN-74, well differentiated adenocarcinoma; MKN-45, poorly differentiated adenocarcinoma).[11] These cell lines exhibit variable response to exogenous TGFβ. The two cell lines from scirrhous type carcinomas HSC-39 and HSC-43 were strongly growth inhibited by TGFβ1 at a concentration of 1ng/ml, and this effect was abrogated by anti-TGFβ neutralizing antibody. By contrast, the cell lines derived from nonscirrhous adenocarcinomas, MKN-7, MKN-28 MKN-74 and MKN-45, were relatively insensitive to TGFβ1. There was a progressive reduction in viability following exposure to TGFβ1 with a dose-dependent response in these scirrhous carcinoma cell lines up to a concentration of 4ng/ml. Failure of these cells to increase [^{3}H] thymidine uptake after removal of TGFβ indicated a nonreversible action upon these cells. Morphological analysis of cells using techniques of fluorescence microscopy together with electron microscopy revealed cellular changes characteristic of programmed cell death, rather than those of a nonspecific necrotic process. Moreover, these features of DNA fragmentation and chromatin condensation were partially prevented in a dose-dependent manner by treatment of cells with the protein inhibitor cycloheximide.[11] This observation is consistent with TGFβ1 activating specific biochemical pathways leading to apoptosis. Programmed cell death within different cellular systems and in response to a variety of stimuli (including cytotoxic agents, radiation and hormones) may involve a common final pathway, perhaps involving activation of a Ca^{2+} and Mg^{2+} dependent endonuclease within the nucleus, which in turn hydrolyses DNA with ladder formation.[12] TGFβ is thought to be involved in processes of programmed cell death in hormonally sensitive tissues such as the prostate where levels of TGFβ expression correlate with degrees of apoptosis.[13]

Yamamoto and colleagues have recently examined TGFβ1 induced apoptosis in gastric cancer cells in more detail.[14] Employing the cell lines MKN-1, MKN-28, MKN 45 and MKN-74 together with the scirrhous carcinoma cell line KATO-III,[15] these authors assessed apoptotic response in relation to TGFβ receptor I/II expression and p53 status. Of the 5 gastric carcinomas cell lines examined, only KATO-III cells showed apoptotic changes with corresponding ladder formation on gel electrophoresis when exposed to TGFβ1 at a relatively high concentration of 10ng/ml. This cell line expressed both type I and II receptors but no amplification of p53 was evident on reverse transcriptase-polymerize chain reaction (RT-PCR) indicating absent expression of this protein. Therefore TGFβ1 can induce apoptosis in KATO-III cells via a p53 independent pathway. As mutations involving p53 are very common amongst epithelial tumors, this could represent an important mechanism whereby cells lacking wild-type protein can undergo programmed cell death in response to exogenous agents.[14]

The failure of some gastric carcinoma cell lines to show a growth inhibitory response to TGFβ may be a consequence of receptor loss or a defect in postreceptor signaling. Ito and co-workers[16] have studied growth inhibition by TGFβ1 in responsive (TMK-1)[17] and unresponsive (MKN-28) gastric carcinoma cell lines. Specific binding of TGFβ to cell surface receptors was analyzed using affinity binding assays and Scatchard plot analysis. TMK-1 cells possess a relatively small number of high affinity receptors, whilst MKN-28 cells have low affinity receptors, albeit in larger numbers (Kd 16.5pM and 178.4pM respectively). Affinity labeling techniques revealed that TMK-1 cells (TGFβ responsive) in fact possessed only receptor type I compared with MKN-28 cells (TGFβ unresponsive) in which all three receptor types could be detected. This is an unexpected finding as receptors I and II are considered to jointly participate in a coordinated response resulting in generation of an intracellular signal following TGFβ binding (see chapter 2). It is possible that the other receptor subtypes are present on TMK-1 cells but at very low density. Conversely, the absence of a growth inhibitory response to TGFβ in MNK-28 cells may reflect complex interactions between the 3 types of receptor, with the type II receptor exerting inhibitory effects upon phosphorylation of the type I receptor.[16] Whatever the events occurring at the type I receptor in TMK-1 cells, TGFβ growth inhibition is associated with arrest of growth at the

G1 phase of the cell cycle and failure of cells to progress through S-phase. Furthermore, growth inhibition correlates with increased levels of the unphosphorylated forms of the retinoblastoma (Rb) protein which is considered central to alterations in cell-cycle kinetics.[18] Curiously, levels of expression of the cell cycle protein c-*myc* were increased in these TMK-1 cells in response to TGFβ1, which contrasts with inhibition of growth by TGFβ1 in keratinocytes where transcription of this nuclear oncogene was reduced.[19] Thus reduced c-*myc* expression is not an obligatory step in TGFβ mediated growth inhibition.

That the TGFβ type I receptor may be involved not only in mediation of a TGFβ growth inhibitory response, but also in escape therefrom, comes from further work by Ito and colleagues.[20] In an immunohistochemical study of tumor tissue from 17 gastric carcinomas, 14 (83%) showed a reduction in levels of expression of the type I receptor compared with normal tissue controls. In these experiments, expression was semiquantified using one-dimensional densitometry, and altered expression correlated with depth of tumor invasion. Thus 50% of tumors confined to the muscularis propria, but all tumors invading beyond the serosa showed reduced expression of type I receptor, suggesting that loss of receptor may occur *pari-passu* with tumor progression. Similarly, tumors with reduced expression of type I receptor were more likely to have lower levels of the TGFβ inhibitory element (TIE) binding protein. This is a conserved sequence present in the promoter region of TGFβ inhibited genes and is part of a nuclear binding complex involving the fos protein.[21] It is unknown whether reduced levels of the type I receptor occur secondary to changes in TIE binding protein.

These in vitro studies confirm that some, though not all, gastric carcinoma cell lines are sensitive to the growth inhibitory effects of TGFβ. Work cited above suggests that carcinogenesis may involve loss of a negative autocrine/paracrine loop involving TGFβ. It is possible that cells such as MKN-28 have acquired resistance to the growth inhibitory effects of TGFβ by postreceptor mechanisms. Park and colleagues have found that a high proportion of human gastric cancer cell lines which are resistant to TGFβ have mutations (deletions or amplifications) involving the TGFβ type II receptor gene which are not detectable in cell lines retaining sensitivity to TGFβ.[22]

As emphasized in the introductory section, TGFβ is a bifunctional growth factor and may represent a double edged sword *apropos* neoplastic progression (See chapter 3 section vi; chapter 7, section iv). For it not only is a potent inhibitor of many epithelial cell types,[23-25] but it can stimulate cells of mesenchymal origin[26] and thereby promote stromal consolidation and tumor development.[27] TGFβ also has immunosuppressive properties which may be pertinent to tumor progression.[29] TGFβ produced and secreted by gastric carcinoma cells may therefore either hinder carcinogenesis by acting as an autocrine growth inhibitor or serve as a paracrine growth factor to stimulate neighboring fibroblasts to elaborate extracellular matrix components and accelerate angiogenesis. These latter actions will tend to promote tumor growth.

In vitro studies have confirmed that gastric carcinoma cell lines express TGFβ mRNA and secrete TGFβ into their conditioned media (CM).[14,16,29] Figure 8.1 shows the concentrations of TGFβ1 detected in CM from 5 established gastric carcinoma cell lines using a radioreceptor assay with NRK-49F as an indicator cell. KATO-III and HSC-39 cell lines which are derived from scirrhous carcinomas are responsive to exogenous TGFβ, secrete relatively large amounts of latent TGFβ. By contrast, levels of secretion for nonscirrhous carcinoma cell lines are almost undetectable. However, following transient acidification active forms of TGFβ1 were measurable in the CM of nonscirrhous gastric carcinoma cell lines at levels comparable for KATO-III and HSC-39.[29]

Northern blotting analysis of mRNA extracted from these cell lines revealed expression of transcript in both scirrhous and nonscirrhous gastric carcinoma cell lines, but relatively

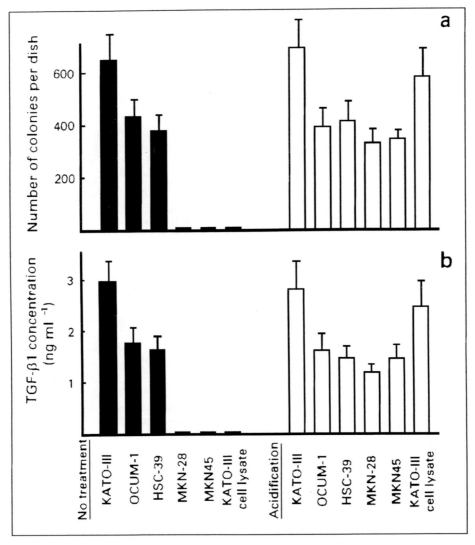

Fig.8.1. TGFβ activity in the conditioned media of 5 established gastric carcinoma cell lines. Activity of TGFβ was estimated using both radioreceptor (a) and colony assay (b). Levels of activity in scirrhous carcinomas (KATO-111; OCUM-1; HSC-39) ranged from 1.63 ng ml⁻¹ to 2.98 ng ml⁻¹, but TGFβ was not detectable at signifcant levels in non-scirrhous cancers (MKN-28; MKN-45) prior to acidification (*solid bars*). However, following activation of latent TGFβ with transient acidification (115 mM HCL) active forms of TGFβ1 were measurable in the CM of both types of gastric cancers (open bars). Reprinted with permission from: Harcourt Brace, Ltd. Mahara K et al. Br J Cancer 1994; 69:777-783.

higher signals were obtained for the former: -KATO-III 5.8; HSC-39 2.6; MKN-28 1.0; MKN-45 0.7.[29] Other authors have confirmed that cell lines from scirrhous cancer have relatively higher levels of expression of TGFβ mRNA.[14,30]

As scirrhous carcinomas are associated with more florid collagen deposition, it seems reasonable to hypothesize that gastric carcinoma cells within these tumors produce and secrete large amounts of TGFβ which in turn evokes a stromal reaction. Immunohistochemical studies of TGFβ expression in both normal gastric tissue and gastric malignancies provide support for this hypothesis.[31,32] Naef and co-workers examined the expression of TGFβ1, TGFβ2 and TGFβ3 in normal human gastric tissue and gastric cancers. They found differential expression of TGFβ isoforms between the various cellular components of the normal gastric mucosa. Though all 3 isoforms are expressed, TGFβ1 is predominantly located in acid secreting parietal cells whilst TGFβ2 is found exclusively in pepsin producing chief cells. TGFβ3 was equally distributed between parietal, chief and mucous producing cells. In tissue sections of gastric cancers, all 3 isoforms were colocalized within carcinoma cells. Some immunoreactivity was evident within fibroblasts, but staining was overwhelmingly epithelial. Northern analysis revealed that transcripts for the β1 and β3 isoforms were present in samples from both normal and cancerous tissues, but levels of expression were much higher in the latter (4.8-fold for TGFβ1 ($p<0.001$); 6-fold for TGFβ3 ($p<0.003$)). Curiously TGFβ2 mRNA was not detected in either normal or malignant gastric tissue. This significantly increased expression of TGFβ in gastric cancer was associated with a 10-fold increase in levels of collagen type I alpha mRNA in samples from malignant gastric tissue. High levels of expression of TGFβ transcript and protein product together with the preservation of cognate receptors and sensitivity to exogenous TGFβ are consistent with the existence of a functional autocrine inhibitory loop in vivo. However, this evidence is circumstantial and addition of anti-TGFβ antibodies alone to cultures of TMK-1 cells in vitro does not result in a proliferative response. Secreted forms of TGFβ within the CM may be diluted such that effective growth suppression by TGFβ does not exist under these culture conditions. Alternatively, secreted forms of TGFβ in vitro may remain in a latent, inactive form, thus interrupting any potential autocrine inhibitory effects.[20]

Therefore irrespective of whether negative autocrine loops involving TGFβ and gastric carcinoma cells are operative or functionally compromised, these cells can produce and secrete TGFβ which stimulates stromal cells and leads to excessive collagen deposition. Submucosal fibroblasts possess all 3 types of TGFβ receptor and are therefore potentially responsive to paracrine sources of TGFβ emanating from neighboring epithelial cells.[33,34] Mahara and co-workers have shown that conditioned media from scirrhous gastric carcinoma cells (KATO-III, OCUM-1 and HSC-39) stimulates synthesis of collagen in fibroblasts. This effect is partially negated by anti-TGFβ neutralizing antibodies suggesting that the active factor in CM is TGFβ.[29]

Whether TGFβ derived from gastric carcinoma cells serves to orchestrate stromal expansion and indirectly enhance tumor growth is unclear. Of interest, Mizoi and co-workers reported that stroma promoting TGFβ derives principally from stromal cells themselves and not from adjacent gastric carcinoma cells, implying that a positive (stimulatory) autocrine loop involving fibroblasts may be operative in vivo.[35] Using antibodies against the TGFβ1 precursor, pro-TGFβ1 and the latent TGFβ binding protein (LTBP), pro-TGFβ1 was found to be localized to the cytosol of cancer cells, but confined within the endoplasmic reticulum and perinuclear cisternae of stromal cells. Furthermore, LTBP was located around and within fibroblasts and smooth muscle cells, but was not seen in carcinoma cells. Taken together, these observations suggest that secretion of the latent TGFβ complex is defective in gastric carcinoma cells and that extracellular forms of TGFβ may originate exclusively from stromal cells.[35]

It might be postulated that deficient production of LTBP by gastric carcinoma cells is *per se* a manifestation of the malignant phenotype which may serve to abrogate any autocrine inhibitory effects of TGFβ. However, as there is upregulation of TGFβ1 in malignant gastric tissue sections, there may be a relative deficiency of LTBP were this to be differentially regulated.[37] Furthermore, abnormal forms of LTBP could restrict the bioavailability of TGFβ1 by interfering with mechanisms of activation once the large latent TGFβ1 complex has been secreted into the extracellular space.

iii) Lung Cancer

Recent research has provided data suggesting that TGFβ plays a significant role as a regulator of growth and morphology in lung cancer. Evidence has emerged from both in vitro and in vivo studies involving human lung cancer tissue and established cell lines as well as developmental studies in lung organ culture and animal models. These data indicate that loss of the tumor suppressive effect of TGFβ might contribute to the malignant pheno-type of lung cancer. Furthermore, TGFβ appears to be implicated in some forms of treat-ment associated morbidity, being a principle mediator of pathological fibrosis in the lung.

The 3 mammalian isoforms of TGFβ, (TGFβ1, TGFβ2 and TGFβ3) are expressed at varying levels and locations during embryonic development as well as in adult murine lung. This specific pattern of temporal and spatial expression probably reflects defined roles in differentiation.[38,39] This diversity of expression is illustrated by data obtained from studies with transgenic mice in which specific genetic alterations of the germline have been intro-duced. Thus transgenic mice expressing constitutively active TGFβ1 in the lungs exhibit arrest of pulmonary morphogenesis as a consequence of perturbation of epithelial differen-tiation.[40] This supported previous results obtained using organ cultures of embryonic mouse lungs, in which a dose-dependent and reversible inhibition of branching morphogenesis by TGFβ1 could be correlated with decreased expression of the transcription factor N-*myc*.[41] Conversely, interference of TGFβ signaling by blocking the TGFβ type II receptor (TGFβ-rII) with antibodies led to stimulation of branching in organ cultures of mouse lung.[42] Since TGFβ-rII was detected in mesenchymal and epithelial cells, this effect may have resulted from altered functional interactions between cells in both compartments. In rat lung, TGFβ-rII is expressed very early in development, peaking postnatally with lower levels in adoles-cence.[43] During this period, expression of TGFβ-rII changed from being located in both stromal and epithelial compartments to being confined mainly to parenchymal and vascu-lar tissue. Testimony to the functional diversity of the different isoforms of TGFβ in lung development comes from studies of knock-out mice, in which transcription and hence ex-pression of TGFβ3 is abrogated. These null mice invariably died shortly following birth. Postmortem studies revealed delayed lung development and defective palatogenesis.[44]

Lung cancer is classified into small cell (SCLC) and nonsmall cell (NSCLC) types. NSCLC is derived from bronchial or mucous epithelium while the precise origin of SCLC cells re-mains to be clarified.[45] Both types are characterized by gross chromosomal rearrangements, of which loss of heterozygosity in the short arm of chromosome 3 is a frequent event.[46,47] Interestingly, the type II receptor gene was reported to map to chromosome 3p22,[48] which led investigators to examine whether mutations involving the TGFβ-rII gene with loss at 3p were present in lung cancers.[49] However, in one study of both SCLC and NSCLC tumors, only one out of 35 specimens harbored a mutation in the TGFβ-rII gene. This tumor showed a replication error (RER+) phenotype in the TGFβ-rII gene with a mutation involving a polyadenosine repeat sequence. In RER+ colon and gastric cancers, this particular region is frequently the site of mutations, thus suggesting that the TGFβ-rII gene has the properties of a tumor suppressor.[50] Although mutations in the polyadenosine repeat seem to be infre-quent in lung cancer,[43,49,51] TGFβ-rII expression is defective in a large number of SCLC lines,[52] which are in consequence resistant to the growth inhibitory effects of TGFβ.[53] By analogy with studies of gastrointestinal malignancy, these SCLC cell lines lacked TGFβ-rII transcript, which in one instant was due to a mutation generating a stop-codon.[51] These data collectively are consistent with the hypothesis that TGFβ-rII acts as a tumor suppressor in lung cancer.[49,51]

Examination of a series of three SCLC cell lines established from a single patient during clinical progression of malignancy revealed interesting data providing further insight and better understanding of the role of TGFβ in disease progression.[54] One of these cell lines, GLC 14, which was established from the tumor prior to instituting any treatment was resistant to exogenous TGFβ and lacked TGFβ-rII. Moreover, these cells did not express TGFβ1. Following treatment with standard chemotherapy, the patient developed recurrent disease at which point a second cell line, GLC 16 was established. Like GLC 14, this cell line also failed to express TGFβ1. Nonetheless, GLC 16 did express TGFβ-rII and exhibited TGFβ1 growth inhibition. Therefore this cell line had acquired sensitivity to TGFβ1 due to expression of TGFβ-rII. The patient subsequently received additional radiotherapy and following a further relapse, a third cell line, GLC 19 was established. This cell line expressed both TGFβ1 as well as its cognate receptor, and was sensitive to growth inhibition by TGFβ1. Thus clinical progression of SCLC was accompanied *pari-passu* by acquired sensitivity to TGFβ.[54] Prima facie, this would seem inconsistent with a role of TGFβ as a tumor suppressor. However, examination of postirradiation DNA repair in SCLC lines demonstrated a correlation between expression of TGFβ-rII and a high capacity for sublethal damage repair.[55] The latter is a radiobiological parameter describing the so-called shoulder of survival curves, and is at least in part ascribed to a cell's capability of repairing DNA damage.[56] DNA repair requires a delay in cell-cycle progression[57] and TGFβ induces arrest in the G1 phase of the cell-cycle.[58] Based on these observations, the following hypothesis can be formulated. Prior to anti-cancer treatment, those cells which are resistant to TGFβ1 due to loss of TGFβ-rII will have a selective growth advantage over neighboring cells in possession of the receptor. However, therapies with either cytotoxic agents or radiotherapy would induce DNA damage which may favor the selection of cells maintaining the capacity for cell-cycle arrest, and which in turn optimizes conditions for DNA repair. Thus cells in which TGFβ-rII is expressed may for this reason be selected out during treatment in preference to those lacking the TGFβ-rII receptor. The emergence of this altered phenotype could be due either to selection of preexisting TGFβ-rII cells or possibly by processes leading to induction of the receptor.

TGFβ probably has a significant role in development of lung fibrosis. It is well-established that TGFβ can stimulate the growth of fibroblasts and induce formation of extracellular matrix (ECM) by increasing expression of ECM proteins and decreasing proteolytic activity.[26] Lung fibrosis is known to be a severe dose-limiting side-effect of certain anti-cancer treatments, including radiotherapy and chemotherapeutic agents.

A number of studies implicate TGFβ as a key mediator in development of pulmonary fibrosis. In animal models, enhanced TGFβ expression appears to be a direct result of irradiation of the lung with both stromal and local immune cells being the source of TGFβ.[59,60] Furthermore, in patients suffering from various forms of nonradiation induced pulmonary fibrosis, examination of lung biopsies showed expression of TGFβ1 in epithelial cells. By contrast TGFβ1 was not expressed in normal lung tissue, whilst TGFβ2 and TGFβ3 were expressed in epithelial, mesenchymal and immune cells of both normal and fibrotic lung tissue.[61] Further support for the role of TGFβ as a mediator of fibrosis comes from studies demonstrating increased levels of TGFβ1 in serum form patients with pulmonary fibrosis following radiotherapy for lung cancer.[62] Elevated levels of TGFβ1 have also been found in broncho-alveolar lavage fluid from patients with other fibrotic disorders such as scleroderma.[63] Interestingly, breast cancer patients receiving radiation therapy after mastectomy in addition to tamoxifen treatment were found to have significantly worse problems with pulmonary fibrosis compared to patients who did not receive anti-estrogen therapy.[64] This suggests that tamoxifen may directly modulate local tissue levels of TGFβ1 and echoes conclusions from data indicating that TGFβ may in part mediate the growth inhibitory effects of tamoxifen in breast cancer (see chapter 7).[65-67]

Fibrosis of the lung is a particular problem with bleomycin and limits the dosage which may be administered. When introduced directly into the trachea of mice, it produces marked pulmonary fibrosis which is associated with a significant increase in TGFβ1 secretion. When isolated lung fibroblasts are treated with anti-TGFβ antibodies, the effect are reversed.[68] The source of bleomycin induced TGFβ appears to be activated immune cells and fibroblasts,[69,70] with minimal contribution from broncho-alveolar epithelium.[68] A putative therapeutic use of TGFβ antibodies was suggested from a study in which it was shown that systemic treatment with such antibodies diminished collagen I deposition in the lungs of bleomycin treatmed mice.[71]

In conclusion, there is evidence that the type II receptor acts as a tumor suppressor in malignant lung tissue in a similar manner to gastrointestinal cancers though precise mechanisms for inactivation of TGFβ-rII may differ. Future research should focus on the clinical relevance of in vitro studies in cell lines in order to determine optimal approaches for therapeutic intervention in the TGFβ system, and in particular to ascertain whether local enhancement of TGFβ levels should have priority over an anti-TGFβ strategy. The former may have an anti-tumor effect, whilst the latter would theoretically minimize morbidity from processes such as pulmonary fibrosis which can severely restrict application of certain chemotherapeutic agents.

iv) Prostate Cancer

The incidence of prostate cancer has risen dramatically in recent years such that currently it is the commonest malignancy in the male population (200,000 new cases per year) and accounts for 35,000 deaths per year in the United States.[72] Efforts have therefore intensified at detecting this disease whilst it remains confined to the prostate for which local therapy will be curative. Autopsy studies reveal that subclinical disease is relatively frequent and microscopic lesions of the prostate have been estimated to occur in up to one-third of men over 50 years of age.[73]

Interest in TGFβ and the prostate gland is based not only on its role in multi-step carcinogenesis, but also in its potential as a biomarker which may permit detection of disease at an earlier if not subclinical stage.[74] As with many tumors of epithelial origin, TGFβ has potent inhibitory effects upon epithelial cell proliferation, but in vivo and in vitro studies indicate a complex functional profile of this growth factor in prostate tissue. Thus in addition to its growth inhibitory effects, TGFβ exerts other biological effects which may serve to promote tumor growth. These include stimulation of angiogenesis,[75] immunosuppression[76] and stromal expansion.[77] Moreover, TGFβ can directly promote mestastases by influencing cell adhesion properties[77] and proteolysis.[78] These functional aspects of TGFβ are elaborated upon in chapter 3.

Stromal-epithelial interactions are particularly manifest in hormone dependent tumors, and the prostate gland provides an excellent example of how endocrine effects can be mediated indirectly upon epithelial elements via paracrine interaction with adjacent mesenchyme. Indeed, much of the seminal work in this field has involved studies with hormone sensitive tissues of the developing genital tract of rodents (see chapter 4).[79-81] Furthermore, recent data from immunohistochemical and other studies have suggested that TGFβ may be a key factor in mediation of these stromal-epithelial interactions within benign and malignant prostate tissues.[72] Androgens may serve to suppress expression of TGFβ, and in consequence ablative androgen therapies may result in enhanced expression of this growth factor together with its cognate receptor.[82] The potential clinical sequelae of such effects are unclear at present, as prostate carcinoma cells may exhibit loss of sensitivity to TGFβ relatively early in the neoplastic continuum.[83] Therefore therapies aimed at boosting either systemic or local endogenous levels of TGFβ within the prostate gland may have limited application as an anti-tumor strategy. Nonetheless, circulating isoforms of TGFβ may be clinically useful as tumor markers to monitor response to more conventional therapies.[74,74,85]

All 3 mammalian isoforms of TGFβ are expressed in human and rodent prostate tissues.[86-91] TGFβ has potent inhibitory effects upon a variety of epithelial cell types in vitro[23,24,65] and is generally stimulatory to cells of mesenchymal origin.[26] These epithelial inhibitory effects of TGFβ include both human and rodent prostate carcinoma cells; LnCaP and PC-3 are cell lines derived from human prostate cancer and both exhibit growth inhibition in response to TGFβ.[92-94] Dunning rat prostate cancer cells are likewise growth inhibited by TGFβ in vitro[91] as are normal rat prostate cells.[95] Furthermore, these prostate carcinoma cells synthesize and secrete TGFβ isoforms and possess corresponding receptors, suggesting that autocrine growth inhibitory loops may be operative in vivo.[96-99] However, the precise role of epithelial sources of TGFβ is difficult to elucidate in these hormone sensitive tissues where some cells have acquired androgen independence and where stromal-epithelial interactions exert a major influence on epithelial cell function in vivo. Both androgen dependent (LNCaP) and androgen independent cells can respond to TGFβ originating from the extracellular space by binding of ligand to surface receptors. Such TGFβ could derive from either epithelial cells themselves or adjacent stromal cells. In androgen sensitive prostatic carcinoma cell lines, androgen treatment results in a proliferative response which has a bell-shaped contour (with a dose-dependent response at lower concentrations and a much reduced proliferative response at concentrations exceeding 10^{-9} M dihydrotestosterone (DHT).[100-102] This proliferative response to androgen stimulation is mediated via mitogenic growth factors of which epidermal growth factor (EGF) and fibroblast growth factor (FGF) probably represent the dominant effectors and may account for as much as 80% of such a response.[103]

In the normal prostate, TGFβ may have a dual role of inhibiting epithelial proliferation, but stimulating stromal cells.[72] As androgen exposure generally evokes a trophic response, this hormonal background may tend under normal circumstances to suppress expression of TGFβ, with levels of androgen being inversely related to those of TGFβ.[72] In normal prostatic tissue, androgen withdrawal leads to decreased expression of EGF, FGF and insulin-like growth factors (IGF's),[95,104-106] whilst levels of their corresponding receptors increase.[107,108] The latter may represent a homeostatic response to reduction in levels of mitogenic growth factors which together with enhanced binding affinity will tend to maintain rates of proliferation. Conversely, expression of both TGFβ and its receptor increase following castration, an observation which is consistent with the above proposal that TGFβ expression is normally 'capped' by androgens.[109] In animal models, these changes in growth factor expression following androgen ablation occur *pari-passu* with shrinkage of the gland, and may be reversed by administration of replacement hormone. Following androgen withdrawal, expression of TGFβ mRNA together with TGFβ1 binding sites are increased in the rodent ventral prostate, with peak levels at 4 days postcastration. Similarly, levels of transcript and receptor are normalized by addition of androgen.[90,109] Thus growth of the normal prostate gland appears to be controlled by a balance of positive and negative growth factors. TGFβ1 inhibits growth of ventral prostate explants by 25%, but androgen deprivation cannot be mimicked by exogenous TGFβ in the intact organism. The observed regression of prostatic tissue appears to result from a combined modulation of stimulatory (EGF, FGF) and inhibitory growth factors (TGFβ) in response to androgen ablation.[110]

As for normal prostate tissue, TGFβ1, TGFβ2 and TGFβ3 have been detected in human[93,101,111-113] and rodent[20,18,47] prostate cancer. Steiner and Barrack reported high levels of expression of TGFβ1 mRNA in rodent prostatic adenocarcinoma cell lines (Dunning 123327) compared to normal prostate cells. Levels of transcript were higher in sublines from fast growing anaplastic tumors (AT2 and MAT LyLu) than in cell lines from slower growing, well differentiated ones (H and HIS), with expression not being directly regulated by androgens in the conditioned medium.[114] Furthermore, when the highly aggressive, androgen insensitive Dunning R3327 subline MAT LyLu was transfected with the TGFβ gene, transfectants could be subcloned which over-produced TGFβ1. When these were grown as xenografts in vivo, they yielded tumors which were 50% larger with greater metastatic potential.[91] Similarly, in the mouse prostate reconstitution model system, transfection of prostate cells with ha-*ras* or c-*myc* results in a marked elevation in TGFβ1 mRNA expression.[116] Thus the tumor promoting effects of TGFβ1 appear to dominate in these poorly differentiated, aggressive tumors in which prostatic adenocarcinoma cells may be resistant to the growth inhibitory effects of TGFβ. Indeed, these MAT LyLu cells are resistant to exogenous TGFβ when grown on monolayers in vitro. Furthermore, though the cell lines LnCaP and PC-3 have generally been reported to possess receptors for TGFβ and to be sensitive to its growth inhibitory effects, results of these in vitro studies are not consensual; both the androgen insensitive cell lines DU145 and PC-3 together with the androgen sensitive line LnCaP have been reported to be responsive to TGFβ1 in vitro.[93,96,101,116] These conflicting results may be attributable to phenotypic drift or nuances of culture conditions, including cell density, presence of serum and duration of exposure to TGFβ. However, prostate carcinoma cell lines derived from poorly differentiated lesions consistently fail to exhibit an inhibitory growth response to exogenous TGFβ. In fact, TGFβ has been found to stimulate DNA synthesis in the T1 and T5 rat adenocarcinoma cell lines.[117] In Dunning rodent tumors, loss of growth inhibition to TGFβ occurred with tumor progression and appeared concomitantly with resistance to exogenous androgens.[118]

These data from rodent models suggest that at least in well differentiated lesions, the growth inhibitory effects of TGFβ1 upon epithelium are operative in vivo. TGFβ1 may act partially to overcome the mitogenic effects of growth factors such as FGF, and in turn the growth inhibitory effects of TGFβ can be attenuated by FGF.[95] Immunohistochemical studies have shown widespread expression of TGFβ1 protein in normal prostate tissue, benign prostatic hyperplasia (BPH) and prostatic cancer. Levels of expression are generally greater in BPH and malignant compared with normal prostate tissue, with highest levels in prostate cancer specimens.[119,120] Truong and co-workers employed antibodies against both the extracellular (CC) and intracellular (LC) forms of TGFβ. Immunoreactivity for the extracellular peptide was more intense in malignant prostate tissue, whilst there was differential staining between stromal and epithelial compartments with the LC antibody. Intracellular staining of fibroblasts was more intense in BPH specimens, but intracellular immunoreactivity was most evident within the epithelial compartment of prostate cancer specimens. Animal studies with the transgenic mouse reconstitution model have also revealed enhanced extracellular staining for TGFβ1 in prostate cancer tissue and this has been correlated with malignant progression.[120] Levels of TGFβ2 appear unchanged in malignant compared to normal prostate tissue, but androgen withdrawal results in increased expression of TGFβ2 in LNCaP cells.[121] Curiously, levels of the β3 isoform are decreased to almost undetectable levels, with signals in prostate cancer approximately one-tenth those in BPH.[73] TGFβ2 mRNA levels have been reported to be markedly elevated in BPH but not all studies involving Northern analysis have confirmed this.[87,73] Moreover, Glynne-Jones and colleagues found no difference in mRNA expression in prostate biopsy specimens taken from 32 patients with BPH and 66 patients with carcinoma of the prostate, with representative samples of curettings from transurethral resections being analysed.[122] Similar findings for mRNA expression of the β1 isoform were reported by Mori and workers.[87] However, notwithstanding sampling bias, these data on mRNA levels are difficult to interpret as the origin of transcript (stromal versus epithelial) cannot be assessed, and *in situ* hybridization studies are increasingly being employed to identify sites of TGFβ synthesis.

As previously alluded to, stromal-epithelial interactions are particularly important within hormonally sensitive prostate tissue. TGFβ is likely to be a central player in such interactions with its precise role very much dependent upon the stage of carcinogenesis and degree of differentiation of tumors. The changing nature of stromal-epithelial interactions as a tumor evolves may be crucial to understanding malignant progression and devising effective therapeutic strategies.

Studies by Cunha and co-workers on the hormonally sensitive tissue of the developing genital tract have provided evidence not only for mesenchymal determination of epithelial differentiation, but also for mediation of hormonal effects upon epithelium indirectly via stromal elements.[79-81] Thus prostatic differentiation can be induced in tissue recombinants of either wild-type or androgen insensitive epithelium (testicular feminization syndrome (Tfm)) by wild-type mesenchyme. By contrast, Tfm mesenchyme cannot direct male pattern differentiation presumably because it is insensitive to circulating androgens which are considered to direct epithelial differentiation via mesenchymal influences. Androgen receptors appear sequentially during development, being first detected within mesenchymal tissue at which time epithelium remains unresponsive to hormonal stimulation. However, adjacent mesenchyme can potentially respond and indirectly influence epithelial growth and differentiation by secretion of soluble factors induced by androgen stimulation of fibroblasts. TGFβ isoforms are widely expressed in developing tissue and are candidates for mediating this intercompartmental signaling. Of interest, bladder carcinoma cells are inhibited by conditioned media from urogenital sinus explants, and this growth inhibitory activity has been identified as TGFβ.[123,124] These stromal influences may persist in tissues of the adult organism; wild-type urogenital mesenchyme can elicit a proliferative response in a single adult prostatic duct[79] and induce wild-type or Tfm adult bladder epithelium to undergo prostatic differentiation. This prostatic tissue atrophies when androgen is withdrawn and is restored by administration of testosterone to host animals. Once again, adult bladder epithelium is devoid of androgen receptors and this response is mediated indirectly via hormonal stimulation of adjacent mesenchyme.[125]

This paracrine theme has been further explored in coculture studies of prostatic adenocarcinoma cells and fibroblasts. These have generally demonstrated stimulation of clonal growth by stromal cells,[126,127] but Kooistra and co-workers have shown that prostatic stromal cells can inhibit growth of either androgen dependent (LnCaP) or independent (PC-3) prostatic carcinoma cells in coculture.[128] Furthermore, conditioned media from prostatic fibroblasts could mediate this anti-proliferative activity upon carcinoma cells, and recent characterization of this soluble factor reveals it to be a protein distinct from TGFβ.[129] In particular, unfractionated conditioned media or partially purified inhibitor had no effect upon either MCF-7 cells or mink lung carcinoma (indicator) cells and the inhibitory response was not abrogated by neutralizing antibodies.[130] This putative inhibitory growth factor has been termed 'prostate-derived epithelium inhibiting factor (p-EIF), and potential problems of coprecipitation have hitherto obviated complete characterization.[131]

These growth inhibitory characteristics of fibroblasts derived from prostatic tissue were not shared by skin fibroblasts. The phenotypic expression of fibroblasts within individual tissues may be determined by local epigenetic influences from adjacent malignant epithelial cells (see chapter 4). Prostatic stromal cells produce a spectrum of polypeptide growth factors, some of which are growth stimulatory and appear related to basic FGF.[132] These findings emphasize the complex nature of stromal epithelial interactions both within normal tissues and derangements thereof in malignant states.

Epithelial sources of TGFβ can act upon epithelial cells in a negative autocrine manner, and can stimulate stromal cells via a paracrine mechanism to elaborate extracellular matrix proteins and synthesize mitogenic growth factors such as EGF, TGF alpha and FGF. The precise nature of reciprocal interactions between fibroblasts and epithelial cells within the prostate is less clear. Kooistra and colleagues performed Northern blot analyses on 2 strains of stromal cells derived from benign prostatic hyperplasia, and both these strains contained TGFβ mRNA. Other studies analyzing mRNA expression in prostatic tissue have used samples containing both stromal and epithelial cells which do not permit identification of the site of synthesis.[73,87] Immunohistochemical studies of prostate cancer specimens have revealed stromal staining for TGFβ1,[120,133] though some have revealed TGFβ1 immunoreactivity to be confined to epithelial cells.[136] Of interest, in well differentiated tumors, TGFβ1 is expressed predominantly in the stroma, whereas in poorly differentiated tumors immunoreactivity is seen throughout the extracellular matrix around both stromal and epithelial cells.[135] This observation is consistent with the findings of selectively increased stromal staining for the intracellular form of TGFβ1 in BPH compared with prostate cancer where epithelial staining is more pronounced.[120] Thus increasing expression of TGFβ1 could either accompany or be a determinant of a more malignant phenotype in prostatic tissue. Urogenital mesenchymal cells can produce and secrete active forms of TGFβ,[123] but data for synthesis and secretion by prostatic stromal cells in vitro is lacking. As discussed above, p-EIF has been identified as the predominant anti-proliferative activity in conditioned media from such cells.

Despite the failure to identify the molecular features of any stromal inhibitory activity within prostatic tissue, the concept is emerging of stroma acting as a 'brake' upon adjacent prostatic epithelium and so restricting rates of proliferation.[129] This would therefore constitute an important component of the reciprocal interaction between fibroblasts and epithelial cells, counteracting potent growth promoting signals upon stroma which emanate from epithelial cells. Release of this stromal brake may lead to the so-called "embryonic awakening" of prostatic cells in benign prostatic hypertrophy.[136] Modulation of both TGFβ and FGF appear to be significant events in development of BPH. Reduced inhibitory signals from stromal cells could lead to enhanced epithelial proliferation which in turn would augment positive paracrine stimuli to stromal cells with increased production of FGF. Transgenic mice with the mouse mammary tumor virus (MMTV) fused to the *int*-2 gene have excessive production of the int-2 protein (related to FGF) and develop florid BPH.[137] However, results of such experiments involving genetic manipulation do not imply obligate malignant transformation.

In hormone sensitive tissues of the prostate, androgens appear to mediate a growth response by changes in levels of positive and negative growth factors which constitute proximate effectors. Androgen withdrawal in normal tissues is associated with decreased expression of EGF and FGF[105] and enhanced expression of TGFβ1 together with its receptor.[109] Thus regression of prostate tissue (involution) results in part from increased expression and activity of TGFβ1. Under normal circumstances, androgens may suppress TGFβ1 levels within fibroblasts and thus indirectly control epithelial proliferation by limiting the capacity of any 'stromal brake'.

This hypothesis is consistent with the observed upregulation of TGFβ1 within specimens of prostatic cancer following various methods of androgen ablation, including orchidectomy, stilboestrol (DES) therapy or administration of luteinising hormone releasing hormone (LHRH) analogs.[82] In this immunohistochemical study of Muir and colleagues, samples of prostate tissue from patients with hormonally responsive and unresponsive tumors were stained with anti-TGFβ1 antibodies recognizing extracellular (CC) and intracellular (LC) forms of the peptide. Marked upregulation of extracellular TGFβ1 was observed between and around stromal fibroblasts with little enhanced immunoreactivity in the immediate vicinity of epithelial cells. This induction was confined to the β1 isoform and only extracellular forms of the peptide demonstrated significantly increased immunoreactivity. This pattern of induction was observed in 3 out of 5 hormonally responsive and 6 out of 7 tumors showing a clinical response.

This increased expression of TGFβ1 therefore appeared to be a general response to androgen withdrawal, and not to specific direct effects of either DES or LHRH analogs on prostatic tissue. These agents have direct cytotoxic effects upon prostate cancer cells in vitro,[138,139] but like many hormonal therapies are considered to act via the hypothalamo-pituitary-gonadal axis. The distribution of extracellular TGFβ suggested that stromal cells were the source and site of increased synthesis. Therefore according to the above hypothesis, androgen ablation would remove any suppressive effects upon stromal expression of TGFβ and augment growth inhibition of adjacent epithelial cells via a negative paracrine effect—'applying the brakes'. It is unclear to what extent such a proposed mechanism will quantitatively contribute to the anti-proliferative effects of androgen ablation. Furthermore, upregulation was observed in some nonresponding tumors, suggesting that the functional sequelae of this TGFβ induction can be counteracted by other mechanisms leading to growth stimulation. Moreover, extracellular forms of TGFβ may in fact be acting as a growth promoter in some of these more advanced lesions by stimulating production of extracellular matrix proteins, angiogenesis and metastatic potential.[140,141]

However, the growth inhibitory effects of TGFβ upon epithelium could be exploited in early prostate lesions and may present a therapeutic strategy for chemoprevention of prostate cancer. By analogy with breast cancer (see chapter 7), local tissue levels of TGFβ could be boostered to shift the balance of growth factors within the local micro-environment of prostatic tissue, such that net epithelial regression is favored. Stromal cells may represent a realistic target, though as discussed above, it is unclear to what extent stromal sources of TGFβ can be harnessed for therapeutic gain. Anti-tumor effects could also be achieved by enhancing inhibitory autocrine loops; androgen deprivation may increase TGFβ expression through dual modulation of both autocrine and paracrine inhibitory loops.

Of interest, retinoids have anti-tumor effects in rodent models, and this suppressive activity may result in part from induction of TGFβ.[142,143] In animal models of breast cancer, a combination of anti-estrogen with retinoids acts synergistically to suppress growth of breast tumors.[144] This could be attributable to selective induction of TGFβ in stromal and epithelial cells by anti-estrogens and retinoids respectively.[27] Retinoids have been shown to exert direct inhibitory effects upon prostatic epithelium at relatively high concentrations, whilst lower concentrations are actually stimulatory.[145] As in breast tissue, retinoids are likely to play a central role in maintenance of epithelial homeostasis. Epidemiological studies have confirmed an association between high intake of the retinoid derivative lycopene and a low incidence of prostatic carcinoma.[146]

Loss of potential responsiveness to the growth inhibitory effects of TGFβ may be a more widespread phenomenon in tumors of the prostate compared with breast cancer. TGFβ resistant clones, which would have a relative growth advantage, may be selected out as a tumor evolves. Conversely, TGFβ sensitive cells would be suppressed in response to local elevated levels of TGFβ with reduced rates of proliferation and increased apoptotic activity.[73] Cell lines derived from advanced, poorly differentiated prostatic lesions are resistant to growth inhibition by TGFβ[91] and in animal models cell lines established from metastatic foci of prostate cancer are often unresponsive to TGFβ.[147] Tumor xenografts from MAT LyLu cells which over-express TGFβ1 yield larger primary tumors with increased number of metastases.[91] In some cell lines, receptor expression is preserved despite resistance to TGFβ, and it is unclear to what extent recently identified defects in the type II TGFβ receptor are applicable to prostate cancer. Postreceptor signaling defects would appear to be more important as a mechanism for acquired resistance to the growth inhibitory effects of TGFβ.

This issue of TGFβ resistance in prostatic epithelium casts doubt over strategies aimed at boosting local endogenous levels of TGFβ and thus of successfully exploiting paracrine/autocrine inhibitory loops. Identification of receptor defects may permit complementary approaches involving gene therapy which could restore epithelial cell responsiveness to TGFβ. This therapeutic approach is potentially valuable not only because of the growth inhibitory effects of TGFβ upon prostatic epithelial cells, but also on account of induction therein of programmed cell death. In the rodent prostate, androgen ablation results in apoptosis of more than 70% of epithelial cells at 7 days, and much of this effect is mediated by TGFβ.[6,90,109] Moreover, TGFβ directly induces apoptosis in human and rodent prostatic epithelial cells in vitro.[90,148] Agents which can activate pathways leading to apoptosis represent a powerful tool for combating cancerous growth. Elimination of cells is preferable to growth arrest of finite duration, and in particular ensures that cells which acquire oncogenic mutations do not propagate.

As prostate carcinoma cells can respond to TGFβ irrespective of their sensitivity to androgen, local induction of this growth factor could overcome the problem of cellular heterogeneity within hormone-dependent tumors whereby only a proportion of cells will respond to hormonal manipulation. Interestingly, androgen withdrawal may induce increased stromal expression via mechanisms independent of the androgen receptor; it is unknown whether androgen receptors are present on stromal cells adjacent to hormone sensitive prostate carcinoma cells in the adult organism.[82] Stromal cells from breast tumors respond to tamoxifen with increased synthesis of TGFβ, yet no estrogen receptor is demonstrable in these cells.[67] Gossypol, an anti-fertility agent in males, exerts inhibitory effects upon the androgen independent prostate cancer cell line PC-3 with a dose-dependent increase in expression of TGFβ1 mRNA.[149] This induction of TGFβ1 mRNA correlated with the growth inhibitory effects of glossypol, and such agents might therefore be used in conjunction with orthodox methods of androgen ablation for treatment of prostate cancer. Furthermore, these agents may in combination with a retinoid be employed in a chemopreventive capacity. Such combined approaches can maximize induction of TGFβ and offer a greater clinical efficacy.

TGFβ has been invoked as a potential prostate cancer biomarker; however, the relationship between plasma TGFβ levels and tumor stage (and differentiation) is uncertain. Ivanovic and colleagues found that plasma TGFβ1 levels were elevated in 12 patients with prostate cancer relative to controls (normal prostate or BPH), though others have been unable to confirm such an association. Thus Perry and coworkers found no correlation between plasma TGFβ1 levels and prostate cancer according to stage, grading and prostatic specific antigen (PSA) levels. Of interest, urinary TGFβ1 and TGFβ2 levels were higher in patients with prostate cancer, with a 3- to 5-fold difference in urinary TGFβ1 levels being observed between prostate cancer patients and controls. Moreover, there was a trend toward higher urinary TGFβ1 and TGFβ2 levels with advancing stage of disease and tumor grade (though this did not reach statistical significance). Ideally, a tumor marker should be expressed at an early stage in tumor development, preferably when the disease remains subclinical. It should predict both response to therapy and disease relapse and have a degree of sensitivity and specificity. Further studies are required to evaluate the potential role of TGFβ urinary and plasma levels in this context.

References

1. Saeki T, Salomon D, Normanno N et al. Immunohistochemical detection of cripto-1, amphiregulin and transforming growth factor alpha in human gastric carcinomas. In J Oncol 1994; 5:215-223.

2. Sporn MB, Roberts AB. Autocrine growth factors and cancer. Nature 1985; 313:745-747.
3. Tahara E. Molecular mechanism of stomach carcinogenesis. J Cancer Res Clin Oncol 1993; 119:265-272.
4. Markovitz S, Wang J, Myeroff L et al. Inactivation of the type II TGFβ receptor in colon cancer cells with microsatellite instability. Science 1995; 268:1336-1338.
5. Ito M, Yasui W, Kyo E et al. Growth inhibition of transforming growth factor β on human gastric carcinoma cells:receptor and postreceptor signalling. Cancer Res 1992; 52:295-300.
6. Rotello RJ, Lieberman RC, Purchio AF, Gerschenson LE Coordinated regulation of apoptosis and cell proliferation by transforming growth factor β1 in cultured uterine epithelial cells. Proc Natl Acad Sci (USA) 1991; 88:3412-3415.
7. Martikainen P, Kyprianou N, Isaacs JT. Effect of transforming growth factor β1 on proliferation and death of rat prostatic cells. Endocrinol 1990; 127:2963-2968.
8. Oberhammer F, Bursch W, Parzefall W et al. Effect of transforming growth factor β on cell death of cultured rat hepatocytes. Cancer Res 1991; 51:2478-2485.
9. Yanagihara K, Seyama T, Tsumuraya M et al. Establishment and characterisation of human signet ring cell gastric carcinoma cell lines with amplification of the c-*myc* oncogene. Cancer Res 1991; 51:381-386.
10. Arteaga CL, Tandon AK, von Hoff DD, Osborne CK. Transforming growth factor β:potential autocrine growth inhibition of estrogen receptor negative human breast cancer cells. Cancer Res 1988 (b); 48:3898-3904.
11. Yanagihara K, Tsumuraya M. Transforming growth factor β1 induces apoptotic cell death in cultured human gastric carcinoma cells. Cancer Res 1992; 52:4042-4052.
12. Wyllie AH. Glucocorticoid-induced thymocyte apoptosis is associated with endogenous endonuclease activation. Nature 1980; 284:555-556.
13. Kyprianou N, Isaacs JT. Expression of transforming growth factor β in the rat ventral prostate during castration-induced programmed cell death. Mol Endocrinol 1989; 3:1515-1522.
14. Yamamoto M, Maehara Y, Sakaguchi Y et al. Transforming growth factor β1 induces apoptosis in gastric cancer cells through a p53 independent pathway. Cancer 1977; 1628.
15. Sekiguchi M, Sasakibara K, Fuji G. Establishment of cultured cell lines derived from a human gastric carcinoma. Jpn J Exp Med 1978; 48:61-68.
16. Ito M, Yasui W, Kyo E et al. Growth inhibition of transforming growth factor β on human gastric carcinoma cells:Receptor and postreceptor signalling. Cancer Res 1992; 52:295-300.
17. Ochiai A, Yasui W, Tahara E. Growth-promoting effect of gastrin on human gastric carcinoma cell line TMK-1. Jap J Cancer Res 1985; 79:1064-1071.
18. Laiho M, De Caprio JA, Ludlow JW et al. Growth inhibition by TGFβ linked to suppression of retinoblastoma protein phosphorylation. Cell 1990; 62:175-185.
19. Pientenpol JA, Stein RW, Moran E et al. TGFβ1 inhibition of c-myc transcription and growth in keratinocytes is abrogated by viral transforming proteins with pRB binding proteins Cell 1990 (b); 61:777-785.
20. Ito M, Yasui W, Nakayama H et al. Reduced levels of TGFβ type I receptor in human gastric carcinomas. Jap J Cancer Res 1992; 83:86-92.
21. Kerr LD, Miller DB, Matrisian LM TGFβ1 inhibition of transin/stromelysin gene expression is mediated through a fos binding sequence. Cell 1990; 61:267-278.
22. Park K, Kim SJ, Bang YJ et al. Genetic changes in the transforming in the transforming growth factor β type II receptor gene in human gastric cancer cells:correlation with sensitivity to growth inhibition by TGFβ. Proc Natl Acad Aci (USA) 1994; 91:8772-8776.
23. Roberts AB, Anzano MA, Wakefield LM et al. Type β-transforming growth factor :a bifunctional regulator of cellular growth. Proc Natl Acad Sci (USA) 1985; 82:119-123.
24. Arteaga CL, Tandon AK, von Hoff DD, Osborne CK. Transforming growth factor β:potential autocrine growth inhibition of estrogen receptor negative human breast cancer cells. Cancer Res 1988; 48:3898-3904.

25. Knabbe C, Lippman ME, Wakefield LM et al. Evidence that transforming growth factor-beta is a hormonally regulated negative growth factor in human breast cancer. Cell 1987; 48:417-428.

26. Roberts AB, McCune BK, Sporn MB. TGFβ: Regulation of extracellular matrix. Kidney International 1992; 41:557-559.

27. Benson JR, Colletta AA. Transforming growth factor β: Prospects for cancer prevention and treatment. [Leading Article] Clinical Immunotherapeutics 1995; 4:No.4 249-258.

28. Morisaki T, Katano M, Ikubo A. Immunosuppressive cytokines (IL-10, TGFβ) genes expression in human gastric carcinoma tissues. J Surg Oncol 1996; 63:234-239.

29. Mahara K, Kato J, Terui T et al. Transforming growth factor β1 secreted from scirrhous gastric cancer cells is associated with excess collagen deposition in the tissue. Br J Cancer 1994; 69:777-783.

30. Yoshida K, Yokozaki H, Nimoto M et al. Expression of TGFβ and pro-collagen type I and type III in human gastric carcinomas. Int J Cancer 1989; 44:394-398.

31. Hirayama D, Fujimori T, Satonaka K et al. Immunohistochemical study of epidermal growth factor and transfroming growth factor β in the penetrating type of early gastric cancer. Hum Path 1992; 23:681-685.

32. Naef M, Ishiwata T, Freiss H et al. Differential localisation of transforming growth factor-β isoforms in human gastric mucosa and over-expression in gastric carcinoma. Int J Cancer 1997; 71:131-137.

33. Quaglino D Jr, Nanney LB, Kennedy R, Davidson JM. Transforming growth factor β stimulates wound healing and modulates extracellular matrix gene expression in pig skin. Lab Invest 1990; 63:307-319.

34. Tahara E, Sumiyoshi H, Hata J et al. Human epidermal growth factor in gastric carcinoma as a biological marker of malignancy. Jap J Cancer Res 1986; 77:145-152.

35. Mizoi T, Ohtani H, Miyazano K et al. Immunoelectron microscopic localisation of transforming growth factor β1 and latent transforming growth factor β1 binding protein in human gastrointestinal carcinomas: Qualitative difference between cancer cells and stromal cells. Cancer Res 1993; 53:183-190.

36. Miyazano K, Hellman U, Wernstedt C, Heldin C-H. Latent high molecular weight complex of transforming growth factor β1. J Biol Chem 1988; 263:6407-6415.

37. Moses HL, Yang EY, Pietenpohl JA. TGFβ stimulation and inhibition of cell proliferation:new mechanistic insights. Cell 1990; 63:245-247.

38. Pelton RW, Moses HL. The beta-type transforming growth factor. Mediators of cell regulation in the lung. Am Rev Resp Dis 1990; 142:S31-S35.

39. Pelton RW, Johnson MD, Perkett EA et al. Expression of transforming growth factor-β1, β2 and β3 mRNA and protein in the murine lung. Am J Resp Cell Mol Biol 1991; 5:522-530.

40. Zhou L, Dey CR, Wert SE et al. Arrested lung morphogenesis in transgenic mice bearing an SP-C-TGF-β1 chimeric gene. Dev Biol 1996; 175:227-238.

41. Serra R, Pelton RW, Moses HL. TGFβ1 inhibits branching morphogenesis and N-myc expression in lung bud organ cultures. Dev 1994; 120:2153-2161.

42. Serra R, Moses HL. pRB is necessary for inhibition of N-myc expression by TGFβ1 in embryonic lung organ cultures. Dev 1994; 121:3057-3066.

43. Zhoa Y, Young SL. Expression of transforming growth factor-β type II receptor in rat lung is regulated during development. Am J Physiol 1995; 269:419-426.

44. Kaartinen V, Vonchen JW, Shuler C et al. Abnormal lung development and cleft palate in mice lacking TGFβ3 indicates defects of epithelial-mesenchymal interaction. Nature Genetics 1995; 11:415-421.

45. Kristensen CA, Jensen PB, Poulsen PB et al. Small cell lung cancer. Biological and therapeutic aspects. Critical Reviews in Oncology/Hematology 1996; 22:27-60.

46. Mitsudomi T, Oyama T, Nishida K et al. Loss of heterozygosity at 3p in nonsmall cell lung cancer and its prognostic implication. Clin Cancer Res 1996; 2:1185-1189.

47. Todd S, Franklin WA, Varella-Garcia M et al. Homozygous deletions of human chromosome 3p in lung tumors. Cancer Res 1997; 57:1344-1352.

48. Matthew S, Murty VS, Cheifetz S et al. Transforming growth factor β receptor gene TGFβ RII maps to human chromosome band 3p22. Genomics 1994; 22:114-115.
49. Tani M, Takenoshita S, Kohno T et al. Infrequent mutations of the transforming growth factor β type II receptor gene at chromosome 3p22 in human lung cancers with chromosome 3p deletions. Carcinogenesis 1997; 18:1119-1121.
50. Markowitz S, Wang J, Myeroff L et al. Inactivation of the type II TGFβ receptor in colon cancer cells with microsatellite instability. Science 1995; 268:1336-1338.
51. Hougaard S, Norgaard P, Moses HL et al. Mutations of the transforming growth factor β type II receptor in human small cell lung cancer cell lines. AACR Special Conference; Growth factors, signalling and cancer. 1997 (Abstract).
52. Norgaard P, Spang-Thomsen M, Poulsen HS. Expression and autoregulation of transforming growth factor β receptor mRNA in small cell lung cancer cell lines. Br J Cancer 1996; 73:1037-1043.
53. Norgaard P, Damstrup L, Rygaard K et al. Growth suppression by transforming growth factor-β1 in human small cell lung cancer cell lines is associated to expression of the type II receptor. Br J Cancer 1994; 69:802-808.
54. Norgaard P, Damstrup L, Rygaard K et al. Acquired sensitivity and TGFβ1 expression in cell lines established from a single small cell lung cancer patient during clinical progression. Lung Cancer 1996; 14:63-73.
55. Krarup M, Poulsen HS, Spang-Thomsen M et al. Cellular radiosensitivity of small cell lung cancer cell lines. Int J Rad Oncol Biol Phys 1997; 38:191-196.
56. Joiner MC. Models of radiation cell killing. In: Steel GS, ed. Basic Clinical Radiobiology. Edward Arnold Publishers, Ltd. 1995:40-47.
57. Kaufmann WK, Paules RS. DNA damage and cell cycle checkpoints. FASEB J 1996; 10:238-247.
58. Alexandrow MG, Moses HL. Transforming growth factor β and cell cycle regulation. Cancer Res 1995; 55:1452-1457.
59. Yi ES, Bedoya A, Lee H et al. Radiation-induced lung injury in vivo:expression of transforming growth factor β precedes fibrosis. Inflammation 1996; 20:339-352.
60. Rubin P, Johnston CJ, Williams JP et al. A perpetual cascade of cytokines postirradiation leads to pulmonary fibrosis. Int J Rad Oncol Biol Phys 1995; 33:99-109.
61. Khalil N, O'Connor RN, Flanders KC et al. TGFβ1, but not TGFs2 or TGFβ3 is differentially present in epithelial cells of advanced pulmonary fibrosis:an immunohistochemical study. Am J Resp Cell Mol Biol 1996; 14:131-138.
62. Kong F-M, Washington MK, Jirtle RL et al. Plasma transforming growth factor β1 reflects disease status in patients with lung cancer after radiotherapy:a possible tumour marker. Lung Cancer 1996; 16:47-59.
63. Ludwika A, Ohba T, Trojanowska M et al. Elevated levels of platelet derived growth factor and transforming growth factor β1 in broncho-alveolar lavage fluid from patients with scleroderma. J Rheumatol 1995; 22:1876-1883.
64. Bentzen SM, Skoczylas JZ, Overgaard M et al. Radiotherapy related lung fibrosis enhanced by tamoxifen. J Natl Cancer Inst 1996; 88:918-922.
65. Knabbe C, Lippman ME, Wakefield LM, Flanders KC, Kasid A, Derynck R, Dickson RB. Evidence that transforming growth factor-beta is a hormonally regulated negative growth factor in human breast cancer. Cell 1987; 48:417-428.
66. Perry RR, Kang Y, Greaves BR. Relationship between tamoxifen-induced transforming growth factor β1 expression, cytostasis and apoptosis in human breast cancer cells. Br J Cancer 1995; 72:1441-1446.
67. Benson JR, Wakefield LM, Baum M, Colletta AA. Synthesis and secretion of TGFβ isoforms by primary cultures of human breast tumor fibroblasts in vitro and their modulation by tamoxifen. Br J Cancer 1996; 74:352-358.
68. Kumar RK, O'Grady R, Maronese SE et al. Epithelial cell derived transforming growth factor β in bleomycin-induced pulmonary injury. Int J Exp Pathol 1996; 77:99-107.
69. Zhang K, Flanders KC, Phan SH et al. Cellular localisation of transforming growth factor β expression in bleomycin-induced pulmonary fibrosis. Am J Path 1995; 147:352-361.

70. Khalil N, Corne S, Whitman C et al. Plasmin regulates the activation of cell associated latent TGFβ1 secreted by rat alveolar macrophages after in vivo bleomycin injury. Am J Resp Cell Mol Biol 1996; 15:252-259.
71. Giri SN, Hyde DM, Hollinger MA. Effect of antibody to transforming growth factor β in bleomycin-induced accumulation of lung collagen in mice. Thorax 1993; 48:959-966.
72. Steiner MS Transforming growth factor β and prostate cancer. World J Urol 1995; 13:329-336.
73. Merz VW, Arnold AM, Studer UE. Differential expression of transforming growth factor-β1 and β3 as well as c-fos mRNA in normal human prostate, benign prostatic hyperplasia and prostate cancer. World J Urol 1994; 12:96-98.
74. Ivanovic V, Melman A, Davis-Joseph B et al. Elevated plasma levels of TGFβ1 in patients with invasive prostate cancer. Nature Med 1995; 1:282-284.
75. Yang EY, Moses HL. Transforming growth factor β1 induced changes in cell migration, proliferation and angiogenesis in the chick chorioallantoic membrane. J Cell Biol 1990; 111:731-741.
76. Fontana A, Constam DB, Frei K et al. Modulation of the immune response by transforming growth factor-β. Int Arch Allergy Appl Immunol 1992; 99:1-7.
77. Newman MJ. Transforming growth factor-β and the cell surface in tumor progression. Cancer Mets Rev 1993; 12:239-254.
78. Desruiseau S, Ghazarossian-Rigni E, Chinot O, Martin P-M. Divergent effect of TGFβ1 on growth and proteolytic modulation of human prostatic-cancer cell lines. Int J Cancer 1996; 66:796-801.
79. Cunha GR, Bigsby RM, Cooke PS, Sugimura Y. Stromal-epithelial interactions in adult organs. Cell Diff 1985; 17:137-148.
80. Cunha GR, Donjacour A. Stromal-epithelial interactions in normal and abnormal prostatic development. Prog Clin Biol Res 1987; 239:251-272.
81. Cunha GR, Alarid ET, Turner T et al. Normal and abnormal development of the male genital tract:role of androgens, mesenchymal-epithelial interactions and growth factors. J Androl 1992; 13:465-475.
82. Muir G, Butta A, Shearer RJ et al. Induction of TGFβ in hormonally treated human prostate cancer. Br J Cancer 1994; 69:130-134.
83. Steiner MS. Review of peptide growth factors in benign prostatic hyperplasia and urological malignancy. J Urol 1995; 153:1085-1096.
84. Perry KT, Anthony KT, Case T, Steiner MS. Transforming growth factor β as a clinical biomarker for prostate cancer. Urol 1997; 49:151-155.
85. Steiner MS. Role of peptide growth factors in the prostate: A review. Urol 1993; 42:99-109.
86. Derynck R, Goeddel DV, Ullrich A et al. Synthesis of messenger RNA's for transforming growth factors alpha and β and EGF by human tumours. Cancer Res 1987; 47:707-712.
87. Mori H, Maki M, Oisho K et al. Increased expression of genes for bFGF and transforming growth factor β2 in human prostate cancer. Prostate 1990; 16:71-80.
88. Madisen L, Webb NR, Rose TM. Transforming growth factors β2: cDNA cloning and sequence analysis. DNA 1988; 7:1-8.
89. Matuo Y, Nishi N, Takasuka H et al. Production and significance of TGFβ in AT-3 metastatic cell line established from the Dunning rat prostatic adenocarcinoma. Biochem Biophys Res Comm 1990; 166:840-847.
90. Kyprianou N, Isaacs JT. Expression of transforming growth factor β in the rat ventral prostate during castration-induced programmed cell death. Mol Endocrinol 1989; 3:1515-1522.
91. Steiner MS, Barrack ER. Transforming growth factor β1 over-production in prostate cancer:effects of growth in vivo and in vitro. Mol Endocrinol 1992; 6:15-25.
92. Schuurmans AL, Bolt J, Mulder E. Androgens and transforming growth factor β modulate the growth response to epidermal growth factor in human prostatic tumor cells (LNCaP). Mol Cell Endocrinol 1988; 60:101-104.
93. Wilding G, Zugmeier G, Knabbe C et al. Differential effects of transforming growth factor β on human prostate cancer cells in vitro. Mol Cell Endocrinol 1989; 62:79-87.
94. Goldstein D, O'Leary M, Mitchen J et al. Effects of interferon β and transforming growth factor β on prostatic cell lines. J Urol 1991; 146:1173-1177.

95. McKeehan WL, Adams PS. Heparin-binding growth factor/prostatropin attenuates inhibition of rat prostate tumor epithelial cell growth by transforming growth factor β. In Vitro 1988; 24:243-246.

96. Ikeda T, Lioubin MN, Marquardt H. Human transforming growth factor β2:production by a prostatic adenocarcinoma cell line, purification and initial characterisation. Biochemistry 1987; 26:2406-2410.

97. Danielpour D, Dart LL, Flanders KC et al. Immunodetection and quantitation of the two forms of transforming growth factor β (TGFβ1 and TGFβ2 secreted by cells in culture. J Cell Physiol 1989; 138:79-86.

98. Sehy DW, Shao LE, Yu AL et al. Activin-A-induced differentiation in K562 cells is associated with transient hypophosphorylation of RB protein and the concomitant block of cell cycle at the G1 phase. J Cell Biochem 1992; 50:225-256.

99. Chomczynski P, Saachi N. Single step method of RNA isolation by acid guanidinium thiocyanate-phenol-chloroform extraction. Anal Biochem 1987; 162:156-159.

100. Sonnenschein C, Olea N, Pasaen ME, Soto AM. Negative controls of cell proliferation :human prostate cancer cells and androgens. Cancer Res 1989; 49:3474-3481.

101. Schuurmans AL, Bolt J, Mulder E. Androgens and transforming growth factor β modulate the growth response to epidermal growth factor in human prostate tumor cells (LNCaP). Mol Cell Endo 1988; 60:101.

102. Lee C, Sutkowski DM, Sensibar JA et al. Regulation of proliferation and production of prostate specific antigen in androgen-sensitive prostatic cancer cells, LNCaP, dihydrotestosterone. Endocrinol 1995; 136:796-803.

103. Jacobs SC, Story MT, Sasse J, Lawson RK. Characterisation of growth factors derived from the rat ventral prostate. J Urol 1988; 139:1106-1110.

104. Fiorelli G, DeBellis A, Longo A et al. Insulin-like growth factor I receptorsin human hyperplastic prostate tissue:characterisation, tissue localisation and their modulationby chronic treatment with a GnRH analog. J Clin Endocrinol Metab 1991; 72:740-746.

105. Hiramatsu M, Kashimata M, Minami N et al. Androgenic regulation of epidermal growth factor in the mouse ventral prostate. Biochem Int 1988; 17:311.

106. Katz AE, Benson MC, Wise GJ et al. Gene activity during the early phase of androgen-stimulated rat prostate regrowth. Cancer Res 1989; 49:5889-5894.

107. Traish AM, Wotiz HH. Prostatic epidermal growth factor receptors and their regulation by androgens. Endocrinol 1987; 121:1461.

108. St-Arnaud R, Poyet P, Walker P, Labrie F. Androgens modulate epidermal growth factor levels in the rat ventral prostate. Mol Cell Endo 1988; 56:21-26.

109. Kyprianou N, Isaacs JT. Identification of a cellular receptor for transforming growth factor β in rat ventral prostate and its negative regulation by androgens. Endocrinol 1988; 123:2124-2131.

110. Martikainen P, Kyprianou N, Isaacs JT. Effect of transforming growth factor β1 on proliferation and death of rat prostatic cells. Endocrinol 1990; 127:2963-2968.

111. Derynck R, Goeddel DV, Ullrich A et al. Synthesis of messenger RNA's for transforming growth factors alpha and β and the epidermal growth factor receptor by human tumours. Cancer Res 1987; 47:707-712.

112. Thompson TC. Growth factors and oncogenes in prostate cancer. Cancer Cells 1990; 2:345-354.

113. Thompson TC, Truong LD, Timme TL et al. Transforming growth factor β1 as a biomarker for prostate cancer. J Cell Biochem 1992; 16:54-61.

114. Steiner MS, Barrack E R. Expression of transforming growth factors (alpha and β) and epidermal growth factor in normal and malignant rat prostate. J Urol 1990; 143:240A.

115. Merz VW, Miller GJ, Krebs T et al. Elevated transforming growth factor β1 and -β3 levels are associated with ras and mys-induced carcinomas in reconstituted mouse prostate:evidence for a paracrine role during progression. Mol Endocrinol 1991; 5:503-513.

116. Wilding G. Response of prostate cells to peptide growth factors: Transforming growth factor β. Cancer Surv 1991; 11:147-161.

117. Shain S, Lin A, Koger J, Karaganis A. Rat prostate cancer cells contain fuctional receptors for transforming growth factor β. Endocrinol 1990; 126:818-825.
118. Steiner MS, Anthony CT, Moses HL. Mutation of the retinoblastoma susceptibility protein correlates with resistance to TGFβ inhibition in prostate cancer (abstract). Proc Amer Ass Cancer Res 1994; 35:127.
119. Truong LD, Kadmon D, McCune B et al. Association of transforming growth factor β1 with prostate cancer. An immunohistochemical study. Human Path 1993; 24:4-9.
120. Thompson TC, Truong LD, Timme TL et al. Transgenic models for the study of prostate cancer. Cancer Suppl. 1992; 71:1165-1171.
121. Knabbe C, Klein H, Zugmaier G, Voigt KD. Hormonal regulation of transforming growth factor β2 expression in the human prostate. J Steroid Biochem Mol Biol 1993; 47:137-142.
122. Glynne-Jones E, Harper ME, Goddard L et al. Transforming growth factor β1 expression in benign and malignant prostatic tumors. Prostate 1994; 25:210-218.
123. Rowley DR. Characterisation of a fetal urogenital sinus mesenchymal cell line U4F:secretion of a negative growth regulatory activity. In Vitro Cell Dev Biol 1992 (a); 28A:29-38.
124. Rowley D.R. Glucocorticoid regulation of transforming growth factor β activation in urogenital sinud mesenchymal cells. Endocrinology 1992 (b) 131:471-478.
125. Shannon JM, Cunha GR. Characterisation of androgen binding sites and DNA synthesis in prostate like structures induced in testicular feminised mice. Biol Reprod 1984; 31:175-183.
126. Sherwood ER, Fike WE. Kozlowski JM, Lee C. Stimulation of epithelial cell growth by stromal cell secretory products (abstract) Biol Reprod 1988; 38:86.
127. Kabalin JN, Peehl DM, Stamey TA. Clonal growth of human prostatic epithelial cells is stimulated by fibroblasts. Prostate 1989; 14:251-263.
128. Kooistra A, Konig JJ, Romijn JC, Schroder FH. Negative control of epithelial cell proliferation by prostatic stroma. Anticancer Res 1991; 11:1495-1500.
129. Kooistra A, van der Eijnden-van R, Klaij IA et al. Stromal inhibition of prostate epithelial cell proliferation not mediated by transforming growth factor β. Br J Cancer 1995 (b); 72:427-434.
130. Kooistra A, Konig JJ, Keizer DM. Inhibition of epithelial cell proliferation by a factor secreted specifically by prostatic stroma. Prostate 1995 (a); 26:123-132.
131. Konig JJ, Romijn JC, Schroder FH. Prostatic epithelium inhibiting factor (PIEF):organ specificity and production by prostatic fibroblasts. Urol Res 1987; 15:145-149.
132. Story MT, Livingston B, Baeften L, Swartz SJ et al. Cultured human prostate-derived fibroblasts produce a factor that stimulates their growth with properties indistinguishable from b-FGF. Prostate 1989; 15:355-365.
133. Eklov S, Funa K, Nordgren H et al. Lack of the latent transforming growth factor β binding protein in a malignant but not benign prostatic tissue. Cancer Res 1993; 53:3193-3197.
134. Tu H, Jacobs SC, Borkowski A, Kyprianou N. Incidence of apoptosis and cell proliferation in prostate cancer: Relationship with TGFβ1 and bcl-2 expression. Int J Cancer 1996; 69:357-363.
135. Steiner MS, Zhoo ZZ, Tond DC, Barrack ER. Expression of transforming growth factor β1 in prostate cancer. Endocrinology 1994; 135:2240-2247.
136. McNeal JE. Anatomy of the prostate and morphogenesis of bening prostatic hyperplasia. Prog Clin Biol Res 1984; 145:27-53.
137. Muller WJ. Lee FS, Dickson C et al. The int-2 gene product acts as an epithelial growth in transgenic mice. EMBO J 1990; 9:907-913.
138. Shultz P, Bauer HW. Evaluation of the cytotoxic activity of diethylstilboestrol and its mono-- and diphosphate towards prostatic carcinoma cells. Cancer Res 1988; 48:2867-2870.
139. Qayum A, Gullick W, Clayton RC et al. The effects of gonadotrophin releasing hormone releasing analogues in prostate cancer are mediated through specific tumor receptors. Br J Cancer 1990; 62:96-99.
140. Ignotz R.A, Massague J. Transforming growth factor β stimulates the expression of fibronectin and collagen and their incorporation into the extracellular matrix. J Biol Chem 1986; 261:4337-4345.